Penguin Books

NO CONCEIVABLE INJURY

Robert Milliken is a journalist who began working for the *Sydney Morning Herald* and later joined the *National Times* for which he reported on a wide range of news and feature stories, including nuclear energy and the arms race. He has worked as a journalist in Britain and the United States and has written for the *Sunday Times*, the *Guardian* and the *New Statesman* of London, and the *Los Angeles Times*.

Robert Milliken

NO CONCEIVABLE
INJURY

PENGUIN BOOKS

Penguin Books Australia Ltd,
487 Maroondah Highway, PO Box 257
Ringwood, Victoria, 3134, Australia
Penguin Books Ltd,
Harmondsworth, Middlesex, England
40 West 23rd Street, New York, NY 10010, USA
Penguin Books Canada Limited,
2801 John Street, Markham, Ontario, Canada L3R 1B4
Penguin Books (NZ) Ltd,
182-190 Wairau Road, Auckland 10, New Zealand

First published by Penguin Books Australia, 1986

Typeset in Goudy Old Style by Leader Composition Pty Ltd
Made and printed in Australia by
The Dominion Press-Hedges & Bell, Maryborough, Victoria

CIP

Milliken, Robert
No conceivable injury.

Bibliography.
Includes index.
ISBN 0 14 008438 X (pbk.).

1. Atomic bomb – Australia – Testing. 2. Atomic bomb –
Australia – Physiological effect. 3. Australia –
Foreign relations – Great Britain. I. Title.

623.4'5119'0994

CONTENTS

ACKNOWLEDGEMENTS

The British nuclear tests of the 1950s covered almost every aspect of relations between Britain and Australia – political, military, diplomatic, scientific – and impinged on many aspects of life inside Australia as well, not least Aboriginal welfare and public health. At every level, there was a fundamental drive by those in the know in the governments of both countries to keep the execution of the events as secret as possible, understandable, perhaps, given the world outlook of the time, but often absurd in hindsight. Much the same sort of secrecy surrounds the more sophisticated nuclear defence projects, domestic and foreign, in both countries today.

The Australian government's decision in 1984 to appoint a royal commission into the British nuclear tests in Australia made it possible to write this book. Many of the documents relied upon were among the thousands declassified by the British and Australian governments during 1985 for the royal commission's inquiry – documents which would otherwise have remained secret for many more years. I am grateful to the staff of the royal commission, and to the lawyers who appeared before it, for their help and patience over many hours. I acknowledge my particular thanks to Peter McClellan, QC, who was the counsel assisting the royal commission, and to Dr John Symonds, the scientific consultant to the royal commission.

My thanks, also, to the staffs of the following libraries: the *Sunday Times*, London, the Public Record Office, Kew, London, the Library of Congress, Washington, the *Sydney Morning Herald*, the Australian Archives, Canberra, the National Library, Canberra.

Many other people assisted with research, provided helpful ideas and guidance, or generally helped to make my task easier – although any opinions and errors in the text are mine alone.

In Britain: Mark Mildred, Joan Smith, David Greason and Dimity Torbett; Professor Margaret Gowing, of Oxford University, and Lorna Arnold, of the United Kingdom Atomic Energy Authority, whose two volume official history of the British atomic project up to 1952 was an essential guide to understanding many of the events which followed; John Sprange and George Pritchard of Greenpeace.

In Australia: Bruce Palling and Sonia Rothbury, who researched the Maralinga story for Film Australia during 1985 and were particularly generous with their help and comments; Andrew Collett, Geoff Eames and Maggie Brady, who provided much assistance with material on the Aborigines' story; Robert Cavanagh, Harold Crosbie, Sue Hobley, Greg James, QC, Frank Muller, Dennis O'Rourke, Tim Sherratt, Jefferson Penberthy, Rosemary Meares and Tania Tench.

My special thanks to Bruce Sims and Cilla Davidson of Penguin Books Australia, for their patience, Timothy Fraser, who edited the manuscript, and Brian Johns, the publishing director of Penguin, who suggested the project and gave it his support and enthusiasm.

Robert Milliken,
Sydney, December 1985.

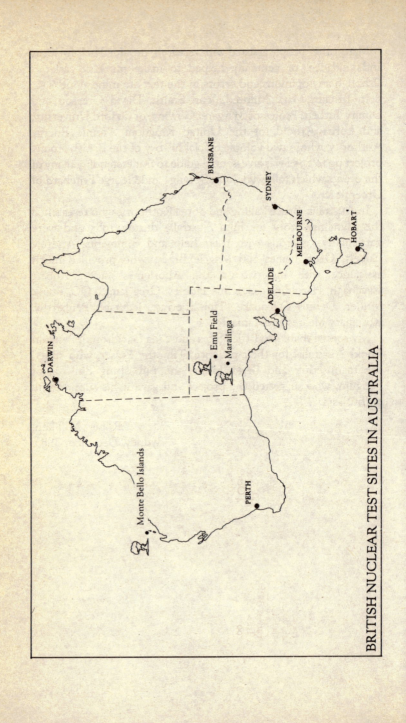

BRITISH NUCLEAR TEST SITES IN AUSTRALIA

BRITISH NUCLEAR TESTS IN AUSTRALIA

Operation	Date	Place	Type	Yield
Operation Hurricane	3 October 1952	Monte Bello Islands	Ocean burst (ship)	25 kilotons
Operation Totem				
Totem One	15 October 1953	Emu Field	Tower	10 kilotons
Totem Two	27 October 1953	Emu Field	Tower	8 kilotons
Operation Mosaic				
Mosaic G1	16 May 1956	Monte Bello Islands	Tower	15 kilotons
Mosaic G2	19 June 1956	Monte Bello Islands	Tower	60 kilotons
Operation Buffalo				
One Tree	27 September 1956	Maralinga	Tower	15 kilotons
Marcoo	4 October 1956	Maralinga	Ground burst	1.5 kilotons
Kite	11 October 1956	Maralinga	Aircraft-drop	3 kilotons
Breakaway	22 October 1956	Maralinga	Tower	10 kilotons
Operation Antler				
Tadje	14 September 1957	Maralinga	Tower	1 kiloton
Biak	25 September 1957	Maralinga	Tower	6 kilotons
Taranaki	9 October 1957	Maralinga	Balloon-suspended	25 kilotons

One kiloton is equal to 1000 tons of conventional explosive, TNT.
One megaton is equal to one million tons of TNT.

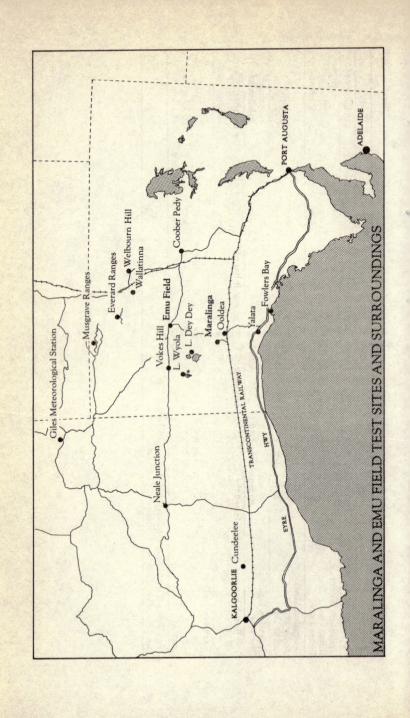

MARALINGA AND EMU FIELD TEST SITES AND SURROUNDINGS

Giles Meteorological Station
Musgrave Ranges
Everard Ranges
Welbourn Hill
Wallatinna
Coober Pedy
Vokes Hill
Emu Field
L. Dey Dey
L. Wyola
Maralinga
Ooldea
Fowlers Bay
Yalata
PORT AUGUSTA
ADELAIDE
Neale Junction
TRANSCONTINENTAL RAILWAY
HWY
EYRE
KALGOORLIE
Cundeelee

BRITISH NUCLEAR TESTS IN THE PACIFIC OCEAN

Operation	Date	Place	Yield
Grapple	15 May 1957	Malden Island	megaton range
	31 May 1957	Malden Island	megaton range
	19 June 1957	Malden Island	megaton range
Grapple X	8 November 1957	Christmas Island	megaton range
Grapple Y	28 April 1958	Christmas Island	megaton range
Grapple Z	22 August 1958	Christmas Island	kiloton range
	2 September 1958	Christmas Island	megaton range
	11 September 1958	Christmas Island	megaton range
	23 September 1958	Christmas Island	kiloton range

The British government has released the yields for the weapons tested in Australia. It has not released the yields for the hydrogen bombs tested in the Pacific. All the Pacific weapons were either dropped from aircraft over the ocean or suspended from balloons over land.

INTRODUCTION

Britain exploded her first nuclear weapon in the Monte Bello Islands off the northwest coast of Australia on 3 October 1952. It was a particularly crude device by the sophisticated standards of today's nuclear arsenals and their delivery systems – a bit like comparing the original steam engine with the bullet train. But it gained Britain her much sought-after place among the nuclear nations – an exclusive club then composed of just two members, the United States and the Soviet Union, and later expanded with the addition of France, China and India.

None of these nations was invited to join the nuclear club, in the sense that the other members assisted them with technological know-how on building and testing nuclear weapons. Instead, it was very much a case of every nation for itself, a fiercely contested race to acquire the weapons from their own scientific resources – and, through the weapons, international power and prestige. Nowhere was this the case more than with Britain. Today, it seems somewhat strange that Britain, such a close ally of the United States, should have been competing against her special relation for nuclear defence capability. But, for reasons explained in the following pages, Britain – alone among the eventual nuclear nations – found herself at the end of the Second World War in the peculiar position of running a desperate, three-cornered nuclear race against both the emerging superpowers, the US and the Soviet Union.

Australia became the testing ground for Britain's nuclear weapons. Over the next five years, after the first Monte Bello test, Britain sought to refine her hard-won nuclear capability by exploding 11 more bombs at Monte Bello and at Emu Field and Maralinga, in South Australia. As such, Australia was cast in the role of silent partner in a drama which often resembled a *folie à deux*, asking few questions and being told only as much as Britain considered she needed to know. Both countries were driven by the relentless Cold War fever of the fifties, a decade when testing nuclear weapons on friendly people's territory was considered more acceptable than not testing them at all.

In the mid-eighties, the Australians set up a royal commission into the British nuclear tests. Australia was no longer the compliant ally of the fifties, when the prime minister, Robert Menzies, held on tenaciously to the country's British origins. At the head of the royal commission was James McClelland, a publicity-conscious judge, former Labor government minister, and a staunch Australian nationalist of Irish origin, who resented almost everything Britain stood for politically in Australian history. Australia may have been a willing, not to say eager, host to the British nuclear venture. But Britain, not Australia, became the defendant in the dock at McClelland's royal commission.

Through thousands of specially declassified documents, and the accounts of those involved, the anatomy of these events of the fifties, so pivotal to defence policy in the eighties, was at last laid bare. The fact that the British civil service had been prepared, if reluctantly, to divulge for the Australian royal commission its secrets of the recent past, without fear of Britain's present defence capability disintegrating, showed starkly how a totally new set of defence secrets had taken over today.

Maralinga had always been a secret and sacred place to the Aborigines. From 1956, for ten years, it became a secret and sacred site to the British defence planners and their Australian hosts. The Suez crisis, the Soviet invasion of Hungary, the Olympic Games in Melbourne, the launch by the Russians of Sputnik, the world's first space satellite – all these events of 1956 and 1957 helped to keep it out of the newspapers at the time.

When McClelland's royal commission delivered its report 30 years later, in December 1985, it recommended, not unexpectedly, that Britain should shoulder most responsibility for the secrecy of the past: Britain should clean up the Maralinga test sites, where tens of thousands of metal fragments contaminated with radioactive plutonium were still scattered around the range. In return, Australia should compensate the Aborigines who were kicked off their lands where the tests happened. It was clear that if both governments accepted these strictures, thus implicitly acknowledging guilt by their predecessors, they would face a flood of compensation claims from British and Australian servicemen who alleged that radiation exposure at the nuclear tests had caused cancer, and from the families of others who linked the radiation to their deaths.

But both the British and Australian governments took just seven weeks to shelve the royal commission's main recommendations. In late January, 1986, they agreed to pass the problem of the contaminated range on to yet another body, to be called the technical assessment group, and gave it 18 months to report on options for decontaminating and cleaning up the range.

What had begun as an innocent show of support from a loyal former colony to the mother country had become a long-running source of legal, political and moral tension between two allies whose national paths had since radically diverged.

Chapter One
FROM HIROSHIMA TO HURRICANE

'For what war are we supposed to be preparing?' – Sir Henry Tizard, 1947.

In June 1879, an English explorer called William Henry Tietkens set up camp at a spot in the central desert of South Australia about 60 kilometres north of where the transcontinental railway now runs. It was desolate, featureless and covered in mulga and spinifex. Yet Tietkens had a grand vision for this land. He was convinced that if water could be found it would support life on a prodigious scale: the flat plains that stretched incessantly in every direction would soon be opened up to homesteads, towns, mines and sheep stations.

Already there was a thriving Aboriginal life. Tietkens had glimpsed it when, four years earlier, he passed through a settlement called Ooldea, on the Nullarbor Plain, on an expedition with the famous explorer, Ernest Giles, from Adelaide to Perth, in Western Australia. Now that he was back in Ooldea, with a mission to find water for white pioneers, Tietkens became closely involved with the Aboriginal tribes whose antecedents had lived there for centuries. He quarrelled with the blacks: at one point he shot and wounded one man brandishing a spear in a bid to frighten him. But in the end they got on. The Aborigines smeared their naked bodies with white ochre, donned coronas of black feathers and performed tribal corroborees night after night. In the mornings, they would visit Tietkens' camp to show themselves off. Tietkens concluded: 'They most certainly were noble looking and handsome men . . . endowed with the qualities of wonderful patience and powerful endurance.' [1]

He could not say the same for his own men. Tietkens had brought up two workers to the spot 60 kilometres north of Ooldea, which he saw as the centre of a new, white civilisation, and told them to start digging for water. It was a disaster. After a month the men had sunk a well 13 metres deep and struck nothing but loose, dry sand through which they could dig no further. They grumbled about the diet of bread and horsemeat and refused to work any more. A row broke out and Tietkens sacked the men, dismissing them contemptuously in his diary later as 'the clods of infamy'.

He trekked almost 200 kilometres south to Fowler's Bay, on the South Australian coast, where he picked up two new workers from the sheep shearing teams. Back at the site they started digging another well, but by Christmas Eve, two months later, the hole was 30 metres down and still dry. Tietkens somewhat glumly celebrated Christmas Day in the mulga, inviting the local Aborigines to join him for a meagre feast of egg puddings, damper and a large baked pumpkin. Next day the men struck water – not fresh, but still good enough for sheep, horses and cattle. Tietkens was overwhelmed. He was convinced his dream of a new frontier in this remarkably inhospitable desert would soon become reality. He packed up and took his men back to Fowler's Bay, where he celebrated New Year's Day 1880, with what he believed to be the greatest success of his life so far.

Tietkens was destined to be one of those supreme optimists whose hopes were cruelly dashed, the sort of person with which Australian exploration history is littered. Refreshed and reinvigorated, he returned to the well a few months later. The men reinforced its walls with timber 42 metres down. Soon afterwards, the upper timbers collapsed. Fine sand started pouring through the rest of the timber beams as fast as the men could dig it out. There was no more water. The water they had found at Christmas proved to be a mere soak. Tietkens had been supported all along by a rich couple in England, a Mr and Mrs Leisler; but by now he had spent two years looking for water and the money had run out. He could not face asking the Leislers for more, so he abandoned the enterprise and returned to Adelaide. It was, he remembered, 'the most bitter part of my life's history'.

For the next 73 years few people, if any, ventured into this lonely landscape apart from the Aborigines who lived there. Tietkens's well, with its roughly hewn timber shafts, survived as a monument to the explorer, as it does to this day. Then in 1953, a modern explorer called Len Beadell arrived at Tietkens' well in a Land Rover. Beadell was Australian, a bushman of the true sort. He, too, was on a mission for Britain. He had been charged with finding a site where Britain could test atomic weapons, possibly for many years to come. Already Britain had fired its first atomic device off the northwest coast of Australia, and was about to explode two more in the remote Great Victoria Desert of South Australia; but a permanent site was needed for future blasts, close to the transcontinental railway.

When Beadell decided that the plains around Tietkens' well were exactly what he was looking for, he and his men built a makeshift runway so that Sir William Penney, the British scientist in charge of the tests, could fly down in a Bristol freighter to inspect the site. There was nothing public about this expedition, as there had been with Tietkens'. It was conducted in the utmost secrecy. While Penney was there, the public in Britain and Australia were told he was somewhere else. But Penney was well satisfied with Beadell's find. 'It's the cat's whiskers', he pronounced.

Over the next three years a large, sprawling township grew out of the desert supporting thousands of people. The water that had eluded Tietkens was pumped from the ground and desalinated or brought in by train. But their work was of a kind beyond the wildest dreams even of William Tietkens. Thirteen years after Beadell found the site, Britain, with Australia's agreement, had detonated seven more atomic bombs and hundreds of smaller devices leaving the land littered with plutonium, a dangerous radioactive product that would contaminate the land for thousands of years.

The Aborigines later called this place Maralinga, or Field of Thunder. To the scientists who set off the bombs it was, as Len Beadell later described it, 'a lot of hard work coming to a climax in a millionth of a second – a very exciting climax'. To the Aborigines and the thousands of British and Australian servicemen involved, it was something else.

More than 30 years after Britain exploded her first nuclear device in Australia, two questions remain. Why did Britain want nuclear weapons in the first place, and why did Australia allow itself so willingly to become the testing ground? From the standpoint of the 1980s, when the enormous nuclear arsenals of the United States and the Soviet Union overshadow those of every other nuclear nation, it seems somewhat remarkable that Britain, a country whose power, influence and economic performance have all steadily declined since the Second World War, should have been determined for so long to acquire its own nuclear deterrent.

The short answer is that British scientists, and refugee scientists living in Britain during the Second World War, were responsible for discovering how the atomic bomb could be made. That is why Britain was so resolute in seeking its own bomb after the war. By then, the United States had stolen the initiative from Britain in atomic technology and had embarked on what was soon to be a nuclear arms race with the Soviet Union. The Americans, typically competitive, did not want the British, or anyone else, to be part of this race. They froze British scientists out of any collaboration on atomic weapons whatsoever. But Britain was not willing to allow the Americans simply to slam the door in its face. The British believed they were entitled to nuclear power status because of, among other things, their key role in the bomb's invention – a role which has always been overshadowed by the enormous effort of the Manhattan project in the US, which actually produced the world's first atomic bombs. This is how it came about.

By 1933, the year William Tietkens died at the age of 89 in the quiet New South Wales town of Lithgow, scientists in Britain and Europe were engaged in a race to unlock the secrets of nuclear physics. The 1930s were an exciting decade in the development of atomic theory, with physicists in the great laboratories of Britain, France and Germany eagerly exploring each other's discoveries in a bid to take them one step further. But the real breakthroughs did not start to take shape until the eve of the Second World War. The first of these came in 1938 when two Germans, Otto Hahn and Fritz Strassmann, discovered the theory of nuclear fission, the essential process in the atomic bomb.

For years scientists had known that atoms, the miniscule entities that make up all matter, contained enormous amounts of potential energy; but the key to actually releasing this energy had managed to elude them. Hahn and Strassmann had been building on the experiments of other scientists, like the Italian, Enrico Fermi, and the Hungarian, Leo Szilard, both of whom, as refugees in the US from fascism during the war, were to play important early roles in alerting the American authorities to the military significance of the atomic bomb.

Hahn and Strassmann experimented with uranium, a radioactive material considered fairly worthless up to then. Their work proved that when an atom of uranium is bombarded with neutrons, the nucleus (or heart of the atom) splits – or, literally, explodes – releasing huge amounts of energy. This process was later called fission.

The nucleus of every atom consists of subnuclear particles, of which protons and neutrons are the most important. The number of protons in a nucleus ranges from one, in a light element such as hydrogen, to 92 in uranium, the heaviest element occurring in nature. The proportion of neutrons to protons in a nucleus also varies: in the lighter elements, they are just about equal; but in heavier elements the number of neutrons increases until in uranium, the heaviest element of all, there are more than 140 neutrons to the 92 protons. This neutron surplus in uranium is a crucial factor in the next stage of the fission process.

That next stage was discovered in Paris, a few weeks after Hahn and Strassmann announced their findings. It was the result of studies by Frederic Joliot-Curie, the French Nobel prizewinner and son-in-law of Marie Curie, the woman who, some years earlier, had helped to discover the nature of radioactivity. Frederic Joliot-Curie found that when a uranium atom is split, it throws out some free neutrons which are capable, in turn, of bombarding other uranium nuclei in a self-sustaining chain reaction. This implied that at each stage of the chain reaction, when another uranium atom undergoes fission, the amount of energy released would multiply many times.

The chain reaction theory had been around for some years, but only now had the radioactive substance, uranium, been isolated as the element in which it could actually be made to happen. These remarkable discoveries caused uproar in the world of physics and a frantic outpouring of work in laboratories all around the world as scientists sought to duplicate them. By now, thanks largely to experiments conducted in the Paris laboratories, scientists also knew of another essential condition which was needed before fission could take place. This was the notion of 'critical mass'. It centred on the fact that some neutrons, released when a uranium nucleus is split, will not fly off and cause fission. They may be absorbed or simply lost. A critical amount, or mass, of the fissile uranium was therefore needed – enough to ensure that the net rate at which neutrons are produced exceeds the rate at which they are lost – before a self-sustaining chain reaction could occur.

So the exciting discoveries of 1939 had shown scientists in several countries that uranium fission may be a source of heat and power far greater than anything yet known. Already, many were speculating about the possibility of it being used to make a super bomb. Some, indeed, soon feared that this might be precisely the secret weapon that Hitler was planning. The British scientific establishment became particularly alarmed at this possibility. Once the potential applications of fission had sunk in, the British moved quickly to buy up the world's known uranium supplies, then located principally in the Belgian Congo, in a bid to keep them out of German hands.

But even though the fission theory was now developing rapidly, there were still some special problems which dampened down the high hopes in some quarters that a uranium bomb could be built soon. The most outstanding problem had to do with the nature of uranium itself. Natural uranium in the ground exists in two main forms, or, in scientific language, isotopes – uranium 235 and uranium 238, the numbers standing for the atomic weight of each isotope. Niels Bohr, the Danish Nobel prizewinner, and one of the greatest physicists of the twentieth century, argued that fission was more likely to happen with uranium 235 atoms than with uranium 238 atoms. Bohr set out this analysis in a paper which he published with an American colleague just two days before the Second World War broke out.

The significance of Bohr's contribution was that it showed just how complicated and expensive it was going to be to build a bomb. Uranium dug out of the ground contains less than 1 per cent of uranium 235 – the 'fissile' atoms, or those capable of undergoing fission. More than 99 per cent of natural uranium consists of the non-fissile uranium 238 atoms. This implied one of several things. Huge amounts of natural uranium would have to be piled on top of each other in the hope of the neutrons finding the right uranium 235 targets, and sparking off a chain reaction. No-one knew how much uranium would be needed – and, in any case, it might be so much that the final bomb would be too heavy and cumbersome to be worth the trouble. Alternatively, the uranium 235 atoms would somehow have to be extracted from the uranium 238 – a process which most scientists on the eve of the Second World War dismissed as totally impractical.

The big discoveries of 1939 were international: they all took place outside Britain, although British scientists had played a significant role in the rapid development of nuclear physics that had gone on right through the thirties. Professor James Chadwick, who was later to lead the British team of scientists working on the first atomic bomb in America, had, in 1932, discovered the neutron, the fundamental particle of atomic fission. As the war broke out, the British set up a series of experiments with uranium under Professor George Thomson at Imperial College, London, and Professor Mark Oliphant, an Australian, at Birmingham University. For the most part, though, scepticism about the atomic bomb had set in, as British efforts were suddenly poured into more urgent projects of conventional land, sea and air warfare, where scientists could actually foresee quick results.

Then in April 1940, two refugees from Nazism, who had been working at Birmingham University when the war started seven months earlier, produced a paper which was to change dramatically the entire pace and scope of atomic bomb research. The physicists were Otto Frisch, an Austrian, and Rudolph Peierls, a German. In a remarkably short paper, just three pages long, Frisch and Peierls presented three lucid arguments. First, they suggested that a lump of pure uranium 235 would, indeed, undergo the fantastically fast chain reaction needed for an atomic bomb. Second, they suggested a way of extracting the uranium 235 from a lump of natural uranium. If that was done, the amount of uranium which one had to assemble to get a 'critical mass' would be nothing like what everyone had thought: a 5 kilogram bomb, said the two physicists – that is, one weighing no more than a bag of potatoes – would liberate the same amount of energy as several thousand tonnes of dynamite. Finally, Frisch and Peierls gave a sombre warning:

In addition to the destructive effect of the explosion itself, the whole material of the bomb would be transformed into a highly radioactive state. The energy radiated by these active substances will amount to about 20 per cent of the energy liberated in the explosion, and the radiations would be fatal to living beings even a long time after the explosion.

Most of the radioactive material, they thought, would probably be blown into the air and carried away by the wind. 'This cloud of radioactive material will kill everybody within a strip estimated to be several miles long. If it rained the danger would be even worse . . .'[2]

The Frisch-Peierls Memorandum, as their paper was eventually called, still stands as one of the most crucial documents in the entire history of the atomic bomb. It was, as Margaret Gowing, the official historian of the British atomic project, described it,

a remarkable example of scientific breadth and insight . . . the first memorandum in any country which foretold with scientific conviction the practical possibility of making a bomb and the horrors it would bring.[3]

Frisch and Peierls showed their memorandum to Oliphant, their colleague at Birmingham, who in turn showed it to higher authorities in the British scientific establishment. As a result of the memorandum, the British government's desultory interest in the bomb idea rapidly changed. In early 1940, the government set up a special committee, the Maud committee, to examine whether an atomic bomb was possible on present knowledge, and how quickly it could be made. The Maud committee was, in Gowing's assessment, 'one of the most successful committees this or any other country has ever seen'.[4]

By mid-1941, after working at a frantic pace, it reported that a bomb, indeed, was possible certainly with uranium 235 and possibly with plutonium. The government gave the project the go-

8

ahead. It also sent a copy of the Maud report – titled, in uncharacteristic direct language, 'Use of Uranium for a Bomb' – to the United States, where atomic research still lagged significantly behind that in Britain. When they read the Maud report, American scientists persuaded their government to take the atomic bomb seriously, and the huge Manhattan project was the eventual result.

The British, indeed, did not realise at the time just how big an impact their work was to have in the US – and what a great deal of pain in their atomic relations with the Americans was to follow for many years to come. In October 1939, just after the Second World War broke out, and almost two years before the Maud report found its way across the Atlantic, President Franklin Roosevelt had himself taken the first tentative steps towards a US atomic project. Leo Szilard, with another refugee scientist, had persuaded the great Albert Einstein to write to Roosevelt drawing his attention to the huge military potential of a uranium bomb, and the dangers if Germany should build one first. As a result, Roosevelt set up an advisory committee on uranium.

The American work ground along at a fairly slow pace. The fear that Hitler might be building a bomb was not as immediate in the US as it was in Britain because the Americans, at this stage, had still not joined the war. By early 1941, American scientists were experimenting with slow neutron reactions in ordinary, unseparated uranium. They had also demonstrated, through experiments in Chicago and Berkeley, California, that a new element, plutonium, was capable of undergoing fission. It was the French who had, almost simultaneously, suggested that a new substance unknown in nature – and later given the name, plutonium – would be formed from slow chain reactions in ordinary uranium.

Two French scientists involved in these slow neutron experiments in Paris had fled to England in 1940, just as France fell to the Nazis. They brought with them, in 26 cans, the world's entire stock of heavy water, which was used to slow down, or moderate, neutrons in fission experiments with ordinary, plentiful uranium 238. The neutrons in these experiments had to be slowed down to give them a better chance of hitting the fissile uranium 235 atoms. By now, most scientists knew these experiments would not give the fantastically fast chain reaction needed for a bomb: that could only be achieved with pure uranium 235. But they did hold hope of providing domestic, non-military nuclear power possibly using ordinary uranium 238.

The British settled the Frenchmen at the Cavendish Laboratory in Cambridge, where two of their colleagues correctly forecast that plutonium produced from the slow neutron experiments would behave in exactly the same way as uranium 235, and would be a usable fuel for bombs. In fact, plutonium was to comprise the fuel for one of the two atomic bombs dropped on Japan five years later.

The British were now faced with a real dilemma. The war made it too expensive and dangerous to build the enormous plants in Britain for 'Tube Alloys', the obscure and misleading name which the British atomic energy project had been given as a security cover. Some of the British scientists and politicians thought it would be better if the whole thing was moved to North America; but others were reluctant, fearing the British might eventually lose control if that happened. The actual building of a bomb was still several years off, but even at this early stage it was clear that atomic weapons and atomic energy were going to be the new keys to national power and status after the war.

By late 1941, as we have seen, the Americans had suddenly rejuvenated their interest in atomic weapons. When the Japanese bombing of Pearl Harbour in December that year catapulted them into the war, they threw their full scientific and technological weight into building a bomb. At first, realising how far ahead the British were, the Americans suggested a joint project, controlled by both countries. The British declined: they wanted to keep the Americans at arms length, although they were keen to continue full collaboration through exchange of information.

The American project moved ahead with astonishing speed – far quicker than the British realised. British scientists visiting the United States six months later became alarmed not just at how the Americans had caught up with the British but were about to leave them behind. By mid-1942, the British discovered – less than a year after the Americans had been alerted by the British Maud report – there were more than four times as many scientists working on the bomb in the United States as there were in Britain. The British became desperate and tried to resurrect the idea of a joint project.

But the Americans were no longer interested. They took the view that they had originated much of the development work themselves, and that to take in a partner now – even one like Britain, to whom they owed an earlier debt in the atomic business – would hinder rather than help them. They even became suspicious about sharing atomic data with Britain, and for the next nine months the flow of information from the United States all but dried up.

It was revived only on the insistence of Winston Churchill, the British prime minister, who, after a great struggle, succeeded in extracting from Roosevelt the Quebec Agreement of August 1943. This said that Britain and the US would never use the atomic bomb against each other; that they would not use it against third parties without each other's consent; that neither country would communicate information about 'Tube Alloys' (taken here to mean atomic energy in general, not just bombs) to third parties without each other's consent; and that any postwar commercial advantages of atomic energy would be dealt with 'on terms to be specified by the President of the United States to the Prime Minister of Great Britain'.

The Quebec Agreement enabled British scientists to join the American bid to build an atomic bomb, the Manhattan Project. Several of the British, however, were discontented by the one-sidedness of the agreement which appeared to sign away Britain's independence over its atomic affairs after the war. The secrecy clause, too, was partly a reaction to the Americans' distrust of the French scientists working with the British and their fear of any information leaking to the Russians.

Already, the British and French scientists from Cambridge working on slow neutron reactions with heavy water moderators had installed themselves in Canada because it was clear the Americans would not have the French. Now, after the Quebec Agreement, the rest of the work in Britain closed down for the duration of the war and its scientists moved to the United States. There, they learned of the existence of Los Alamos, the top secret laboratory in New Mexico where more than 300 scientists were already secluded away working on the actual fabrication of the bomb.

The biggest contingent in the British team went to work at Los

Alamos, the holy of holies, or, as it was referred to in hushed tones by insiders, Shangri La or simply Y. Others, like Mark Oliphant, joined the Berkeley team of Professor Ernest Lawrence, the Nobel prizewinner who had invented the cyclotron, or atom smasher, and who was now working on an electromagnetic method of separating uranium 235 from ordinary uranium. Oliphant had worked with Lawrence at Berkeley before the war, and the two were close friends. It was Oliphant who later told Lawrence about the British Maud committee work, an account which deeply impressed Lawrence and which helped galvanise the Americans to the true possibilities of using uranium for a bomb. The Americans, as we shall see, were later to regard Oliphant with the utmost suspicion when he turned against the atomic bomb; for this reason his great talents were ignored during the British bomb project in Australia.

A great friendship was formed between James Chadwick, the leader of the British scientific team in America, and General Leslie Groves, the tough, brash US army officer who was put in charge of the Manhattan Project. Nobel prizewinner though he was, Chadwick was a shy and modest man who had never been to the US before. His health played havoc with him, and he preferred to spend most of his time in Washington than in the confines of Los Alamos. He and Oliphant, his deputy, were particularly diplomatic and got on well with most of the Americans, especially Groves. Most of the scientists, by contrast, tended to resent Groves – a military man with military ways and a military obsession with secrecy which he took to extraordinary lengths – being head of the show.

So the Anglo-American collaboration and flow of information resumed, but against a background of latent suspicion. For one thing, the Americans and British always had a nagging worry about security standards in each other's camps – the Americans quite rightly so, in view of the later British spy scandals. And, as we shall see, American distrust of Australian security was to play a role in restricting the flow of information between Britain and Australia when the British eventually went, reluctantly, to Australia to test their bombs.

Groves was particularly paranoid in this regard, and often preferred to discuss secret information with colleagues while walking outside in the open for fear of being bugged. Once, while visiting Lawrence and Oliphant at Berkeley, he demonstrated a point by doing a quick calculation on a scrap of paper, which he then promptly tore up. 'Why did you do that?' Oliphant asked him. 'Because I am determined that there will be the fewest possible records of this project', he shot back. 'I don't want anything on paper that needn't be on paper.'

It was at this stage, even before the first bomb was built, that the first abortive bid was made to control the spread of nuclear weapons. It came through Niels Bohr, the brilliant if diffident Danish scientist whose crucial article on the eve of the Second World War had explained the fundamentals of uranium fission. Bohr had stayed in Denmark after it was occupied by Germany in 1940, but had conducted a clandestine correspondence with Chadwick who was keen for him to join the British atomic work. By late 1943, when it was clear that Bohr and his family were in danger of arrest, they were smuggled out of Denmark. Bohr himself arrived in England hidden in the empty bomb rack of a Mosquito bomber. He was astounded to learn how far and how fast the Americans and British had moved towards making a bomb, and he now became one of the first scientists to grasp the real meaning of the atomic bomb for the future of the world.

Bohr realised that unless, even now, atomic energy was placed under some form of international control, the implications could be horrendous. He became desperate to see Churchill and Roosevelt. At first Churchill refused to see him. The prime minister had other preoccupations: the Allied invasion of Europe was imminent and, besides, Churchill had a somewhat lofty disdain for scientists, even those as outstanding as Bohr, getting involved with politics. (The reverse did not necessarily hold: with the atomic bomb, it was the politicians and their advisers in the military and the civil service who were rapidly taking over the labours of science.)

Among those who implored Churchill to give Bohr a hearing, however brief, was Sir Henry Dale, president of the Royal Society, the most prestigious scientific body in the country. Dale had been a member of the original Tube Alloys consultative council, and he wrote Churchill an impassioned letter putting the question in the starkest possible terms: 'I cannot avoid the conviction that science is approaching the realisation of a project which may bring either disaster or benefit on a scale hitherto unimaginable to the future of mankind.'[5]

Dale's entreaty worked, for it helped to persuade Churchill to receive Niels Bohr in May 1944. The meeting was a disaster. Churchill did not want to hear Bohr's fundamental argument: that the Russians would inevitably build their own bomb after the war; that this would lead to a terrifying arms race; and that one way of avoiding this would be to take the Russians into confidence about the Manhattan Project, so the problems of future control of atomic weapons could be confronted here and now – to wait until after the war, when the fragile Soviet-Western alliance would surely disintegrate, would be too late.

This argument was anathema to Churchill, who already regarded the Russians with the gravest suspicion. It simply lacked political realism. Moreover, Bohr's manner irritated Churchill. Indeed, Sir Henry Dale's worst fear – that Bohr's 'mild, philosophical vagueness of expression and his inarticulate whisper' may fail to make an impact on the prime minister – proved to be right. As Bohr took his leave, depressed and demoralised, he asked gingerly if he could write to Churchill and explain his views further. The prime minister replied that, of course, he would always be honoured to receive a letter from Professor Bohr, as long as it was not about politics.

Bohr fared somewhat better with Roosevelt, whom he met three months later, in August 1944. The president was not as cursory as Churchill, and listened to Bohr for an hour and a half. He shared the professor's concern about the political problems raised by the bomb; Bohr's spirits lifted immensely when Roosevelt undertook to raise with Churchill the possibility of an early approach to the Russians about it.

In fact, just the opposite happened. When Churchill and Roosevelt met in America the following month, they signed another accord, known as the Hyde Park Agreement, which consolidated the secrecy surrounding the atomic bomb. It rejected the notion that the world should be informed about the Tube Alloys project (as it was still coyly called) with a view to international control over its use. Moreover, a final paragraph specifically called for inquiries to be made about Bohr's activities, and for steps to be taken 'to ensure that he is responsible for no leakage of information, particularly to the Russians'.

The Hyde Park Agreement appeared to give the British all they were looking for: it also said that full Anglo-American atomic collaboration 'should continue' after the war. This was at the heart of Churchill's outlook. He was determined to keep the whole atomic business as secret as possible, and he regarded the earlier Quebec Agreement as the very bedrock of British atomic policy. It was not just that Britain could benefit from the great technical strides the Americans had made during the war years; for Churchill, atomic co-operation would be just one part of an Anglo-American partnership that would help to provide stability in the postwar world. Churchill's faith was all-embracing on this point. He told Lord Cherwell, his principal adviser: 'Our associations with the United States must be permanent and I have no fear that they will maltreat or cheat us'. [6]

Like many political agreements, before and since, the Hyde Park Agreement turned out to be worthless. Within six months of its signing, Roosevelt was dead. When the British sought to discuss the agreement after the President's death, they were alarmed to discover that none of the atomic energy people in Washington had heard of its existence. In fact, they had to ask the British to supply them with a copy.

If British hopes of an atomic partnership with the Americans were shot down by this incident, they were dealt a final blow just over a year later, in August 1946, when the US Congress passed the McMahon Act. Sponsored by Brien McMahon, a robust Senator from Connecticut, this legislation was born in an expanding mood of nationalism in the United States over the economic and military superiority with which the Americans had emerged from the war, and the need to protect this dominance from its obvious emerging competitor, the Soviet Union. The McMahon Act outlawed the passing of any classified atomic information to any other country, including the US's wartime allies, Britain and Canada. The penalties included life imprisonment and death.

The McMahon Act was a symptom of a new gung-ho attitude towards the atomic bomb in the United States, the view that the

Americans must keep a monopoly over this terrifying new technology in order to maintain their new superpower role. McMahon himself was later on record as saying that strategic bombing with nuclear weapons must be 'the keystone of our military policy and a foundation pillar of our foreign policy'. The act was to have a profound effect on Britain's nuclear role over the next decade.

Less than a year before the McMahon Act, in July 1945, the world's first atomic bomb, with a plutonium core, was exploded in a test above the desert at Alamogordo, in New Mexico. Groves and the other scientists at the centre of the Manhattan Project heaved a great sigh of relief: the bomb had cost $2 billion to build, and it worked. Churchill, the Soviet leader, Joseph Stalin, and Roosevelt's successor, President Harry Truman, were meeting at the last of the great wartime Allied summits in the Berlin suburb of Potsdam when the news was flashed in secret code to Truman from Los Alamos. Truman and Churchill had wondered whether to tell Stalin about the bomb. In the end, Truman mentioned briefly and obliquely to Stalin that the US had a new weapon of unusual destructive force. The words atomic bomb were never mentioned. Stalin's response was equally casual, Truman noted later. The whole question of international control of the bomb had been neatly avoided.

The following month, the two atomic bombs dropped on Hiroshima and Nagasaki brought the Second World War to a sudden end. The bomb which hit Hiroshima killed 64 000 people within four months of impact, and the Nagasaki bomb another 39 000. Almost 100 000 more people in both cities were injured. More than half the deaths at Hiroshima were caused by burns – many from the flash from this totally new kind of weapon, rather than from flames. Eighteen per cent died from the blast. Thirty per cent died from a new cause: radiation. The radioactive contamination was lower than it might have been because the bombs, delivered by aircraft, were detonated from a height above the ground designed to cause the maximum amount of damage from blast.

So five and a half years after Frisch and Peierls at Birmingham University had produced their memorandum explaining how an atomic bomb could be made, the terrible nature of these weapons had been demonstrated, and Neils Bohr's vision of a world irrevocably changed was about to unfold. But the bombs had foreshadowed something else – the shift of strategic power away from Europe to the United States. Although the bomb had begun largely as the venture of a brilliant group of scientists working in Britain, the British had ended up as junior partners in the Manhattan Project. It was the Americans' decision to drop the bombs on Japan, even though Britain's consent had been sought, as a matter of course, and given.

Britain ended the war with plenty of knowledge on how to produce fissile material, uranium 235, but less knowledge, and fewer resources, on how to actually turn this material into a bomb. The war had drained the country economically and emotionally. John Maynard Keynes, the Cambridge economist whose theories were to govern Western economies for the next 25 years, told the newly elected Labour government of Clement Attlee on the day Japan surrendered, in August 1945, that Britain was 'virtually bankrupt, and the economic basis for the hopes of the public non-existent'. The Attlee government had come to power almost completely ignorant about the wartime atomic project. Almost none of the new Labour ministers had heard of atomic bombs before 1945. This was because Churchill had rigidly insisted on the whole thing being kept secret, and had allowed only a select few in his coalition war cabinet to be told about it. Neither Attlee, the deputy prime minister in the war cabinet, nor Ernest Bevin, his future foreign secretary, had been told.

There was, moreover, a great deal of confusion about where Britain now stood in atomic matters. The McMahon Act, at least, soon put paid to any hopes of resuming work with the Americans. But among the British military chiefs, and most scientific luminaries, there had always been an implicit assumtion that Britain would have a bomb of her own. Some, indeed, saw the McMahon Act as something of a blessing if it would prove to be a catalyst for the British getting their own act together. Chadwick, Britain's greatest living nuclear physicist, put it this way as the immediate postwar soul searching began: 'Are we so helpless that we can do nothing without the United States?' Cherwell, the scientific adviser to

Churchill, was adamant that Britain should press ahead and assemble a stockpile of atomic bombs. He disparaged the idea, proposed in some quarters, that Britain would be better off letting the Americans build the bombs and then buying them ready made. He argued:

If we are unable to make bombs ourselves and have to rely entirely on the United States army for this vital weapon we shall sink to the rank of a second class nation, only permitted to supply auxiliary troops, like the native levies who were allowed small arms but not artillery.

Cherwell's atomic nationalism was based not just on the bomb; he also saw great British industrial potential in atomic energy. The country's prosperity in the Victorian era, he pointed out, was due largely to the men who had the imagination to put and keep England ahead for 60 to 80 years in the use of steam power for industrial purposes. Cherwell wrote to Churchill: 'It is quite likely that our prosperity in the coming century may depend on learning how to exploit the energy latent in uranium (1 pound = 1000 tons of coal)'. [7]

Indeed, the idea of a flexible atomic project, one that could be used both to make bombs and build power stations to provide electricity to the homes and factories of Britain, had found growing support as the war drew to a close. By 1946, therefore, the government had authorised the building of a reactor to produce plutonium. Britain was able to get its head start in plutonium production thanks to the earlier work of the refugee French scientists who had joined the British team during the war. (Ten years later Britain opened Calder Hall, the world's first nuclear plant designed to feed electricity into the national power system). There was no doubt in anyone's mind in 1946, however, that the most immediate and pressing purpose of the plutonium was to build a bomb; the first plutonium reactor approved was anticipated, on full capacity, to be capable of producing enough material for 15 bombs a year.

The actual, formal, decision to build a bomb was made in January 1947, not by parliament, not even by cabinet, but by a top secret committee of ministers handpicked by Attlee, the prime minister.

· NO CONCEIVABLE INJURY

Ever since August 1945, there had been an inner ring of six senior ministers who gathered together to discuss atomic energy policy. It was known simply as Gen (for 'general') 75. It kept few records and met in dire secrecy, which meant that other cabinet ministers could well have been completely ignorant that it existed at all.

Among those in the know, Attlee jokingly referred to Gen 75 as 'my atom bomb committee'. But by the time of its last meeting, in December 1946, no explicit decision about a bomb had been taken. The decision was made a month later, not, ironically, by Gen 75, but by another ad hoc committee set up especially, and known as Gen 163. The composition of Gen 163 was even smaller: three of the Gen 75 ministers were pointedly excluded from it – including, significantly, Hugh Dalton, the chancellor of the exchequer, and Sir Stafford Cripps, the president of the Board of Trade, the two economic ministers who had earlier worried about the huge cost of a large-scale atomic program at a time when Britain was struggling to get back on its feet.

Gen 163 met for the first, and last, time in early January 1947, and made the vital decision that Britain would build and test an atomic bomb. This inner sanctum of ministers discussed a paper explaining Britain's bomb options written by Lord Portal, the former chief of the air staff. It was Portal whom Attlee had persuaded in March 1946 to delay retirement and take on the key new job of controller of atomic energy – a post which initially involved being in charge of plutonium production, but which soon placed Portal at the centre of the bomb project. Such was the obsession with secrecy at this meeting, that Portal's paper was shown individually to each of the ministers present – and then quickly withdrawn. Parliament, as we shall see, did not hear of this decision, and then only obliquely, until almost 18 months later, and it was to be many years before the public learned about what was really going on.

If Churchill had covered the whole Tube Alloys business up from the very beginning, then Attlee continued and extended the tradition of atomic secrecy. During the six years of Attlee's government, as Margaret Gowing has reported, atomic energy or bombs appeared less than ten times on the cabinet agenda. Even then, it was rarely discussed: on most occasions, cabinet was simply being informed:

Apart from Mr Attlee's two, partly 'atomic', visits to Washington (in 1945 and 1950), the cabinet as a body was completely excluded from all the major decisions on atomic policy in these years. [8]

The government actively encouraged ignorance about the bomb, even – indeed, particularly – among the ranks of its own Labour party, where there was at the time growing dissension about Britain's foreign policy. The independent nuclear deterrent was kept right out of these Labour party debates. Even among the closed circle of those who did know about the bomb, there was almost no questioning. [9]

The first British bomb, a crude, Nagasaki-type device, would eventually be codenamed Hurricane and ignited in the Monte Bello Islands off the northwest coast of Australia in October 1952. It would be a full seven years after the first detonations produced from the Manhattan Project. Most humiliatingly, it would be three years after the Soviet Union had tested its first atomic bomb, in 1949, proving, if further proof was needed, that Britain was no longer in the great power league. Indeed, by the time of Hurricane, Britain's first bomb, the US had tested 29 more atomic bombs and was about to leap a stage further in the bomb stakes by exploding its first thermonuclear device in the Pacific Ocean.

And yet, Britain doggedly persisted with its own bomb project. It did so from a variety of motives: a genuine belief, as the Cold War set in, that its defence strategy was best served by an independent nuclear deterrent; an understandable feeling that Britain, as the midwife of the world's first atomic bomb, had a proper role to play in future atomic weapons technology; national pride and a reluctance to accept that the power configurations in the postwar world were irretrievably different from those in the prewar world; and Churchill's earlier determination, supported by Chadwick, the leader of Britain's wartime scientific team in the US, that the bomb must not stay in American hands alone – that if Britain was to have a voice in determining policy on its future use, then Britain ought to be in on the act. Perhaps most important were the British hopes, which never dimmed, that someday, somehow, the Americans would take them back into their confidence on atomic matters; if, in the meantime, the British could demonstrate they meant business by assembling and exploding a British bomb then, the reasoning went, the day of reconciliation may be that much closer.

It was to be a long and bitter wait: almost ten years. And it was, almost alone, Sir Henry Tizard, the chief scientific adviser to the British Ministry of Defence, who warned of what he saw as the futility of embarking on such a painful course. By 1949, two years after the government had made the secret decision to build a bomb, Tizard had come to the view that atomic bombs should have no place in Britain's postwar plans. To him, economic reconstruction of the country was far more important. He set out his reasons in a cogent memorandum:

We persist in regarding ourselves as a Great Power, capable of everything and only temporarily handicapped by economic difficulties. We are not a Great Power and never will be again. We are a great nation, but if we continue to behave like a Great Power we shall soon cease to be a great nation. Let us take warning from the fate of the Great Powers of the past and not burst ourselves with pride (see Aesop's fable of the frog).

Tizard's plea was tersely ignored (he himself had been excluded as a consultant from the secret committee which decided on the bomb). As the full weight of Whitehall was thrown behind the bid to explode a British bomb as soon as possible, the story became one of Britain fighting an intense battle of strategy and wits with the Americans. To be sure, as the scene of the action shifted to Australia over the next ten years, the overt theme became one of Anglo-Australian relations. But the real and dominant theme was Britain's relationship with the United States. It was because of this relationship, and the frustrations the British constantly encountered in it, that Britain in the 1950s was obliged to test its bombs in Australia.

Nevada was Britain's first choice as a test site: it would have been cheaper, more efficient and, most important, it would have given the British access to the vast array of nuclear know-how the Americans had built up in a very short space of time. But when the trust on atomic matters broke down between Britain and the US,

Australia became, literally, the final outpost. And if not Australia, where? As William Penney, the man who was to take charge of the British bomb project, said, 'If the Australians are not willing to let us do trials in Australia, I do not know where we should go'. [10]

The Australians were willing, in stark contrast to the Americans' reticence. And in spite of the way the testing was dressed up, particularly by the Australian government at the time, to be a significant venture in Commonwealth atomic co-operation, Australia was, in the final analysis, merely the place to test the British bombs.

Chapter Two
PENNEY

'I said that these terrible weapons were going to stop war.' – Lord Penney, 1985.

Even in his mid-seventies, there was still a trace of youth in his face. It was the face of a man who had clearly spent many years pondering and worrying. The sandy hair had turned almost completely grey. He smiled as he spoke, in a friendly rather than a cocky way. There was no arrogance or smugness, as there can be with some scientists of his eminence. He sat at a microphone in a room in London, on a bitterly cold day in January, 1985, trying to remember. An Australian royal commission, inquiring into the effects of the British nuclear tests in Australia, had gone to London especially to question him and others about the strange events of the past. He wore a grey suit, a white shirt, a nondescript tie and a pullover – exactly the same combination he had on when he stepped off an aeroplane in the middle of the South Australian desert 30 years earlier to give the orders for the firing of Britain's first atomic bombs tested on land. All that was missing now was the felt hat. Clearly, he was not well. His interrogators, a bevy of smart lawyers half his age, frequently had to break off so the old man could have a rest. It was, he muttered later, 'an ordeal.' Neither he nor his scientific colleagues had ever dreamed in their younger years, at the height of their powers, that they would one day be called upon to explain themselves. And in a rare flash of impatience, as if to try to shut the snapping lawyers up, Lord Penney, formerly Sir William Penney, the father of the British atomic bomb, told exactly why he took the task on:

'I thought we were going to have a nuclear war. The only hope I saw was that there should be a balance between East and West. That is why I did this job, not to make money. I did not make any money. What I really wanted to do was to be a professor.' [1]

When the Attlee government decided, in January, 1947, that Britain must have its own atomic bomb, it chose William George Penney as the man to build it. The decision was kept so secret that Penney himself did not learn of it for another five months, until the following May.[2] Penney at least was ahead of the public in this regard. The government agonised over when, how or even whether an announcement should be made. In the end, A.V. Alexander, the minister of defence, simply alluded to it casually in the House of Commons in May 1948, in reply to a planted question from George Jeger, a Labour MP, 16 months after the actual decision:

Jeger: 'Is the minister satisfied that adequate progress is being made in the development of the most modern types of weapons?'

Minister: 'Yes, Sir. Research and development continue to receive the highest priority in the defence field, and all types of weapons, including atomic weapons, are being developed.'

Jeger: 'Can the minister give any further information on the development of atomic weapons?'

Minister: 'No. I do not think it would be in the public interest to do that.'

This was how the British public learned that their country had begun building atomic bombs, and it was the only information they were given on the subject for the next four years. Even within the bomb project itself an elaborate cover plan was devised in order to prevent the many people who would be obliged to contribute, at many levels, to know the real object of their activities. Penney himself was imbued with this secrecy from an early stage. When, in November 1946, two months before the bomb decision, he sent a scheme to Lord Portal outlining how the bomb could be built in Britain, it was on a piece of paper Penney had carefully typed out himself so that no-one else could see it.

In later years, the newspapers called him H-Bomb Penney, and in one particularly fulsome article in 1957, the Daily Express solemnly declared: 'Never before in history has the British government placed such reliance on one man's word'. It was true that Penney became indispensible to the bomb project, and it was not just because of his brilliant technological expertise. His modest, unassuming personal manner, with its mixture of heartiness and privacy, enabled him to command respect across a broad range, from the most temperamental cabinet ministers and civil servants to the casual and easy going servicemen who carved out the sites in the Australian desert where most of the bombs were eventually detonated. He liked to be called Bill rather than doctor or Sir William, and when he visited the bomb sites he would don a slouch Australian 'digger's' hat and sometimes follow the lead of the servicemen by stripping down to his shorts in the stifling desert heat.

Penney was by no means the unrelenting, categorical champion of nuclear weapons that some popular accounts have painted him. In this sense, he was not the British equivalent of America's Edward Teller, the 'father' of the hydrogen bomb, or Australia's Sir Ernest Titterton, men whose lofty superiority on the subject of the morality of nuclear weapons has made them targets of anti-nuclear campaigners. Penney, by contrast, did question at various stages the implications of his work, and was more prepared than either of these men to display a degree of humbleness towards it. When his contribution to the tests in Australia was over he became, among other things, a chief British negotiator at the Geneva talks on atmospheric weapons test bans, a period when, he later told a colleague, he never worked so hard in his life.

Penney was born in Gibralter, where his father was stationed as an army warrant officer. His education began at Sheerness Technical School in England, by which time it was clear that he possessed extraordinary mathematical skills. His career at the universities of Wisconsin and Cambridge came through scholarships, and by 1936, at the age of 27, he had become an assistant professor of mathematics at Imperial College, Cambridge. During the war Penney made his name as an expert on explosives when he performed for the Home Office and the Admiralty a series of outstanding experiments to help predict the effect of underwater blasts on the transportable harbours to be set up for the Allied invasion of Normandy.

So when, during 1944, the British scientists working on the Manhattan Project were asked to produce some experts on explosives, Penney was one of the first men they turned to. He went to Los Alamos where he played a key role in calculating the damage from blast and shock waves from the Alamogordo bomb trial and from the bombs dropped on Japan a few weeks later. Penney and Group Captain Leonard Cheshire, VC, who had great experience of British bombing raids over Germany, were the two British representatives in the observation plane above Nagasaki when the bomb fell. Later, Penney went into Hiroshima and Nagasaki with the teams measuring the bombs' effects.

His reports so impressed the Americans that a year later, in June 1946, they implored Penney to come back and take part in their first postwar atomic weapons trials at Bikini, in the Pacific – even though the McMahon Act was about to descend, and even though the Bikini trials would yield so much secret military information that many leading American scientists had been excluded from them. Penney had struck such a chord with the Americans, professionally and personally, that General Groves, the US atom bomb supremo, had come to regard him as the one man on whom he could rely.

In many ways Penney's work had a remarkable degree of simplicity, of which there is no better example than his famous petrol tin experiments. At Nagasaki, while the American scientists were earnestly recording measurements and taking photographs, Penney had noticed that empty petrol tins strewn about the town were bent and damaged to different intensities, clearly depending on their distance from the blast. He collected a lot of the debris and personally humped it back to England to make his own calculations. At the Bikini tests the following year, he arranged for several hundred army petrol tins, which he had carefully helped to fill with water, to be strategically placed so they would register the blast pressure at different points. The elaborate, sophisticated instruments which the Americans had trained on point zero, where the bomb was calculated to burst above the ocean, failed to do the job properly because the bomb fell wide of the mark; Penney with his petrol tins was able to calculate the bomb's power more accurately.

During the first British atomic bomb trials on land, at Emu Field in South Australia, seven years later, Penney used the same method, somewhat refined: he set up in special frames around the range thousands of toothpase tubes which had been flown out from England, minus the paste.

When Britain decided after the war to pursue its own atomic project, the work was set up under three separate sections: a research establishment built on a wartime airfield at Harwell in Berkshire, near London, an organisation to design and construct the plants which would produce the fissile material, plutonium, and an establishment at Aldermaston, also in Berkshire, to actually produce the bomb. John (later Sir John) Cockcroft, a Cambridge physicist, was appointed to run the Harwell research establishment. Cockroft had been a member of the great New Zealand born physicist, Ernest Rutherford's, Cavendish laboratory at Cambridge. In 1932, Cockroft and a colleague had been the first scientists to split an atom by artificial means, an achievement awarded by a Nobel prize in 1951. Christopher (later Lord) Hinton, an outstanding engineer, was responsible for the plutonium plants. And Penney was put in charge of the Aldermaston atomic weapons plant, an establishment inaugurated, of all dates, on 1 April, 1950, although work there did not actually begin until later.

Forty years later, Penney at the Australian royal commission described himself and his two brilliant colleagues, Cockcroft and Hinton, as 'the three lunatics' whom the civil service chiefs, knowing nothing about nuclear matters, were put in the impossible position of trying to control. More seriously, there is little doubt that the talents and personalities of the three men, and their abilities to cut through a miasma of government bureaucracy, were key elements in the project's fruition.[3]

Penney's work on making and testing the atomic bomb was given the official title High Explosives Research, another of those euphemisms, which abound in this story, designed to convey precisely nothing about its true nature. As Penney later put it: 'We always had words which had nothing to do with the subject.' Penney, along with Cockroft and Hinton, believed Britain should build its atomic bombs as soon as possible, partly from national prestige and an unwillingness to concede monopoly over the bomb to the United States, but also because the military chiefs of staff were strenuously pushing for a stockpile of weapons to be produced over the next five years. But there was a definite limit to Penney's enthusiasm. He recognised that Britain was embarking on testing a Nagasaki-type plutonium bomb which the United States already regarded as obsolete, and that even this was placing enormous strains on the country's resources. Could it afford an entrenched bomb program, which would inevitably mean continually refining the design of the weapon as well as producing and testing it? By 1952, the year of Britain's first atomic test, Hurricane, the US was building its first device for a super, or hydrogen bomb. Lord Cherwell, the dour adviser to Churchill, who by then had returned to power, forcefully argued that work begin at once on Britain's own H-bomb. Penney did not share his eagerness.

Penney has been described as a reluctant weaponeer, a man who was roped into the role of Britain's bomb chief when, as he says, he would have preferred the life of a mathematics professor. Certainly there was no shortage of offers: he could have taken several university chairs, including one at Oxford, and named his own price in the US. He stuck with the bomb project not because he believed in the intrinsic superiority of nuclear weapons, but out of a sense of national duty and a genuine belief at that time that the arms race was containable if second ranking countries like Britain were able to have a say in the way these terrible weapons were deployed. During the bomb trials in Australia in the fifties, he said:

'Since I was asked to lead this work I have repeatedly asked myself if I was right to do what I have done. In all humility I can say that I have never wavered in the belief that I was right. To claim that I have never been worried about my action would, however, be very far from the truth.' [4]

Penney and the British team of scientists had returned from Los Alamos with a good knowledge of the scientific theory behind the bomb, at least the American bomb of 1945. As Penney explained:

'The way the British agreed to go to work in America during the war was that nobody would make any notes, nobody would try and steal documents. So we had no documents. But what we had in our minds could

• NO CONCEIVABLE INJURY

not be expunged.'[5]

The British were able to list the bomb's components and principles, and they knew about the apparatus necessary for its testing. But the Americans had deliberately kept them ignorant about certain other key matters, including plutonium production and the actual weapon assembly and design.

The rush to overcome these gaps and to test the first British bomb as early as possible was spurred on by several factors. Until 1947, no-one seriously considered that another major war was imminent. The military chiefs of staff had tried to persuade the Labour government that British defence planning should assume the possibility of war with the Soviet Union, but Attlee and Ernest Bevin, his foreign secretary, would have none of it. They argued that to paint Russia as the enemy could prejudice Britain's outlook and provoke the Russians to take exactly the sort of belligerent steps that could lead to war. In 1947, the main thing threatening Western Europe with collapse was not war but economic failure.

The outlook changed dramatically a year later. There had been a series of disputes between East and West during 1947, and in October of that year the Cominform Declaration from the communist countries had proclaimed the doctrine of a world divided into two opposing and conflicting camps. In June 1948, the Soviet Union imposed its blockade on Berlin, signalling the onset of the Cold War. By then, Bevin had abandoned his reluctance to name the Russians as the enemy. In March, he had grimly told the cabinet: 'It really has become a matter of the defence of Western civilisation or everyone will be swamped by this Soviet method of infiltration'. Rearmament and defence, until now second in priority to economic restoration, were suddenly given new importance. As late as September 1952, a month before the first atomic test in Australia, the military chiefs of staff in Britain produced a secret report which concluded: 'Our whole standard of living stems in large measure from our status as a Great Power and our military strength is a visible indication of our greatness'. It was certainly important to restore Britain's economic independence if it was to regain its place as the major partner with the US in world affairs, the chiefs said; but this would be insufficient unless Britain could also maintain its role as a strong military power in Nato, the Middle East and Asia.

Even before they produced this philosophical report, the military chiefs had been galvanised by the growing East-West tension building up in 1947 to think beyond the mere goal of an independent nuclear deterrent, and to put down on paper precisely how many bombs they wanted and why. This could not necessarily speed up Britain's atomic program, because the earliest target date for the first bomb test, given current knowledge and economic constraints, was five years from 1947 (a timetable which was eventually met with remarkable efficiency). In any case, the defence chiefs confidently calculated that the Russians would not have atomic bombs of their own for several years and that they would not be in a position to use them in a war before 1957 – an extraordinary miscalculation, since the first Soviet atomic test, in 1949, was just two years away.

Acting on the chiefs of staff's conclusion that the only way to deter the Russians was to confront them with similar large-scale weapons of mass destruction, an interservices subcommittee drew up Britain's stockpile goals. It forecast that 600 atomic bombs would be needed to target effectively the Soviet Union by 1957; of these, 400 would come from the United States, leaving 200 bombs to be made in Britain by that year. It was a totally arbitrary figure, reflecting the haphazard process of the decision-making. Even by the end of 1952, after the first British atomic device had been successfully tested, there was still no real plan for future requirements. It was all too often as if Britain's demonstrated ability to build atomic weapons was what mattered most, regardless of how many were needed or the capacity to actually fire them at the Soviet Union. The inconsistency finally became too much for Sir Frederick Morgan, the hapless army general who, in 1951, took over from Lord Portal as controller of atomic energy. Morgan fired off a rash of memoranda to Penney and his colleagues, complaining that the whole business was becoming hog-wild and demanding that some sort of order be brought into it:

'As I understand it, the output figure for weapons ... was arrived at originally by some sort of process akin to that known as a Dutch auction. It seems to me that the requirement has never been keyed in any definite way to any plan of strategy or tactics. This is in a way understandable, since we know that the atomic bomb, ever since the original mishandling of publicity over Hiroshima and Nagasaki, has been regarded as a political far more than as a military weapon.' [6]

Perhaps a more significant reason why the bomb project was able to rush ahead unhindered was that it was almost completely devoid of public controversy. There had been, indeed, a good deal of public concern over the political and moral questions of atomic weapons after Hiroshima and Nagasaki. But this soon faded, as public attention turned to the preoccupations of reconstructing lives dislocated by six years of war. The 'ban the bomb' protest movements, revolving around the Campaign for Nuclear Disarmament, did not begin to build up until the mid-fifties when the hydrogen bomb, an infinitely more powerful weapon than the atomic bomb, with a yield measured in megatons rather than kilotons, came to symbolise the horror of nuclear weapons to a new generation just coming of age.

Once the government had decided to build the atomic bomb, it surrounded the project with a lead shield of secrecy. The Attlee Labour government and, after late 1951, Churchill's Conservative government, were indistinguishable in this respect. Initially there were tangible reasons for the secrecy: to stop any information leaking to the Russians, to avoid the charge from the Americans that the British were bad keepers of secrets and to allow the fledgling efforts at atomic energy control through the United Nations to get under way without being prejudiced. But secrecy quickly became an obsession, and it was often taken to staggering and irrational lengths. It dominated the British atomic project and Britain's atomic relations with other countries, particularly Australia.

Atomic energy was never debated in parliament during the life of the Attlee government. When, on one occasion, a group of MPs sought to put on the notice paper a motion asking for an international conference on atomic weapons control, Bevin tersely told Foreign Office officials: 'Keep it off'. [7] In February, 1951, almost three years after the oblique disclosure in parliament that

Britain was engaged in research and development of atomic weapons, an MP asked whether Britain now had the technical knowledge to build a bomb. This seemingly logical and legitimate question produced an extraordinary flurry of paper work in Whitehall over how it should be answered. Officials advised the government there were only two possible answers: 'Yes, sir', or 'It would not be in the public interest to answer the question'. The reply finally given, in writing, was: 'Yes'. On another occasion, one MP complained that if anyone asked questions about the atomic bomb, 'the prime minister looks at him as if he had asked about something indecent'. Another MP suggested, in the same vein, that the press was as aloof on the subject of the bomb and atomic energy as it had been on sex in the past.

The press in both Britain and Australia, at least initially, did not probe at all into the political, scientific, moral, economic or any other aspect of the atomic project. They allowed themselves to be bound by a series of D-notices, a system of self-denying but non-legally binding ordinances whereby the government secures the agreement of newspapers and broadcasters not to mention subjects whose non-disclosure the government deems to be in the national interest. In London, D-notices were issued over such things as the movement of uranium within the United Kingdom, the location of atomic plants and the identification of people working in them. Even right up to the Hurricane explosion at Monte Bello, only the most bare information was released, in press statements that were usually meaningless. The press were left to speculate, and the result was often a mish-mash of half-truths, inaccuracies and fantasies that sometimes ventured into the realms of science fiction.

Some newspapers said the Hurricane bomb was more powerful than the American atomic bomb, others that it was smaller. Most reported that the bomb had been exploded on a tower built on one of the Monte Bello Islands, when in fact it had gone off in the hull of an old warship, the *Plym*, a fundamental item which the government did not announce until weeks after the event. Some journalists wrote that animals were used in bizarre experiments at Monte Bello, as one reported, 'in tests of anti-atom dust suits designed for air raid wardens'. Another newspaper suggested that scientists at the test were experimenting with special injections on humans designed to build up immunity against radioactivity.

The serious newspapers in Britain tried to discuss this, Britain's first atomic explosion, in the context of renewing the bid for atomic co-operation with the Americans. The popular press, by contrast, took the opportunity to engage in an uninhibited bout of jingoistic chest-thumping, suggesting that the atomic age was about to herald for everyone a brave new world of wealth, luxury and leisure beyond human dreams. The Daily Graphic, for example, published in servile tones an open letter to Penney after the Monte Bello test, headed: 'Thanks, Penney, for the Bomb'. It began:

'Any moment you will be walking through the door of your modest home at West Norwood, London, S.E., into the arms of your family, safely back from the successful test of Britain's first atom weapon. In fact, you might be there this morning to read this because your life is so important to Britain that the greatest secrecy is kept about your movements. Britain and the Commonwealth owe a debt – almost impossible to repay – to you . . . The fact that you and your team have made it possible for Britain to make and store atom bombs has made the country a world power once again.'

When government leaders were asked questions, they replied dismissively. In Australia, Robert Menzies, the prime minister, announced: 'I cannot assist the test – except by keeping quiet.' Howard Beale, his minister for supply, who, as we shall see, became a key figure in Australia during the 1950s testing, did not treat seriously the bewildered alarm expressed by photographers and others that radioactivity which drifted across the mainland from the Monte Bellos might damage sensitive equipment. Beale retorted that Australians were not likely to receive warning of the explosion, and if anyone wanted to protect his goods against radioactivity he should make his own arrangements.[8] In London, Churchill assured the House of Commons, amid loud laughter, that the only animal life reported on the Monte Bello Islands, where the forthcoming bomb was to be ignited, were some lizards, two sea eagles and what looked like a canary sitting on a perch. Later, the scientist in charge of collecting flora and fauna from the islands before the explosion presented a paper listing more than 400 different species of plants and animals, including over 270 kinds of insect. The collection was a significant one, since 20 species of insect, six plants and a subgenus of lizard were totally new to science.[9]

An aura had been carefully allowed to build up around atomic weapons. The public indifference and confusion of the time were a product of government-sponsored ignorance, secrecy and mystery. People were not quite sure whether to expect magic or mayhem from nuclear power. The mood was later summed up by James Cameron, the distinguished British journalist who was among the observers at Operation Crossroads, the two American atomic tests at Bikini in 1946, where Penney used his petrol tins. 'The public,' wrote Cameron, 'vaguely resentful that neither bomb had started a tidal wave or a mass outbreak of the gamma-ray heeby-jeebies, refused to be shocked.' [10]

During this postwar period leading up to Britain's first atomic explosion, there were three strands to her atomic relations with other countries: her relations with the United States, with Europe and with the Commonwealth. The American atomic relationship, as we have seen, was the most significant to Britain, and she was not prepared to jeopardise it by entering into any atomic relationship that involved sharing important information with any other country. If this meant disappointing wartime supporters like Canada and France, or keeping in the dark Commonwealth friends like Australia, it was the price that had to be paid for keeping open her hopes and options with the Americans.

To take Europe first, Britain felt she owed a debt to Belgium, from which the wartime supplies of uranium had been secured, and particularly to France, whose refugee scientists had played such a key role in the development of the Anglo-Canadian heavy water nuclear reactor project during the war.

As for the Commonwealth, Canada had emerged from the war in a special position because of her involvement in the wartime atomic project and was able to go on to develop her own heavy water reactor system for domestic energy independent of British involvement. As a member of the tripartite wartime atomic alliance, she had been able to share much classified information with the other partners, the British and the Americans. Australia was not in such a privileged position. She had not contributed to the Anglo-American atomic project, although three Australian-born scientists, including Oliphant, had been part of the British team working in North America. But by the end of the war, Australia (and New Zealand) had been told nothing about Britain's plans to become a nuclear power. At that stage, neither country appeared to Britain to be of any consequence as a supplier of technology, scientific know-how or raw materials.

During a visit to Australia in 1947, before returning there for good a few years later, Oliphant had suggested to the Australian government the possibility of building an atomic reactor in Australia. He was keen for Australia to pursue nuclear energy for domestic power, and wanted Britain to help. The Labor government in Australia agreed, but saw the proposal in somewhat broader terms as possibly being used to produce plutonium for some future Commonwealth defence program. In 1948, Australia gingerly approached Britain for advise, and suggested that Sir John Cockcroft might visit Australia for talks. The proposal came to nothing partly because Britain, still feeling bound by its wartime agreements with the United States, was worried about passing on classifed atomic information without guarantees of security from Australia. The Americans then, as later, particularly regarded Australia as not terribly security conscious.

The idea was revived three years later by the conservative Liberal government under Menzies, which unseated Labor at the 1949 elections. The difference this time was that the proposed Australian atomic reactor would be fuelled by Australian uranium, whereas a complicating factor of the earlier proposal had been that Australia would have had to get the uranium – as well as the information – from Britain. By early 1951, promising uranium deposits had been discovered at Radium Hill in South Australia and further discoveries were to follow there and at Rum Jungle in the Northern Territory.

Menzies cabled to Attlee that Australia wanted to exploit these uranium deposits for industrial power and urged that co-operation with the UK 'would be of very great assistance to any Australian undertaking'. Attlee replied , in effect, that there was little Britain could offer Australia. There would be no point in Oliphant discussing the proposal with Cockroft, as Menzies had suggested. Attlee explained that the Australian plan would involve the use of classified information which Britain could not pass on, under existing rules, without the consent of the US and Canada. 'Complete separation of power and military programs for the use of atomic energy is not possible', Attlee wrote.

This was at the heart of the emerging atomic relationship between Britain and Australia. At every step of that relationship over the next decade, Britain's stand was governed by the attitude of the Americans or what it perceived or feared would be the American attitude. Britain had been unwilling to allow the McMahon Act to be the end of the matter. It continued to seek a reopening of atomic collaboration with the Americans over the next ten years, but for the most part its efforts came to nothing. There was a brief flutter of hope in 1948 when American and British officials negotiated, again in total secrecy, an arrangement known as the *modus vivendi*. This appeared to offer some areas of technological collaboration, but the British ended up giving away more in this agreement than they gained from it. In any case, no-one in Washington was quite sure how binding it was or for how long. Significantly, the British agreed under American pressure during the talks for the *modus vivendi* to abandon the principle in the Quebec Agreement that neither country would use the atomic bomb without the other's consent – a clause which had outraged American senators when they learned of it after the war. This was to cause the British much anguish soon afterwards when they agreed, during the Berlin airlift, that American aircraft capable of carrying atomic bombs could be based in Britain. When the Korean war broke out two years later, in 1950, there seemed a real possibility that the Americans would use atomic weapons. Britain was suddenly faced with the intolerable situation of risking annihilation in retaliation for atomic attacks launched from bases on its soil over which it had no control. It sought from the Americans a restoration of Britain's right to consent before atomic bombs were used from bases in Britain, but was only partly successful in this.

The door to renewed atomic collaboration was finally slammed by Washington in February 1950, when Klaus Fuchs, the German-born, naturalised British physicist, who had worked at Los Alamos during the war, was arrested in Britain and convicted of spying for the Russians. Fuchs confessed that he had passed over a great deal of important material about the bomb, including the make-up of the plutonium bomb tested at Alamogordo in July 1945. He had also told the Russians all he knew about the principles of the hydrogen bomb, as they were discussed at Los Alamos. This was not the first spy case to rock Anglo-American relations, nor was it to be the last. In 1946, Alan Nunn May, a member of the British scientific team in Canada during the war, had been convicted of spying. Six months after Fuchs's conviction, Bruno Pontecorvo, another eminent physicist who had worked with Fuchs at Harwell, disappeared and surfaced with his family soon afterwards in Russia. The following year, 1951, Donald Maclean, who had been a senior diplomat with access to atomic secrets in the British embassy in Washington during 1947 and 1948, also fled to Russia. The British spy scandals confirmed the worst fears among some Americans about British security.

The plain fact was that the US was determined to keep its monopoly over atomic energy, for both military and industrial power. In spite of the close and special relationship the British and Americans were forging at this time in foreign affairs, through NATO, the Americans insisted on keeping the atomic question as a world apart. They were unimpressed by Britain's unrelenting bid for renewed atomic collaboration, and by its arguments that separate atomic programs would be a waste of resources, manpower and money. To the Americans, there was something of the poor relation about Britain. Despite the illusions among the British military and civil service chiefs about the need to maintain Britain's great power status, British affairs now seemed of only marginal importance to the Americans. Yet despite the agonies and disappointments, the British stood ready to work for Anglo-American atomic collaboration as the first priority; and they were prepared to forego close collaboration and information-sharing with other friendly countries, including Australia, to achieve it.

It was a traumatic time for Britain for other reasons. In August 1949, the Russians exploded their first atomic bomb. This was a shattering moment of truth for the British, the realisation that the

Soviet Union was, indeed, the world's second superpower. Although the British had helped invent the atomic bomb, the Russians, starting from scratch, had beaten them. Many atomic scientists in Britain simply could not believe it, and were convinced it was the work of spies (something which has since been open to dispute). In any case, Britain's own nuclear deterrent, still three years away from testing, would now look far less impressive. Already, British officials had been dismayed to learn in 1949 of the huge strides the Americans had made in weapon technology and manufacture since the end of the war. Recent events, not least the Berlin blockade, the Soviet atomic explosion and the communist victory in China had convinced the Americans that bigger and better weapons were needed if what they perceived as a monolithic advance by communism around the world was to be stopped. In January 1950, President Harry Truman announced that the United States was to start work on a thermonuclear weapon, the super or hydrogen bomb. As the British correctly saw, this would make their chances of collaboration with the Americans even more distant.

So the British went ahead with their own bomb. When Churchill returned to Downing Street as prime minister after the elections of October 1951, he was momentarily stunned by the size of the outgoing Attlee government's atomic program. Churchill discovered, with a mixture of surprise and the foxy admiration of a good parliamentarian, that the previous government had managed to spend almost 100 million pounds on atomic energy without informing parliament. He demanded to know how this had been hidden in the accounts, and muttered that if he had done the same thing he would have been branded a warmonger. He then proceeded to do the same thing, reluctantly agreeing with the argument of Lord Cherwell, his chief adviser, that for Britain to publish its figures on atomic expenditure would not impress the Americans and would give everything away to the Russians.

Cherwell was a significant figure in the British atomic bomb story because of his considerable influence over Churchill, and his undivided support for the bomb project. He was born Frederick Lindemann in Germany in 1886, the younger son of a wealthy German father and an English mother who settled in England when he was a boy. He had a comfortable, English county upbringing, studied physics and mathematics and by his mid-thirties had been offered a chair of physics at Oxford, where he lived alone in rooms in Christ Church College for much of his life.

Despite his privileged surroundings, his political toughness and his unhidden pleasure at being a regular guest in some of the smartest homes in England, Cherwell was a man of some complexity who, in many ways, led an austere life. He did not drink or smoke and was a lifelong vegetarian. He also had extraordinary personal inhibitions. His biographer, Lord Birkenhead, has reported that Cherwell's fear of being thought ridiculous was almost overwhelming. He felt it necessary to retire behind a curtain before mopping the sweat from his brow, and he could not bear to be seen in a dressing gown.

Cherwell's long friendship with Churchill stemmed from the interwar years, so that when Churchill became prime minister after the outbreak of the Second World War it was perfectly natural that he should take on his old friend as his personal assistant. Before long, Churchill made him a baron. Cherwell stalked the corridors of power as Churchill's *eminence grise* on most matters, but particularly scientific and atomic affairs. Many civil servants resented him because of his remarkable position of power without responsibility, a situation Churchill later regularised by making Cherwell a member of his cabinet as paymaster general.

When Churchill returned to 10 Downing Street as prime minister in 1951, he again called in Cherwell and reappointed him paymaster general with the same advisory role. Cherwell by this time prided himself on knowing more about the bomb project than Churchill: during the Attlee government Cherwell had been kept on as a member of Lord Portal's technical committee and he took a deep and abiding interest in the bomb and its problems. There were no inhibitions about his views here: Cherwell fervently believed that Britain should build the bomb, and as soon as posssible. He just could not contemplate the thought that Britain might 'rank with other European nations who have to make do with conventional weapons'. Moreover, he was more realistic than Churchill who, even now, still hoped that the spirit of the Quebec Agreement could be revived and perhaps lead to a reintegration of the British and American bomb projects. Cherwell had no such faith in the Americans changing their minds, and he told Churchill so in blunt terms.

Cherwell approved of the goals drawn up under the Attlee government for Britain to accumulate a stock of atomic bombs by 1957. If he had any criticism, it was that the pace of work was far too slow. He blamed this on the cumbersome administrative structure of the atomic project, which was still run by the civil service in Whitehall. Cherwell was convinced the project could succeed only if it was freed from the usual constraints of civil service accountability. He campaigned vigorously for the whole business to be given its own separate organisation, where talented people could be hired at attractive salaries and civil servants would not be able to poke their noses.

Cherwell was eventually successful when the UK Atomic Energy Authority came into being in 1954. This was the year Britain took the decision to build a hydrogen bomb, a move for which, as we have seen, Cherwell himself had been pushing very early on. Cherwell had no time for scientists getting involved in politics, especially when their views were not the same as his. To him, one scientist in politics, like himself, was enough. He was particularly averse to scientists like Professor Joseph Rotblat, the Polish-born physicist who helped found Pugwash, a peace movement among atomic scientists set up in the wake of the hydrogen bomb tests of the mid-fifties. Rotblat had worked with the British team at Los Alamos, but had left the Manhattan Project abruptly when it was clear that Hitler was not going to build an atomic bomb. Rotblat could see no further justification for the American atomic bomb project, and returned to England to work on radiation medicine. In 1957, shortly before Cherwell died, he attacked the Pugwash scientists in the House of Lords. Cherwell said he could not understand how anyone with a logical mind could argue that Britain ought not to test thermonuclear weapons if it had them. The argument that the tests were a danger to the health of humanity was, said Cherwell, 'unmitigated nonsense'.

By the time Churchill returned to Downing Street, Penney and his team at Aldermaston had almost finished working out the bomb design. But the question of where to test the weapon had been causing them acute anxiety for almost 18 months. It was somewhat ironical that while the Attlee government had been turning down Australia's request for help with a proposed nuclear reactor, it had also been negotiating with Australia quite separately to explode the bomb there. Most of the British team, particularly Penney, wanted to use the well-equipped American test sites in Nevada or the Marshall Islands in the Pacific: it would mean less strain on British resources and it would be in line with the ultimate hope of reviving Anglo-American atomic collaboration. But a British request during the first half of 1950 to use one of the American test sites had not even been answered by Washington (the general atomic talks that had been quietly going on between the two countries had collapsed the previous February after Fuchs' arrest).

A search for alternatives was mounted. Penney went to Canada to survey seven possible sites there, and in London Attlee sent a highly classified message to Menzies asking if Australia would agree in principle to the test being held in the Monte Bello Islands and to take part in a survey of the site. Menzies took just three days to say yes to both requests. The Monte Bellos were a windswept group of islands 80 kilometres off the northwest coast of Australia. They were known mainly by navy people and itinerant pearl fishermen, since no-one lived there and hardly anyone else ever went there. In fact, it was not even certain that Australia owned the islands because no-one had ever laid claim to them. Their inlets had acquired certain swashbuckling names like Claret Bay, Rum Cove and Vodka Beach, but apart from the remarkable wildlife mentioned earlier they were otherwise undistinguished.

One advantage of the Monte Bellos over the other possible sites was that they would be ideal for Penney's preferred option of testing the weapon in the hull of a ship to study the possible effects of an enemy smuggling an atomic bomb into a British port. At the 1946 Bikini trials, Penney had been particularly worried by the phenomenon of the 'base surge': when an atomic bomb was exploded under water it blew the water into an enormous cloud of fine mist, containing the weapon's dangerously radioactive fission products. After the water cloud reached its zenith, it quickly fell down again under gravity rolling out and spreading the radioactivity as it went. How would this sort of occurrence affect navy personnel and surrounding civilian populations?

In February 1951, the British chiefs of staff agreed to Penney's idea of a shipborne bomb in the Monte Bellos, and the following month Attlee formally asked Menzies if the trial could take place there in October 1952. Attlee also asked for Australian help in preparing the site and with logistics. And he warned that the area around the islands was likely to be contaminated with radioactivity for at least three years afterwards, during which time it would be unsafe for human occupation, even for visits by pearl fishermen. Menzies advised that because of an impending election in Australia he could not give a final decision; but the following May, when his government was safely returned at the polls, he cabled his agreement. Far from insisting on some quid pro quo – such as, for example, a bomb test site in exchange for help in setting up an Australian atomic energy program – Menzies agreed to the British request, as Gowing, the official historian, has put it in fine understatement, 'without striking a hard bargain over technical collaboration'.

Yet even though Australia had been lined up, Britain continued to keep its options open on the American sites until almost the last minute. Penney flew across the Atlantic for further agonising talks, but the Americans did, indeed, strike a hard bargain. They wanted to impose so many restrictions and conditions under the McMahon Act for the exchange of information from Britain's bomb test, that the exercise would have amounted, in effect, to a joint test. Penney explained at the Australian royal commission in 1985 what the Americans had proposed:

'They would do the test, and they would want a drawing of exactly what was in it [the bomb], that kind of information. Our government said, 'No, that is unacceptable'. But I would have taken it. The reason was I wanted to get back to Anglo-American collaboration.' [11]

When Churchill took over from Attlee the following October (1951), the chiefs of staff had concluded that, under the circumstances, Monte Bello was the only choice. Cherwell agreed, and implored Churchill to give his approval to the Australian site. One point Cherwell made was that there was always a chance that the bomb might not detonate properly, 'and it would be disastrous if this happens in full view of the United States newspapers'. Churchill, ever hoping for a rapprochement with the Americans, grudgingly gave in.

An announcement of the test, without naming the actual site, was made in Britain and Australia four months later, in February 1952, shortly before the first British ships sailed for Western Australia. 'It will be conducted in conditions which will ensure that there will be no danger whatever from radioactivity to the health of people and animals in the Commonwealth', the statement said. Most newspapers jumped to the conclusion that the bomb would be let off at the Woomera rocket testing range in South Australia. Monte Bello was not revealed as the true site until the following May, and only then after much official soul-searching about whether such a revelation at all before the blast would invite sabotage. The press were forbidden from attending the test, in contrast to the practice at American atomic trials since 1946. But press groups armed with telephoto lenses set themselves up on Mount Potter on the mainland, 88 kilometres from the Monte Bello Islands, outside the prohibited zone around the islands which the Australian government had declared in special legislation.

The bomb itself was very similar in construction and assembly to the first atomic weapon, Trinity, tested at Alamogordo in July 1945 just before the use of the atomic bombs on Japan. Penney had been able to duplicate the implosion technique mastered at Los Alamos. In assembling any atomic weapon the problem is to avoid a chain reaction taking place prematurely. The fissile material therefore has to be kept at below its critical mass until the moment of the explosion. Two or more lumps of fissile material, each smaller than the vital critical mass, are kept separate, then brought together extremely rapidly so that the explosion happens at the moment when the mass becomes supercritical. Unless this assembly takes place very quickly, the energy released through fission will be dispersed and the explosion will peter out.

During the Manhattan Project, scientists initially focused on the gun method of achieving this rapid assembly, using uranium 235 as the fissile material. Two subcritical lumps of the uranium were placed at opposite ends of the barrel of a gun and fired into each other at the right moment. The scientists were so confident this method would work that they used it in the Hiroshima bomb, which they called Little Boy, without testing the weapon first.

They found, though, that while the gun method was fine for uranium 235, it would not work with the other fissile material, plutonium. Because of problems with certain isotopes of plutonium, there was every danger that the chain reaction would be premature and that the explosion would fizzle using this method. The scientists found another technique, called implosion, to detonate a plutonium bomb in a way that would bring the subcritical masses together at a far greater speed than in the gun method. It involved surrounding a sphere of subcritical plutonium with ordinary high explosives. These explosives were then detonated, and the force of their blast directed inwards so that it literally squeezed the plutonium together until it reached criticality. It was a particularly complicated method with many physical problems to be perfected, which is why the scientists decided to test it at Alamogordo first before employing it in the Nagasaki bomb, dubbed Fat Man to distinguish it from the Hiroshima model. The British team at Los Alamos had had more to do with the implosion work than the gun assembly, and they were able to assemble a manual on it when they returned home after the war.

The implosion bomb Penney devised made its way to Australia in the utmost secrecy, and in two different stages. The weapon itself, without its vital radioactive core, was concealed aboard HMS *Plym*, a frigate which was destined to be pulverised by the blast. In early 1952 the *Plym* and the flagship of the expedition, HMS *Campania*, a converted aircraft carrier, held a secret rehearsal with a third ship to simulate the layout of the trial in the Thames estuary. Then in June the *Plym* and the *Campania* sailed for Australia via the Cape, avoiding the Suez Canal. Two other ships, the *Zeebrugge* and the *Narvik*, had already gone as an advance party. None of the seamen was told the purpose of their mission before departure, although many guessed, and no-one knew the bomb itself was in the *Plym*. As the target vessel she was given the initials TV, which most people associated with television; a tangle of antennae was set up on her deck to help reinforce this impression and conceal her true nature.

The bomb's radioactive core, a ball of plutonium inside a container, arrived separately by air two weeks before the blast. It came in a special flying boat and had been entrusted to one W.J. Moyce, from Aldermaston, who had been given blunt and basic instructions to make sure it survived the three-day flight from England. The core had been packed in a cork box, with a bag of dye attached, the idea being that if the aircraft crashed in the sea the bomb core would float and the spreading dye would help a search party to trace it. Moyce had been told that if the aircraft looked like crashing over land, he was to make a parachute jump clinging on to his precious consignment.[12]

Moyce and both sections of the bomb arrived safely, and when it was finally assembled for D-Day it resembled, according to a witness who saw it, a rotary washing machine. Despite the traumas and anxieties of his flight, Moyce probably had the better journey. The sea voyages had been marked by tension and bickering between the navy men and the 'boffins', the civilian scientists, doctors and engineers whose casual and laid-back style, particularly over dress, was completely anathema to the regimented and disciplined ways of the Royal Navy. The uneasy gap between the boffins and the servicemen was never quite bridged throughout the entire weapons test program over the next five years.

For apart from its essentially political purpose, this first British test had certain military and civil defence goals as well. The navy, as we have seen, wanted to test the effect of an atom bomb exploded in the hold of a ship. Other basic experiments were set up on the Monte Bello Islands to measure the effect of blast and shock waves on buildings, paint and clothing. Boxes of fruit and vegetables grown on the voyage out were dotted around the sand dunes to see how much radioactivity they would absorb. Fish were caught after the explosion and their glands taken back to England to probe the uptake of radioactive fission products like iodine and strontium. And there was, of course, the task of tracking the cloud from the blast so that samples of airborne radioactivity could be made, a job for which seven Lincoln aircraft of the Royal Australian Air Force were stationed at Broome on the mainland coast.

At 8 am on 3 October 1952, the Hurricane bomb was detonated about 3 metres below the waterline. The *Plym* was completely blown to pieces and the bits instantly vaporised. The power, or yield, of the bomb was about 25 kilotons, the same amount of energy released in the detonation of 25000 tons of TNT. This was slightly more powerful than each of the bombs which had devastated Hiroshima and Nagasaki, and the second most powerful of the British nuclear weapons to be exploded in Australia. After all that, the spectacle was somewhat disappointing to some of those who watched it. The cloud rose to about 3000 metres, but instead of becoming the familiar mushroom of the American bombs it was quickly torn about by winds at different levels and took on a rather dull Z shape.

Penney, who had arrived at Monte Bello ten days earlier, gave the firing order from the deck of the *Campania* where he was stationed with Rear Admiral A.D. Torlesse, the naval commader of the expedition, and with three Australian scientists, Ernest Titterton, Leslie Martin and Alan Butement. He had been Dr Penney when he arrived in Australia for the event, but, within a few days, Churchill acknowledged the scientific success of his efforts by announcing a knighthood for Penney, at the age of 43. Penney recorded a personal account of the blast, which was broadcast on radio simultaneously in Britain, Australia, New Zealand, Canada, South Africa and the US, and flew back to England a week after the test. He told his millions of listeners:

'The sight before our eyes was terrifying'. 'A great, greyish-black cloud being hurled thousands of feet into the air and increasing in size with astonishing rapidity. A great sandstorm suddenly sprang up over the islands. . . . Mr Churchill has said that the results of our atomic weapon program should be benficial to public safety. As a scientist, I should like most strongly to agree with this view. The energy and enthusiasm which have gone into the making of this new weapon stemmed essentially from the sober hope that it would bring us nearer the day when world war is universally seen to be unthinkable.'

Others were closer than Penney to the blast and had a different experience of it. Henry Carter, a Royal Navy mechanic on the

Plym, was 30 at the time of the test. He was one of the four last people to leave the *Plym* before the explosion, having been charged with the job of taking the final two scientists off the ship and returning them again if the bomb malfunctioned. The party rowed ashore, then transferred to a small power boat with five other people and zig-zagged around the islands before taking shelter behind a ledge about 3 kilometres away from the *Plym*.

'The signal came over the radio to prepare for countdown, and a black, heavy canvas tarpaulin was pulled over the boat so we were now in darkness.' 'We all then draped jungle green towels over our heads and I pressed the palms of my hands into my eye sockets. I was dressed in shorts and a pair of shoes. At zero there was a blinding, electric blue light of an intensity I had not seen before or since. I pressed my hands harder to my eyes, then realised I could see the bones of my hands. It seemed that this light was passing through the tarpaulin and towel for about 10 or 12 seconds and there seemed to be two surges and two detonations with a continued rumbling and boiling sensation. My body seemed first to be compressed, and then billowing like a balloon.'

When the all clear came and the men in the boat removed the towels from their heads, Carter noticed there was sunlight coming through holes in the tarpaulin.

'Several days after the detonation, I was taken by helicopter for a view and saw that everything was black and burned including the sand and rocks right up to the ledge we had been sheltering behind. I believe that the holes in the tarpaulin were caused in the same way as the blackening of the area.'

Thirty years later, Carter had cataracts removed from both his eyes. He tried to obtain a copy of his service medical file, but was told it had been 'stripped.' He said:

'It was well known that no-one had any true idea of the final results to be expected, just as they still have no answer to the particular illnesses still suffered by the veterans.' [13]

There was no precedent in Britain for working out whether there were any radiation exposure levels from an atomic bomb which could be regarded as 'safe', nor was there any legislation to cover this. The Monte Bello bomb was the 33rd atomic weapon test since the war (there had been 29 American and three Soviet trials). But the Americans had been as secretive about the radioactivity aspect of their own tests in Nevada and the Pacific as they had been about almost everything else.

A top secret document prepared in London just a few months before Hurricane, and shown to only a few people in charge of the test, frankly admitted:

'We have no information about the spread of fission products when an atomic bomb is detonated on the surface of the ground or on the surface of the sea. It is, in fact, one of the objects of the experiment to fill to some extent this gap in our knowledge.'

The document warned that about 10 per cent of the fission products could be deposited on the Australian mainland; about 30 per cent would be thrown up in water spray and would settle again quickly, and the remaining 60 per cent would be deposited on condensed metal particles in the cloud, which would be spread over such a wide area that the radioactive contamination would be 'negligible'.

In preparing for this question, the trial planners in the Admiralty were clearly concerned that radiological safety must not be allowed to overshadow everything – or, as another secret pre-trial document put it: 'Some degree of risk must be run by some people if we are to achieve the full purpose of the trial.' Penney was to seek the advice of the British Medical Research Council on radiation exposure levels, but the planners were worried that the council may 'play for safety to such an extent that we might be quite unable to achieve the scientific purpose of the trial'. So they asked in strict confidence that the council should recommend two exposure levels – a general level, and a special, once-only level for volunteers. In the end, Penney put forward for approval by the Admiralty and the Ministry of Supply three maximum permissible levels. The first was a low dosage rate for continuous exposure over normal working. The second was a higher 'integrated dose' received in one or a few exposures. People whose work required them to be exposed to this higher dose would need the permission of the radiation safety officer and would not be subjected to radiation again for the rest of the operation. The third, and still higher level, would be for cases of extreme urgency – for instance, recovery of vital records – and people involved here would be banned from any further radiation for at least a year. The measurements were drawn up in conjunction with trial orders which decreed that everyone in the areas contaminated by the bomb was to wear protective clothing and gas masks; even those outside the contaminated areas were to wear film badges which would measure any possible exposure to the outsides of their bodies. Clothing which was 'badly contaminated' on men returning from the bomb area would be taken off and dumped in the sea, although 'lightly contaminated' clothes were to be sealed up and taken back to England for decontamination (the whole question of radiation safety is discussed further in Chapter Seven).

Not everything went according to plan. The bomb cloud rose to between 3000 and 4000 metres, which was only half the height predicted, and at such levels it was subjected to rapidly varying wind behaviour. 'It was obvious that within a few hours large and rapidly increasing errors in its estimated position were inevitable', a secret report by the naval commander noted later. Contamination did drift over the Australian mainland, where tribal Aborigines lived and for whom no consideration had been made in the trial orders drawn up in London. The vital job of tracking the bomb cloud and monitoring its behaviour was delayed for six hours. There was a mishap in transmitting the monitoring order from the naval fleet at Monte Bello to Broome, on the mainland, where the RAAF Lincolns were standing by to begin the search. The signal was badly sent from the ship and could not be deciphered in Broome. The ship was asked to repeat it again, and again. Four old and experienced operators were brought in at Broome to try to take it down. Finally it was proved that the signal itself was completely wrong, and the whole thing had to start from the beginning.

The safety standards laid down in the trial orders were not always enforced and, generally, were less strict than those at later

British trials. For example, the Australian air and ground crews of the Lincolns involved in tracking the bomb cloud were given neither film badges to measure their own contamination nor dosimeters to record contamination inside their aircraft.

For those on the ground, the weather was so hot that many of the men who went into the danger areas had to remove their protective clothing so they could breathe, and few of them bothered with the radiation measuring devices because they did not know how to read them. Thomas Wilson, who served with the Royal Engineers at Monte Bello, was sent with a group to collect food and other exposed materials from one of the islands a few days after the blast. The men were given overalls, a hat and a gas mask. 'We had to remove the mask time and again,' Wilson the Australian royal commission in 1985. 'The heat was so bad it was very hard to breathe, and we could not see because the condensation impaired our vision. We got covered in sand and grit thrown up by the wheels of the Land Rover'.

Michael Stephens, a navy meteorologist based on the flagship, the *Campania*, needed several showers before he was cleared of external contamination. After the blast, with his meteorological forecasting work over, Stephens was assigned to the crew of a boat taking scientists back and forth for six weeks to study the effects of the bomb on the islands. The usual rig, he remembered, was shorts and sandals. After each trip they would check through the decontamination procedure of showers and geigercounters, but the system was not foolproof. For years afterwards, Stephens kept as a souvenir a pair of sea boots which should have been destroyed.

'Of course I would not have done this if I had known there was any radiation risk. But radioactivity was regarded as a joke by the crew and servicemen. There was no education about any potential danger. The only danger we were warned of was sharks and barracuda.'

As the remnants of the radioactive cloud drifted into the atmosphere, few of the scientists who had helped produce it thought about the horrors of nuclear weapons or the doubts and questioning that lay ahead. They had fulfilled with complete professionalism and efficiency what they had been asked to do: to build a British nuclear deterrent that was adequate, cheap and that worked. Britain was now a member of the nuclear club. Where was she to go from here? As with most clubs, the rules were being written not by the new members, but by the big boys – and they were changing, at a frightening speed.

Chapter Three
MENZIES AND TITTERTON

'Well, actually, Ernest, to be quite frank, you're the worst possible advocate of the truth . . . so aggressive about it'. – Keith Lokan, head of the Australian Radiation Laboratory, to Sir Ernest Titterton, 1981. [1]

Now that Australia had been drawn into the British atomic program, even if by default, some serious questions arose. What role was Australia to play in all of this? What steps was Australia to take to make sure that no-one in the country suffered from radioactive fallout, not least the Aborigines who lived in and around the desert where future bombs were to be exploded? Was Australia to be more than a mere testing ground, insisting on being given a bare minimum of information and a say in the proceedings before allowing them to go ahead; or was she to have faith in the superior scientific knowledge of the British, who had, after all, built the bombs?

These questions were never asked, still less debated, in Australia at the time. There was, instead, a secret conjunction of science and politics at the top level, from the genesis of the tests in Australia in 1951 until the time the British left Maralinga in 1967. It came about largely through a meeting of minds between two men: Robert Menzies, the prime minister, and Ernest Titterton, an eminent nuclear physicist. Both were later made knights. The personalities of these two men, and their respective convictions on such questions as the role of the British Commonwealth in the postwar world and the inherent superiority of science and scientists as providers of answers in that world, were pivotal to the events that followed. Without the unequivocal support of Menzies and Titterton the tests would not have taken place in Australia in the manner that they did, and may not even have taken place in Australia at all.

Menzies was born in 1894, in Jeparit, a small, ordinary town in western Victoria that had little to boast of in the way of the social and political grandeur which marked Menzies' later life. His father was a former member of the state parliament of Victoria. Menzies entered the Victorian bar in 1918 and Victorian state politics 10 years later, then transferred to the House of Representatives in Canberra where he quickly became attorney-general in the conservative government of Joseph Lyons, a post he held until he became prime minister in March 1939. Two years later, after bitter factional fighting, his party, the United Australia Party, dumped him as leader and soon afterwards the Labor party, under John Curtin, came to power. Menzies spent the war years regrouping the forces of conservatism and eventually formed the inaptly named Liberal Party, which took office with him as leader in 1949 and stayed there until the Labor Party's Gough Whitlam unseated it in 1972, Menzies himself having retired from politics in 1965 after a record 16 years as prime minister.

Menzies was a brilliant politician with an uncommonly ascerbic power of oratory which he successfully exploited to keep his enemies at bay. He stood for three things: anti communism, free enterprise and a staunch defence of white Australia's Anglo-Saxon origins. During the 1950s, the Australia of Menzies' era was not a country in which diversity – social, cultural or political – was encouraged. It was a decade of postwar prosperity, in which most Australians responded positively to Menzies' anti communism and support for a continuing defence role for Britain in their part of the world, both being seen as two readily identifiable measures for maintaining security in a period of unprecedented economic boom. In 1951, when the Cold War had set in, the Korean War was under way and communist movements were gaining ground in some of the newly independent countries of South-east Asia, Menzies unsuccessfully held a referendum to ban the Communist Party in Australia; but other forms of censorship, literary, visual and political, were blithely carried on by his government for years without the public taking much notice or interest. The nationalism and self-questioning that characterised Australia after Menzies left the scene still lay more than 20 years in the future.

Menzies – not alone among the Western leaders of his day – worked on the politics of fear at home and abroad, and the biggest threat he portrayed to domestic and international stability was the fear of communism. In 1951, two years after he became prime minister, he warned Australians: 'It is my belief that the state of the world is such that we cannot and must not give ourselves more than three years in which to get ready to defend ourselves. Indeed, three years is a liberal estimate'. Communism was a monolith and the communist forces of the world were preparing to turn the Cold War into a 'hot war', a world war.

The communists could now overrun Europe with the same speed as Hitler had done in 1940 – that was surely clear, 'subject only to atomic reprisals'. In September 1950, Menzies made three radio broadcasts, billed as the 'Defence Call to the Nation'. In the first of them he declared:

Do you think that this Communist enemy would hesitate to overrun Western civilisation if the United States did not have the atomic bomb? Don't let's pretend about the bomb. It's real. It is today keeping the world out of a tragic world-wide war. Horrible as it is (and I saw Hiroshima a few weeks ago), it is today not an instrument of war, but of peace. How many years do you suppose will elapse before the communist has it, in large quantities? Five? Four? Three? Two?

Menzies' attitudes were perhaps nowhere more concentrated than in his perceptions of Australia's role in the world. He persisted in regarding Australia, a country with less than 200 years of history of European settlement, as an extension, if not an appendage of Britain in world affairs. True, there were inevitable divergencies. Australia's military realignment away from Britain towards the United States had begun during the Second World War as an act of sheer national survival in the Pacific war against Japan. The Liberals under Menzies did not follow Britain and recognise Mao Tse tung's communist regime in China after 1949. Instead they followed the United States, whose military involvement in Asia and the Pacific they regarded as the key to Australia's defence policy, and closed the diplomatic door on China for the next 23 years.

But for the most part, Menzies clung to the Britishness of Australia, and he was fond of speaking of the two countries almost as one – of, as he put it, the ancient virtues of their character and institutions. In late 1953, after the first three of 12 British nuclear bombs had been exploded in Australia, Menzies wrote to Churchill:

The basic fact is that we stand or fall together, and that Great Britain will no more need to worry about Australian cooperation in the future than she has in the past. The longer I engage in public affairs the more convinced I am that we must at all times nourish our ancient stuctural unity which remains the best thing in the free world.

Menzies was perhaps more at home than anywhere else sitting at Commonwealth prime ministers' conferences in Downing Street, the British prime minister's official London residence, with a picture of Walpole gazing down from the fireplace. He saw the Commonwealth in terms of old-fashioned family values, in which the younger members had a duty to support and assist the mother country which had given them so much. For Menzies, the white Commonwealth countries, Britain, Australia, New Zealand and Canada, were the ones whose values really mattered. He resisted the inevitable broadening of the Commonwealth with new, non-white countries who had won their independence under the impetus of the nationalist movements in the early post-war years. This made the Commonwealth less comprehensible to Menzies; it put 'unhappy thoughts in my mind'.

In later years he wrote:

I love Britain because I love Australia . . . Our language comes to us from Britain and so does the bulk of our literature. To have no love for a relatively small community in the North Sea which created and handed on these vital matters would be, to my mind, a miserable act of ingratitude . . . We are British subjects because we owe our allegiance to the Queen, an allegiance which so far from weakening our independence gives it pride and strength'. [2]

But at the time of the atomic tests in the 1950s, no one could have captured Menzies' refusal to recognise or come to terms with an order of Britain and Australia that was already thoroughly out of date, more than Menzies himself. As he lamented to parliament in Canberra: 'When we have grown up in a world of a certain pattern and have accommodated ourselves to ideas of a certain kind, it is not easy to adjust ourselves to a new world or to new ideas'. [3]

To Menzies, then, the secret and swift decision to allow Britain to test its nuclear weapons in Australia, a decision taken without consulting his cabinet colleagues, stemmed from two of his pivotal passions, his adoration of Britain and his abhorrence of communism. There was also, as we shall see, a consideration that Australia may gain some knowledge for an atomic energy program of its own, but this was purely secondary to the political overtones just mentioned. Menzies himself said very little publicly about the British bomb, even though he was the man who, almost unilaterally, had agreed to Australia becoming the test site. His cabinet learned of it only after the event. Up to mid February 1952, atomic matters came before the Menzies cabinet only once, and that was an occasion, on 18 February that year, when Menzies informed cabinet he intended to release a press statement announcing the testing of a British atomic device in Australia. At the same cabinet meeting, ministers spent more time discussing the forthcoming coronation of Queen Elizabeth II and the timing of her visit to Australia after she was crowned.

Later that year, Menzies left on a visit to Washington and London, where secret talks were held with members of the British atomic energy committee about security arrangements for the forthcoming trial at Monte Bello. On his return to Canberra in July Menzies reported to cabinet on his overseas talks, but among the detailed official record of the topics on which he briefed ministers, atomic weapons is not listed. From then until the end of 1954, atomic questions were never raised in cabinet, except for ministers to approve, without debate, arrangements already drawn up in secret by civil servants, such as the establishment of the permanent weapons testing ground at Maralinga. By contrast, Menzies initiated a long discussion in cabinet in August 1952, about proposed changes to the royal style and title which would have made the Queen's title different in each country of the

Commonwealth. [4]

There was no dissension from the opposition Labor party in Australia to the holding of the first British atomic tests. If anything, Labor MPs in the 1950s supported an Australian foreign and defence policy directed towards maintaining the military power of Australia's traditional allies, Britain and the United States, reflected through Australia's membership of regional alliances such as ANZUS and the now defunct South East Asia Treaty Organisation, which included both Britain and the US. One of the rare parliamentary debates on atomic energy was initiated not by the government or the Labor opposition but by a backbench Liberal MP, William Wentworth, a descendent of one of Australia's most famous nineteenth century explorers and a man with something of a reputation as an eccentric and a rebel. It took place in Canberra on 15 October 1953 - extraordinarily enough, the day of the first land based British atomic bomb test at Emu Field, in South Australia. The date was purely coincidental, because although the debate revolved around the call for international control of nuclear weapons, no MP raised the subject of the British atomic tests in Australia. Despite the high minded sentiments from MPs of both major parties, it was as if this particular subject was unmentionable, and to question it was tantamount to treason. Among the speakers was Herbert Evatt, the fiery Labor party leader who had been the first chairman of the United Nations atomic energy commission in 1946, at the time of the abortive postwar moves to control the spread of atomic weapons. Evatt did not really become critical of the British nuclear tests for another four years, when Britain was testing its hydrogen bombs on Christmas Island in the Pacific and when Evatt's own career was in decline.

One of Menzies' rare statements came after the first atomic bomb test on land at Emu Field, when an MP asked in parliament that, before any more bombs were exploded, a thorough investigation be made into the atomic bomb's radioactive impact on human, animal and plant life. Menzies' reply is a worthy illustration of his calculated facility with obfuscation and for talking down to a questioner. He said:

It has been stated most authoritatively that no conceivable injury to life, limb or property could emerge from the test. I should like to say that it would be unfortunate if we in Australia began to display some unreal nervousness on this point. The tests are conducted in the vast spaces in the centre of Australia, and if it is to be said, however groundlessly, that there are risks, what will be said in other countries? Are we then to reach the position in which we shall not conduct these experiments? Believe me, the enemy will conduct them. If the experiments are not to be conducted in Australia, with all our natural advantages for this purpose, we are contracting out of the common defence of the free world. No risk is involved in this matter. The greatest risk is that we may become inferior in potential military strength to the potential of the enemy.

Menzies left what few public statements there were to Howard (later, Sir Howard) Beale, his minister for supply. Beale was, if anything, more enthusiastic about the British atomic tests than Menzies. But Beale became a victim partly of the ignorance and secrecy that surrounded the whole affair and partly of his own overenthusiasm. He was born in 1898, the son of a northern New South Wales clergyman, went to the bar in 1925 and entered federal politics when he was elected to the House of Representatives in Canberra for Menzies' newly formed Liberal Party in 1946, at the relatively late age of 48. When Menzies came to power three years later, he took Beale straight into his first ministry. In 1950 he made Beale minister for supply, the portfolio that was to be in charge of Australia's role at the British atomic tests, a post Beale held for the next eight years until Menzies shunted him off to become Australian ambassador in Washington.

Beale drew ribald comments from fellow MPs when he first took his seat in parliament because he insisted on somewhat pompously wearing his barrister's pince-nez, an accessory that may have been acceptable in the cloistered world of the Sydney law but was then considered a bit freakish in the sleepy and isolated capital, Canberra. But he soon established himself as a hardworking minister who earned Menzies' respect, if not his total confidence. Through his role at the later storm centre of the atomic tests, Beale also achieved something Menzies did not like or encourage among his ministers: a high profile.

Menzies is reputed to have irreverently nicknamed him Oliver, but among some of his colleagues and the more outlandish newspaper columns of the day he was known simply as Paddles. 'He is a man with a statesmanlike tread,' one journalist wrote of Beale in 1957, a year before Menzies removed him from the domestic political scene.

He moves with an ease and precision somewhat reminiscent of a stage butler announcing to a titled household that "dinnah is served!" Every movement of the man seems to speak of a sense of superiority, of calm assurance, of the masterful administration of the unseen. For Paddles could take on the mantle of Menzies at a moment's notice and turn out to be just the leader that the Libs are looking for. [5]

Such public notice spelled political death for any minister whom Menzies discerned as the slightest possible rival. Beale joined a gallery of Liberals whom Menzies clinically despatched to Australian embassies around the world, High Court judgeships and chairmanships of public organisations once their political stars began to rise too high.

Steeped as each of them was in the world of the law, Menzies and Beale, from Beale's own account, never really got on. 'He once told a colleague that we were "not on the same wavelength", which was another way of saying he did not like me,' Beale explained years later in his retirement. [6] For Menzies, this took the form of keeping from Beale certain key pieces of information about the atomic tests, and this landed Beale in trouble on more than one occasion. In June 1951, and again the following October, Beale was questioned in parliament about reports that Britain was to use Australia as a testing ground for atomic weapons. Beale dismissed the reports as 'completely false' and 'utterly without foundation'. The previous May, Menzies had secretly cabled his agreement to Attlee for the Hurricane test at Monte Bello to go ahead and for preparations of the islands to proceed. Beale's categorical denials unnerved the Commonwealth Relations Office in London, which sent a top secret letter to the UK high commission in Canberra demanding to know what was going on. 'Mr Beale's statement comes pretty close to being untrue', it said. 'We have assumed that Mr Beale was now more or less in the picture'. The high commission's diplomats reported back to London that, after making discreet inquiries, they had discovered that Beale, indeed, had not been told that Australia was to be the testing ground.

When Beale discovered this, he boiled and fumed with rage, as he later put it, particularly as he learned that his own Department of Supply had already been designated to give the British help. Yet Beale's confusion on the subject could not all be laid at Menzies' door. His political memoirs, written in 1977 after his retirement from public life, contained a chapter on the atomic tests which was notable for its number of fundamental misstatements. [7] Beale told his readers there were nine atomic bombs tested in Australia (there were 12); that four bombs were exploded at Emu Field in South Australia (two were); that a safety committee of Australian scientists attended the Emu Field bombs (the committee was not formed until two years later); that no Aborigines lived near Maralinga, the principal mainland test site, or were ever found there (several were discovered there during the tests); that after Operation Buffalo at Maralinga in 1956, there were never any more tests in Australia (there were three more bomb explosions and several secret minor trials); and that the Hiroshima and Nagasaki bombs were dropped 'a year or more' after the world's first atomic bomb test at Alamogordo, New Mexico (they were dropped three weeks after Alamogordo). Menzies' two volumes of memoirs, by contrast, *Afternoon Light* and *The Measure of the Years*, also written during his retirement, contain no reference at all to the British atomic tests, events whose planning, execution and aftermath occupied 15 of the 16 years of his prime ministership.

Although the Hurricane incident was not the first, or the last, time Menzies kept him in the dark, Beale shared Menzies' essential view that the atomic tests were a vital episode in Commonwealth co-operation and the defence of the Western world. By 1957, when the Australian public began to grow alarmed about the effects of radioactive fallout from the British tests and from American tests in the Pacific (although the Soviet Union was also testing nuclear weapons in the atmosphere, almost nothing was known about them), Beale embarked on a propaganda campaign in a bid to dampen down their fears. He put his name to a long document on the subject, *Why We Hold A-Tests in Australia*, which his office posted to any member of the public who wrote in protest. 'Atomic weapons are absolutely essential to the survival of Great Britain and the Commonwealth in the event of another world war,' it began rather heroically. The document went on to speak of mankind's need to master the new problems of the atomic age just as his ancestors had to master the problems of fire and electricity. And it argued, somewhat incongruously, that atomic weapons tests contributed to the expansion of knowledge about the problems of radiation. 'Up to 1954 tests were carried out in Australia without much comment (except from the communists),' Beale wrote. 'Indeed, there was some general pride that Australia was able to make so valuable a contribution to British Commonwealth defence.'

The atomic tests in Australia were pushed ahead against a background of growing alarm at what Britain and her Western allies perceived as aggressive Soviet intentions. This outlook was contained in a remarkable, top secret defence strategy paper prepared in Canberra for the Australian government in early 1953, when the Cold War was at its height and conflicts between Western and local communist forces were smouldering in Korea and Malaya. The Australian defence paper clearly envisaged the prospect of the Western allies making an atomic first strike against the Russians if full scale war broke out, and it mapped out a scenario of a war using nuclear weapons as a war which could be won – much the same strategy of 'limited nuclear war' adopted by certain American defence strategists in the Reagan administration in the eighties.

'A Moscow controlled communist dominated world is the ultimate Soviet aim', the Australian defence paper warned. A global war would probably begin, it said, with a full scale Soviet attack against Western Europe, the Middle East and sea communications, including heavy air attacks on the UK. The Russians might refrain from using A-bombs first.

But whether or not Russia used the atomic bomb, the allies would undoubtedly launch an all out atomic attack against her and probably against her satellites. The outcome of this two way atomic offensive cannot be foreseen. However both sides would suffer devastation and, even if the Russian regime were to collapse, as it is hoped, conventional operations would still have to be undertaken by the allies.

The document sought to raise the recently exploded first British atomic bomb, Hurricane, at Monto Bello to a level of crucial significance in all of this. The Hurricane bomb, plus the fact that the US had by now exploded 28 atomic bombs, emphasised the growing capabilities of the allies, it argued.

The ultimate result of the next world war may well be decided in the first few weeks, when the atomic onslaught is expected to take place. It is considered, therefore, that Russsia will not precipitate a global war until at least such time as she considers she holds an adequate stockpile of atomic weapons.

Meanwhile, the document concluded, the defence task facing the allies was twofold: to participate in Cold War activities and to prepare for global war. 'Priority should be given to Cold War commitments'.

The philosophy of this document was in stark contrast to the one dissenting argument against the British bomb put forward in government circles during the period leading up to the making and testing of the Hurricane bomb. The lone voice came not from a military man or a politician, but from a scientist, Professor Patrick Blackett, a member of the British government's advisory committee on atomic energy. We have seen how Sir Henry Tizard, chief scientific adviser to the British ministry of defence, had seriously questioned the great power philosophy implicit in the Attlee government's decision to manufacture atomic bombs. Blackett had put his opposition to the British bomb on record much earlier than Tizard, and he argued it strongly but in vain. He had been a member of Britain's wartime Maud committee, the first body to explain the feasibility of making an atomic bomb, and had made an outstanding contribution to Britain's war effort in the development of operational research, later receiving the Nobel prize for physics.

By the end of 1945, when Britain was agonising over its atomic future, Blackett had concluded that the country should not acquire atomic bombs of its own.

Presenting his case in a secret memorandum, Blackett feared that Britain would end up devoting too much of its scarce resources to building up a stock of atomic bombs that would be too small to be of any military value. He advised the government that, given the political situation and military strength in each of Britain, the US and the Soviet Union, for Britain to acquire or build atomic bombs now would tend to decrease rather than increase security. The use of the bombs as a threat would most likely stimulate the Russians to an aggressive military reaction, not necessarily against the UK but elsewhere in Europe. The Russians would certainly assume, said Blackett, that the British bombs were intended for use against them, probably in alliance with the United States. Finally, Blackett put the case that a decision not to manufacture bombs would allow the greatest possible progress in Britain in the industrial application of atomic energy, and would give Britain a chance to retrieve her once leading position in nuclear physics. Once the decision not to build bombs had been made, it should be publicly announced, he said, and Britain's atomic establishments thrown open to international inspection to make sure the rest of the world believed her. [8]

Blackett's thinking was the complete antithesis of the military chiefs' outlook on atomic policy in this period. Attlee dismissed Blackett's memorandum, saying: 'The author, a distinguished scientist, speaks on political and military problems on which he is a layman'. He sent it to the chiefs of staff, who ignored it. In February 1947, soon after Attlee's secret committee of ministers had decided to build the bomb (a decision from which Blackett, like Tizard, was excluded as a consultant), Blackett wrote another paper arguing against the bomb and proposing a neutralist atomic policy for Britain as part of a neutralist foreign and defence policy. He was disturbed by the extreme conservatism he found emerging in the US and by the talk there of preventive atomic war, although he did not believe that such a war would be launched. Blackett spoke to Attlee twice about his plan, but his views had no influence on the government. Bevin, the foreign secretary, wrote contemptuously on Blackett's paper, 'He ought to stick to science.' [9] The paper was never discussed at any ministerial meeting. It is not possible to say how Britain's strategic situation would have been affected if the path Blackett advocated had been followed. But some of what he forecast did come to pass, particularly the deprivation of other areas of industrial research by the enormous scientific and financial effort poured into the bomb project. And by the early 1950s, as the Australian defence strategy document quoted earlier revealed, the arms race had helped to produce such a frenzied Western perception of Soviet expansionism that it was already too late to accommodate the measured caution that Blackett had called for.

When the question of Australian scientific representation at the atomic tests arose, the British and Australian authorities were careful to ensure that no-one was chosen, however eminent, who could be even faintly accused of harbouring the sort of sceptical mind that Blackett had displayed. It was clear from the start that Australia would have to have some representation at the tests held on its soil. But the question of precisely what role the Australian representatives would play was never pursued in detail by Britain or Australia, still less made the subject of a written agreement between them. Menzies was not interested in the tests much beyond the public relations value for Australia's stocks with Britain and the Commonwealth. As for Britain, knowing what low esteem the Americans gave to Australian security, it wanted to give Australia as little information as possible and would have been perfectly happy if Australia had sent no-one to the tests at all. Australia did not press hard on this subject, and left no doubt about how it saw things when Philip McBride, the defence minister, presented to parliament in Canberra in June, 1952, the bill to set up a prohibited area around the Monte Bello islands before the first test, Hurricane.

The executive control of the project rests entirely with the United Kingdom authorities, and the policy on matters such as those relating to the presence at the test of observers, whether they be officials or representatives of the press, is entirely for the United Kingdom authorities to determine.

The British, indeed, kept one step ahead on this subject for it was they, and not the Australians, who first put forward the name of

• NO CONCEIVABLE INJURY

the most controversial Australian scientist to be involved in the tests, Ernest Titterton. At the time of the planning of the Hurricane trial, Titterton was about to take up the chair of nuclear physics at the newly created Australian National University in Canberra from his native England. He was one of two British scientists who went to America to work on the Manhattan project, and who later took up senior academic posts in Australia. The other was Philip Baxter, a chemical engineer who, in 1941, had produced Britain's first uranium hexafluoride, a vital step in the production of fissile uranium, and later played a leading role among scientists working on the atomic bomb at Oak Ridge, Tennessee. Baxter moved to Australia in 1950 to become professor of chemical engineering at the New South Wales University of Technology (later the University of New South Wales), vice chancellor of the university five years later and chairman of the Australian Atomic Energy Commission in 1957. He was knighted in 1965, five years before Titterton. Both men have been Australia's most outspoken advocates of nuclear energy and have urged that Australia embark on its own domestic atomic energy program and consider acquiring nuclear weapons as part of its defence strategy, two options which no Australian government has yet seen fit to adopt.

Titterton's association with the atomic bomb was an intimate and significant one, and it went back almost to the very beginning. He took his degrees at Birmingham University, where he was the first research student to work under Mark Oliphant. In 1941, when he was 25, Titterton joined the research effort spearheaded by the Maud committee in England into the feasibility of making an atomic bomb. He worked in Birmingham with Otto Frisch, co-author of the famous Frisch-Peierls memorandum, who was undertaking measurements aimed at determining as accurately as possible the critical mass of uranium. Two years later, after the Quebec agreement was signed, they formed part of the team of 19 leading British scientists who eventually moved to the top secret Los Alamos for the rest of the war, where Titterton became leader of the group working on the instrumentation and timing involved in actually firing the bomb. Titterton, in fact, was the last of the British to leave Los Alamos. When the McMahon Act, ending Anglo-American collaboration, was passed in 1946, the remaining

British scientists were obliged to pack up and go, but Titterton was kept on for another year, despite the Americans' obsession with security, on grounds of 'irreplaceability.' [10]

At the world's first atomic bomb explosion at Alamogordo, New Mexico, in July 1945, Titterton was a senior member of the timing group; it was he who devised and installed the electronic time signals whose activation detonated the bomb. (Titterton himself has said: 'I had the responsibility of firing the world's first nuclear weapon'. [11] His involvement with the atomic bomb continued after the war when he joined a British team of scientists, including Penney, at the first postwar American atomic trials at Bikini in 1946. Titterton was an adviser on instrumentation, and gave the countdown and detonation order for the tests. His identity, though, was kept secret: the radio operator at Bikini referred to him mysteriously as 'the Voice of Abraham'. It was, however, typical of the Americans' determination to stress a United States monopoly over atomic weapons technology that, in the official US film of the Bikini trials, Titterton's English voice was dubbed over with an American accent.

Back in England, after his four years at Los Alamos, Titterton took up a research post at Harwell until Oliphant invited him to move to the new national university in Canberra. He did not work directly with Penney at Aldermaston on 'High Explosives Research,' although he, like other Los Alamos veterans, certainly contributed valuable advice to the independent British bomb project.

Among the scientists who had worked on the Manhattan Project, there had grown up a certain clubbishness which sprang from the privilege and excitement of being part of the inner sanctum who were present at one of science's most dramatic and awesome events, the birth of the bomb. The secrecy of their work, the professional brilliance involved in its fulfilment and the mind boggling nature of its implications helped to give these men something of a public aura, a feeling that they were the recipients of knowledge, not transferable to other mortals, which literally held the difference between life and death for us all. The public in Australia in the early fifites certainly bestowed this aura on a returning brilliant native son, Oliphant, and on his no less brilliant

British colleague, Titterton, both of whom represented the new wonders of the nuclear age, even though both men by then had diverged sharply on their support for atomic weapons, as we shall see later. Titterton, in particular, cultivated this aura and notion of scientific superiority when he went to Australia, something of which the British authorities were no doubt conscious when they approached the Australians to ask for his services at their own bomb trials.

Titterton's most extensive explanation of his role at the British atomic tests came when he appeared in 1985, before the Australian royal commission set up to inquire into the conduct of the tests. We shall meet the royal commission and its members in Chapter Eight, but at this point it is worth considering Titterton's appearance before the commission, highlighted as it was by a series of volatile clashes with the commission's president and lawyers. The president was James McClelland, a former New South Wales judge who retired from the bench halfway through the royal commission's inquiry, former Labor party member of the Senate, the upper house in Canberra, and former minister in Gough Whitlam's government in the 1970s. McClelland was caustic, pithy and feisty. He prided himself on his terse and articulate use of written and spoken English. In almost every respect, McClelland and Titterton were worlds apart: Titterton, the outstanding nuclear physicist who had helped to invent the atomic bomb, and who harboured no doubts about the efficacy of his life's work; and McClelland, the dandy from the liberal wing of Labor party politics and the law, who maintained a sceptical, not to say touchy, mind towards almost everyone and everything, particularly self assured scientists such as Titterton.

But McClelland and Titterton did have some things uncannily in common. Both men were then aged 69, robust, vain and possessors of particularly sharp and competitive minds. Both intensely disliked criticism or being challenged. If Titterton gave the forthright appearance of a man who had never lost a night's sleep over his work, McClelland projected an assured air of someone who had devoted a considerable part of his energies towards his own personal appearance and wellbeing. The confrontation of these two men had the makings of a showdown, played out before members of the public and the scientific fraternity who packed the Sydney hearing rooms of the royal commission for Titterton's four days in the witness box in May 1985.

McClelland did not wait to release his royal commission's report the following December before he put on record his feelings about Titterton and his evidence.

From the bench, he told another witness, in a voice of despair: 'There came a point, when Sir Ernest Titterton was giving evidence, when there was almost no point in asking him anything because we could not get the facts out of him'. On another occasion during the hearings, he spoke scornfully of Titterton's 'vigorous personality,' his 'habit of railroading his opinions through,' and his 'domineering conduct' which he 'saves up for royal commissions'.

It was Titterton's views on the infallability of scientists which appeared to upset the judge most of all – even more than when Titterton, at one point, inadvisedly accused his honour of 'misuse of the English language'. Titterton is a small, squat man with a healthy tan and a barely lined face that makes him look at least 10 years younger than he is. At the hearings, his lower lip protruded bullishly from his mouth, and his eyes were hard and penetrating. His voice was deep and inflexible and he addressed his listeners, at least on the subject of nuclear science, with an unfortunate and unrelenting air of condescension. 'I was born a scientist,' he told the royal commission. 'Lawyers are a little less fortunate,' McClelland shot back. 'They have to be trained'. Was not scepticism towards his fellow scientists, Titterton was asked, an essential quality for taking part in the tests? Staring at the wall opposite, and leaning back in his chair, Titterton replied: 'I do not have very much scepticism of scientists as a group. I have considerable scepticism of some of them'. Then, turning to cast his eyes across the lawyers at the bar table, he added: 'And I have huge scepticism of pseudo-scientists who learn a little and think they know a lot'. Could he think of any other qualities that may have endeared him to those running the tests? 'Yes, I can think of many other qualities, but I do not wish to scratch my own back in public. That is for others to do'.

When Titterton was presented with evidence that some of his

leading scientific colleagues had criticised some aspects of the British atomic tests before the royal commission, his response was to belittle them or to discredit their views. Penney himself, he was told, had said under cross examination in London that, with hindsight, and taking into account the risk factors, the first land bomb, codenamed Totem One, in October 1953, should not have been fired. 'It sounds to me like the answer of a very tired man', Titterton replied. 'He is getting rather fed up with it. People are prepared to agree to anything for a little mercy . . . He certainly sounds very depressed. And, of course, the man is 75 years old and he does have worries.'

Titterton was reminded that secret documents revealed how the late Sir Leslie Martin of Melbourne University, his fellow observer at the first three bomb tests, and a fellow member of the Australian safety committee set up to monitor the later trials, had forecast as long ago as 1960 that a day would come when a royal commission would be held into what went on at Maralinga. Martin, replied Titterton, was disposed to pessimism and worry. He had 'difficulties'.: 'He was under pressure from his university. He was rather tired. He was prone to making mistakes'.

And, he was told, Keith Lokan, the nuclear physicist who is director of the Australian Radiation Laboratory, had given evidence that, in his view, so-called 'minor trials', which had left Maralinga to this day scattered with an unknown amount of highly radioactive plutonium, should never have been allowed to happen. 'Dr Lokan was one of my students,' said Titterton. 'He knows a great deal about many things. But I am afraid he knows absolutely nothing about nuclear weapons'.

McClelland suggested to Titterton that he was Britain's special agent at the tests, the man they chose to put there as Australia's go-between to make sure the Australians caused no trouble. 'I think you are very clever to be able to interpret what the British thought 30 years ago,' Titterton replied. And Geoff Eames, one of the barristers appearing at the royal commission for the Aborigines, wound up his examination of Titterton with an accusation: 'I am putting it to you, professor, that not only were you a particularly unfortunate choice for a person to be in charge of safety standards, but you were then, and remain now, a biased source as to the effect of those programs with which you were associated'.

'The answer is always plain that the other side is biased,' replied Titterton.

'I do not accept that description myself. The difference between the two is that the so-called pro nuclear (people) deal in facts whereas the antis deal in fiction very largely'. McClelland cut in: 'Sir Ernest, that answer would be more convincing if you had not denigrated before us every person who has criticised you'. Then the judge abruptly adjourned and went to lunch.

The British first appear to have raised the subject of Titterton's involvement in the atomic tests as early as January 1951, almost 18 months before the first bomb trial at Monte Bello. Michael Perrin, a deputy to Lord Portal, the controller of atomic energy, wrote to the Commonwealth Relations Office in Downing Street asking that Menzies, who was then visiting London, be requested to make Titterton available. Titterton, wrote Perrin, 'would be able to make very valuable contributions' to the Monte Bello test. The initiative to secure Titterton sprang from a secret discussion a day earlier between Portal, Cockroft and Penney.

They appear to have been particularly anxious to get Titterton's services, because the following month London instructed the British high commission in Canberra to take the matter up again with Menzies 'in case it should otherwise get overlooked'. Six weeks later the high commission cabled to London that Menzies had entirely agreed that Titterton's services could be made available and that he could well be spared. Menzies, in fact, had not yet put the question to Oliphant, Titterton's boss at the Australian National University.

At this stage, early 1951, Menzies appears to have been conducting the negotiations with the British over the weapons tests single handedly; certainly his cabinet colleagues were not aware of what was going on. The British had told Menzies that several Canadian scientists would also be present as observers at the Monte Bello test, and Menzies raised no objection. What they did not tell him was that the Canadians would be playing a far more significant role than any Australians. The Canadians, as a party to the wartime atomic project with the British and Americans, were to be given classified information about the bomb, but the Australians were not. The Canadians, for example, would receive details of the weapon's design which would help them calculate its effects. Menzies informed the British he saw no problem about Australia being denied the design information since Australia was not interested in acquiring nuclear weapons – as the British in Canberra delicately reported to London, 'He would not be perturbed, nor did he think anyone else would'. But the British did not tell Menzies that, unlike the Canadians, the Australians at Monte Bello would not be allowed close enough to the actual trial to be able to draw any scientific conclusions from it.

There was a definite conflict here on the part of the British. They now depended on Australia for weapons test sites and were starting negotiations for the purchase of Australian uranium for their atomic program. They had shown some sympathy with Australia's wish to gather atomic information for its own possible atomic energy program, and in different circumstances the British may have been willing to assist. But the Australians' desire for information, symbolised by their wish to have scientific representatives at the tests, conflicted with Britain's utmost priority of restarting atomic collaboration with the United States. As Penney has put it:

We had a very clear understanding with the Americans right from the wartime period that certain weapons information was, if not wholly of American origin, very nearly wholly of American origin. We were under a very strict promise, contract or call it what you like, a very strict promise that would be obeyed'. [12]

The doubts which the Americans harboured about Australian security were also a brake on Britain's willingness to share information with Australia. The Australian politicians and bureaucrats in Canberra never seem to have understood the full import of this American dimension to Britain's behaviour, even if the scientists, like Titterton, did.

Apart from Titterton, the British initially did not envisage any Australians of importance being present at Monte Bello. In April 1952, London asked that, in addition to Titterton, the assistance of 'two junior Australian technicians' be provided for low security tasks, such as helping to study blast damage to concrete shelters. The high commission in Canberra was told to ask Menzies if he wanted to nominate the two. The top secret cable from London went on:

For your own information, assistance of two officers of this kind is not really needed by us on practical grounds. But we imagine the attendance of some Australians in this way would be welcomed by Mr Menzies and they can, of course, do useful though junior jobs'.

As well as these junior people there were, in the end, two senior Australian scientists chosen to accompany Titterton as observers at both the Hurricane trial at Monte Bello and the two Totem trials in South Australia a year later: Leslie (later Sir Leslie) Martin and Alan Butement. Martin, a physicist, was a professor at Melbourne University and the scientific advisor to the Department of Defence in Canberra. Apart from a brief stint at Cambridge University's famous Cavendish Laboratory in England, he had spent his whole academic career in Australia, where he was now a significant figure in Australia's plans for atomic energy development. Martin encouraged nuclear physics in his own department at Melbourne University and oversaw atomic energy research groups from government bodies such as the Department of Supply. He was an important focus around which Australian atomic energy research could be developed. Alan Butement, unlike Titterton and Martin, was a professional civil servant. He had begun work for the War Office in Britain in 1928 and later transferred to the Ministry of Supply where he made significant contributions to radar inventions and helped run overall scientific research during the Second World War. After the war he went to Australia in the British team sent out to set up the Woomera rocket range in South Australia for the testing of British guided weapons. In 1949, the Australian government seconded Butement to be chief scientist of the Department of Supply, a position he held for 18 years. [13]

The appointment of all three men, Martin in particular, caused varying degrees of difficulty at the top level of the British government. Lord Cherwell questioned whether Australia should have scientists at the trials at all, and he was deeply worried that the Americans might form an unfavourable impression of British security arrangements. He was prepared to accept Titterton, who had been involved at Los Alamos. He was unhappy about Butement's addition but realised it could not be refused unless, as one official secretly suggested, 'lack of accommodation provides a valid excuse'. Cherwell grudgingly cabled his approval of Butement to Penney only at the last minute, a fortnight before the Hurricane blast, on strict condition that Butement would have no access to vital efficiency data. Titterton's and Butement's appointments, however, were relatively smooth compared with Martin's. By mid-1952, Australian defence officials were becoming disturbed by the lack of senior Australian representation at the forthcoming test and frustrated by the hedging replies they were receiving from Britain on the subject. They believed that, as a minimum, Martin, as the defence scientific advisor, should be an observer at Monte Bello. Martin's official invitation to attend did not come until the last week of September, a week before the trial, and only then after much torrid correspondence during which British officials sought to define his role far more precisely than those of the other two.

Eminent enough as they were, neither Titterton, Martin nor Butement could have been considered technically vital to the Hurricane trial from the British point of view. The British, after all, were sending a big team of their own scientists and they were to be assisted by four Canadians. The three Australians, by contrast, were to have a status no higher than observers. Why, then, were these three men, in particular, chosen? The reason British officials cited for nominating Titterton all along, in their correspondence with the Australians, was that Titterton was attending the trial at the personal invitation of Penney. Clearly, this put Titterton in a more privileged position than the others. As for Titterton's role, London cabled the British high commission in Canberra in April 1952, that it hoped Menzies would make Titterton available 'to help in the field work on telemetry,' adding: 'We would arrange for (Titterton) to be given certain other data (within limits imposed by security rules) which would be of interest and use to Australians in relation to weapon effects from point of view of civil defence'.

When it came to Martin, there were other reasons for Britain's approval which appeared to have more to do with public relations and an investment in future Australian co-operation. At this time, September 1952, Menzies, again without informing cabinet, had given approval for Penney to make a top secret mission before the Monte Bello test to inspect a site about 400 kilometres north west of Woomera which Len Beadell, the surveyor and explorer, was preparing to carve out for the first atomic bomb trials on land the following year. Beadell eventually called the site Emu Field. Penney had suggested to Lord Cherwell that it would be a good idea if he had the support of an Australian scientist when he was making his assessment of this new site's technical possibilities, and the best man would be Martin. Martin had impressed Penney as able, sensible and discreet. Penney also thought Martin should be invited to join the health physics team at the forthcoming Monte Bello trial, where he would be given full details of all weapon effects and of the layout of the site – but no access to the weapon itself or the results of measurements of weapon functioning. Penney suggested there would be an advantage in this course:

'We have not treated the Australians very generously in the way of inviting their scientific help,' he wrote to Cherwell. 'The invitation to Professor Martin would, I think, give them pleasure and would make them feel that we were not attempting to use their land but at the same time were keeping them out'. Penney's reasoning was accepted, and the invitation to Martin went ahead. But before it was issued, a letter from the Ministry of Supply in London to the British Foreign Office revealed the acute apprehension the Whitehall mandarins still felt on two key questions: the independence of any Australian scientists at the tests, and the delicate task of heading off any future Australian opposition to exploding atomic bombs in Australia.

The Commonwealth government are likely to be nervous about allowing the use of a site in the heart of the continent for atomic weapons tests, and may have to face criticism from their own people. It is obviously desirable that one of their own scientists should be able to advise them from first hand knowledge, and it seems right to use the Monte Bello test as an opportunity for indoctrinating such a scientist. The best way to prevent the Australians from feeling that we are 'attempting to use their land but at

• NO CONCEIVABLE INJURY

the same time keeping them out' would be to ask them to make a nomination for this purpose, but we cannot risk their unfettered choice.

The British, then, were concerned for security and political reasons that if they must accept Australia sending its own representatives to the tests then the people chosen should be the 'right kind'. Butement and Martin, unlike Titterton, had had no experience of atomic weapons tests and were not part of that exclusive inner sanctum of atomic scientists like Titterton and Penney, mentioned earlier. But they did have close links with the Australian government and vested interests in government-sponsored defence projects and potential atomic energy projects – Martin through his pivotal position at the centre of atomic energy research in Australia, and Butement through his intimate knowledge of the Woomera rocket range. Clearly, the choice of both men cut both ways: for the British, they were valuable links, if more were needed, with the Australian government and officialdom; and for Australia, they helped to give the project the imprimatur of Anglo-Australian co-operation which Menzies was anxious to promote publicly.

Titterton, Martin and Butement again acted as Australian observers at the second and third atomic bomb trials, which took place at the new Emu Field testing ground in October 1953. Again, the arrangement was entirely informal, although Titterton had a slightly larger role at the Emu Field tests in that he set up some measurements of the fast neutron flux in the weapon at various distances from the explosion. It was not until July 1955, when the principal testing ground at Maralinga was being planned, that the Menzies government sought to put Australia's role on a more formal basis by setting up a body called the Atomic Weapons Tests Safety Committee (the AWTSC) to advise the government on safety aspects of all future trials.

By then the question of radioactive contamination from nuclear bombs was becoming a hot political issue, following the Americans' testing of their first deliverable hydrogen bomb in the Marshall Islands in the Pacific the previous year. Apart from the horrendous destructive potential of these new super bombs, public attention from this American test had focused on the scandal revolving around a boatload of Japanese fishermen who were trawling, undetected by the Americans, in the test zone and who suffered bad doses of radiation sickness after contaminated ash and debris from the H bomb, codenamed Bravo, came showering down on their boat. The yield of the Bravo bomb was 15 megatons, the largest hydrogen weapon the Americans have ever tested, 750 times more powerful than the Hiroshima bomb. Many Marshall Islanders, themselves, suffered appalling illnesses after this bomb, including deaths from leukaemia, some of which the American authorities later admitted were attributable to radiation exposure. But at the time the health impact on the Marshall Islanders, and their medical treatment, was covered up and it was not until years later that the full story emerged. [14]

Even before the hydrogen bomb test helped to galvanise public concern, Menzies and Beale had faced questions in parliament about possible radioactive fallout over Australian cities from the atomic tests at Emu Field. One MP suggested that the Australian people were becoming obsessed by the fear of radioactive clouds. Menzies and Beale shrugged off the questions with their usual bland assurances. 'The tests are quite safe,' Beale impatiently told the House of Representatives. 'If they were not safe they would not be taking place . . . The atomic tests are in the hands of scientists of great skill and experience, and the timing is entirely a matter for them and not for anybody else'.

It was to meet this political need, of being seen to satisfy the public's concern on safety, that the government set up the atomic weapons tests safety committee. But there were other, less public, concerns being voiced as well. Some Australian officials believed Australia had not been told enough about the first three British bomb tests. With the establishment of a permanent test site at Maralinga, it seemed likely that the trials would go on for some time at regular intervals. There was, therefore, a need for Australians to have more control over the actual decisions to ignite these weapons and for Australian scientists to be able to check the safety standards on a more formal – and, it was suggested, independent – basis. Six bombs were due to be exploded in 1956 alone, two at Monte Bello and four at Maralinga. Martin, in particular, agreed with this view.

So the safety committee was set up in July 1955, composed of the original three observers, Titterton, Martin and Butement, and two additions: Cecil Eddy, director of the Commonwealth X ray and radium laboratory in Melbourne, and Philip Baxter, who was vice chancellor of the University of New South Wales and deputy chairman of the Australian Atomic Energy Commission, a body set up by act of parliament two years earlier to oversee all operations involving atomic energy. The size of the committee was later expanded. Martin was appointed chairman, but was replaced by Titterton two years later. The committee was given two functions: to examine 'information and other data supplied by the United Kingdom' to determine whether proposed safety measures for atomic weapons tests were adequate; and to advise the prime minister, through the minister of supply, of their conclusions, and whether extra safety measures were needed.

In fact, the Australians depended completely on the British for information to do their job. A succinct account of this has come from Ronald Siddons, a senior British scientist at the Totem trials in 1953, who returned to attend the final round of bomb trials, Antler, in 1957, where he was in charge of pre shot forecasting of radioactive fallout and briefing the Australian safety committee. Siddons later became a deputy director of the atomic weapons research establishment at Aldermaston, and in London in early 1985 he explained to the Australian royal commission the way the Australian safety committee went about its task. 'The interaction was one of a rather formal briefing,' Siddons said. 'The meteorologists stood up and said, "this is the meteorological information", and I stood up and said "these are our fallout predictions". . . . So it was a fairly formal thing'.

The Australians, then, had almost no independent means of safety assessment apart from what the British told them about expected fallout levels based on meteorological forecasts and expected weapon yields. The brief which set down the safety committee's functions implied that the Australians had a veto power over the firing of any bombs, but this was never written down in any government to government agreement. And in spite of the safety committee's claim in a report to the government to have exercised a veto over firing on at least two occasions, there is now considerable doubt as to whether it actually did so.

After the three Antler bombs in 1957, the safety committe, with Titterton by now its chairman, sent a secret report to Menzies about how things had gone. The report claimed that, in the interests of safety, the committee had vetoed possible firing conditions of the first two bombs 'because they were not considered to be completely satisfactory'. Yet during his evidence to the Australian royal commission in 1985, Siddons denied that this had happened. Geoff Eames, one of the barristers representing the Aborigines, asked Siddons: 'Was there ever a situation during the Antler series where your advice, and the opinion of the British people at the table that a test could be fired, was disputed by the Australian (safety committee)?'

'No', replied Siddons. 'I recollect no such dispute within the committee. The situation was generally fairly clear cut – that everyone was in agreement'. Eames asked: 'Was there ever a situation where the Australian (safety committee) had to apply a veto to stop a test being conducted, which was otherwise going to be conducted?' 'No', said Siddons. John Moroney, who was the scientific secretary of the safety committee at the time of the Antler trials, appeared to agree with Siddons. Moroney told the royal commission: 'The committee held the power of veto over firing; however, I know of no occasion when there was pressure to fire which called for a veto'.

Before the safety committee was announced publicly, Canberra had sent the names of its proposed members to London for comment. Whitehall raised no objections, but it asked for an assurance that each member had received a full security clearance in view of Britain's discussions with the Americans about possible renewed atomic weapons collaboration that were going on in the mid-fifties.

Menzies expressed his approval of the five inaugural safety committee members in somewhat remarkable political terms, given the later debate over the effectiveness of this committee as a safeguard of Australia's interests. Menzies wrote to Sir Philip McBride, his minister for defence:

The committee must include members who are sufficiently well known to command general confidence as guardians of the public interest, and who are not in any way to be identified as having an interest in the success of defence atomic experiments.

Given their professional backgrounds, none of these five people, with the possible exception of Eddy, could have been possibly described as being disinterested in the success of atomic experiments, defence or otherwise. How, then, did their backgrounds, and Britain's approval of them, affect their independence, the ostensible reason for their appointment – and how did they and the British see their own role?

Titterton's account of this again came when he appeared in Sydney before the royal commission in 1985. As Titterton told it, the first he knew of the proposal for the first test at Monte Bello was in April 1952, when Allen Brown, the secretary of the Prime Minister's Department in Canberra, called him in and asked him to work with the British at the trial. A few days later, a meeting was arranged between Titterton and Menzies, at which Menzies – 'the very fine constitutional lawyer,' as Titterton described him – gave the nuclear physicist his brief. Titterton remembered the meeting, and the brief from the prime minister, this way:

In view of your experience of three nuclear weapons tests around the world, which is unique in Australia, I would be glad if you would be prepared to go to the Monte Bellos to lend whatever help you can to Dr Penney's team, and to, well, essentially stick your oar in to make as certain as it is humanly possible to be that there will be no adverse effects on the Australian people, flora and fauna, and in particular the Aborigines. From the first five minutes, a major concern of the Australian prime minister was Aborigines'. [15]

Before that, Titterton was asked, had he ever discussed with Penney or anyone else in England the prospect of being involved in the tests in Australia? 'No, I had not. I had never heard of it, as a matter of fact. The first inkling I had was from Allen Brown'.

This version did not square with an account Titterton himself gave in a letter he wrote to Brown at the prime minister's office in March 1953, a year after the meeting with Menzies. The first Monte Bello trial now over, Titterton was advising the prime minister's office about Australian participation in the forthcoming bomb tests at Emu Field. 'Before coming to Australia, Sir William Penney asked me to act as technical director for the Monte Bello test but, because of my commitments to the Australian National University, I felt unable to accept his offer,' Titterton wrote then. 'However, if it was considered important enough from the Australian point of view and was not too expensive in time, I would be prepared to work closely with one of Penney's teams in the field or, if necessary, take charge of the test program at the (Emu Field) site in Australia'. How, Titterton was asked, could he reconcile this letter with what he had just said about not being approached by the British? 'Well, you cannot. It is quite obvious that that point was forgotten. I simply cannot guarantee that I remember every detail. I have absolutely no recollection of that at all'. [16]

Titterton saw the Australian observers at the trials being 'totally incorporated, with no holds barred, into the entire operation ... There was implicit confidence between the Australian and the United Kingdom governments'. The position of the three Australian observers at the Hurricane and Totem trials, he said, was the same as that of the full safety committee at the later trials: 'It was a team. It was not Australians v British or British v Australians. It was a team to do a job as well as we knew how to do a job.' [17]

Penney had a similar recollection of the Australians' standing: 'In a broad sense they were members of the team ... They would have full access to all the information that was going to be necessary for them to say to me that they were satisfied that it was safe to fire at the time.' [18] He could not recall any periods when the safety committee expressed any concern about the level of information being provided to the Australians.

Yet despite these claims of implicit confidence and total integration between the two sides, there were clear and significant limits on what the Australians were told. At the Hurricane trial at Monte Bello, none of the Australians was given access to the bomb itself or to the results of the measurements of the weapon functioning. They were told, beforehand, the estimated yield, that is, the power of the blast, in this case, 25 kilotons, equivalent to 25000 tonnes of TNT. But this was not sufficient to enable them to make their own detailed calculations of the radioactive fallout pattern. Titterton has described, in fairly dramatic terms, how he learned about the estimated yield:

Quite a bit of the vital information was given to me under top secret conditions in a Hastings aircraft flying from Melbourne to Onslow (Western Australia), roughly over the central Australian desert, when Bill Penney told me in the centre of that aircraft – outside the range of any human ears – the nature of the bomb. [19]

Inexplicably, Titterton could not say whether Martin and Butement were told everything he was told about the bomb. Penney, however, has said he also told Martin and Butement the Hurricane bomb would be about the same explosive yield as the atomic bombs at Alamogordo and Nagasaki and the 1946 bombs at Bikini.

Menzies' special brief to Titterton to look after the Aborigines' safety above all else at the Hurricane trial was to have a curious ring in the light of the standards laid down for radiation exposure from the bomb. Titterton says he had never seen an Aborigine until he arrived in Onslow, the Western Australian coastal town near the Monte Bello Islands, and that he was 'incredibly ignorant of our Aborigines'. In discharging his brief to Menzies, he had not thought it necessary to carry out an investigation, for himself, of the local sources of population near the Monte Bellos. His university, which would rather have had him working in Canberra than being at the bomb trials, was not keen for him to be away doing 'totally unnecessary work', and the university 'would have taken a great deal of umbrage had I suggested that I should become an anthropologist, and start investigating the people living on the north-west corner of Australia'. [20]

In spite of Menzies' concern for the Aborigines, documents secret at the time, but now declassified, reveal that regulations laying down acceptable levels of radiation doses from the Hurricane blast applied to the white population only; they made no special provision for Aborigines who were living in the open in a naked or semi naked state. It was only in 1956, after the first three rounds of bomb trials were over at Monte Bello and Emu Field, that different levels of exposure were laid down for Aborigines.

When Titterton was confronted at the royal commission with the proposition that the earlier regulations, therefore, must have been inadequate for safeguarding the Aborigines, he replied:

I don't give a hoot who wrote what documents . . . The only thing that counts in nuclear weapons tests is whether you did them successfully, with no damage under the terms of reference. In the case of Hurricane, the actual results of the experiment show that there was absolutely no problem from the fallout. [21]

Indeed, as the tests proceeded during the 1950s, political opposition to them, and the job of safeguarding the population against radioactive fallout, appear to have become two intertwined questions, according to Titterton's own account:

No-one on the (safety) committee was apprehensive about the fallout. They were apprehensive about the behaviour of the media and certain people with political objectives using the media in whatever way they could, even by misinformation, to stir up public opinion against the trials. That is what they were apprehensive about. [22]

Titterton may have felt that the Australians were completely integrated with the British, but the reality was different. The British government was particularly nervous about even the slightest details being passed to the Australians. The attitude was illuminated by a letter the British High Commission in Canberra received from the Commonwealth Relations Office in Whitehall in March 1952, a few months before the Hurricane trial, at the time when Australian officials were putting on pressure for more senior Australian scientists besides Titterton to attend the trial. The letter began by referring to Menzies' wish for a categorical and authoritative statement that the bomb's effects would be innocuous, and the fact that the wording of the public statement, to which the British and Australian governments had agreed, had managed to give this assurance. The letter from London to the high commission in Canberra went on:

We hope that, now that the announcement is over, there will be no further pressure from the Australian side for fuller details, or for information about the grounds on which this assurance was given.

For your own information only, it is now felt here that it would be a mistake to pass any detailed memorandum on to the Australian authorities, for this would be of little value to Mr Menzies without the comments on it of his own scientific advisers, and this in itself might lead to an embarrassing situation. For example, the Australians might disagree with the United Kingdom scientists' assessment of the risks, or they might suggest that, in order to ensure that necessary precautions against contamination were in fact taken, Australians should be allowed closer to the scene of the test than we at present propose.

The letter left the high commission with the instruction to 'do your best' to dissuade the Australians from pressing for more information.

Titterton's background, his British birth and education, his early involvement with the Maud committee's atomic research, his important work on the Manhattan Project and the postwar American atomic bomb trials, his postwar research work at Harwell and his high reputation as a nuclear physicist gave him a special relationship with the British that the other members of the Australian safety committee did not have. This was perfectly natural. It was a relationship born of mutual professional respect and understanding, if not personal friendship. If the British must have someone between themselves and the Australian authorities, they could not have hoped for a more accommodating person than Titterton.

Indeed, Titterton became more than a first among equals on the safety committee. His great knowledge on nuclear weapons put him in a privileged position to advise the Australian government and to be used as a conduit by the British to help gain Australian approval for some proposals that were likely to raise political flak in Canberra. One particularly sensitive episode illustrated this. It involved one series of the so called minor trials, the experiments at Maralinga conducted outside the main bomb testing program. and which lasted for six years after the bomb tests had finished. The minor trials were conducted in complete secrecy. They left highly radioactive plutonium littering the test range and a political row 30 years later over how it should be cleaned up. In 1959, the scientists at Aldermaston were planning to begin a series of minor trials at Maralinga called Vixen. They became the most controversial of all the trials because of their use of plutonium. The aim was to assess what would happen if nuclear weapons met with accidents while being stored or transported. Initially the Vixen plan for 1959 at Maralinga included burning and exploding only natural uranium and beryllium. Trials burning plutonium were on the books for the following year, but the scientists decided to bring those forward to 1959 instead.

The decision to include plutonium in the trials raised a sensitive question of tactics, which a secret Aldermaston document posed: 'Since the use of plutonium in assessment tests is unprecedented, and capable of misinterpretation politically, the question of procedure with Australia in laying on these tests needs considering.' Aldermaston decided to get around the problem by asking Penney to approach Titterton directly, explaining the nature of the plutonium tests and the estimates of contamination, and asking Titterton to advise on how best to obtain political clearance. Titterton did obtain Australian government approval, and the trials went ahead, with somewhat alarming environmental and political consequences later on (this episode, and the minor trials generally, are discussed more fully in Chapter Six).

Titterton not only knew more about nuclear weapons than the others on the safety committee; he also, from some accounts, received more knowledge from the British about the tests in Australia. This applied particularly to the minor trials. John Moroney, who became scientific secretary of the safety committee in 1957, the year Titterton became its chairman, and who remained with the committee for ten years, told the royal commission in June 1985, precisely where Titterton stood:

There is no question that Sir Ernest had a greater knowledge than anyone in Australia on the major trials and the minor trials, and that was quite generally recognised . . . Senior officers and ministers recognised that Professor Titterton was in a privileged position as far as sensitive information was concerned.

This also meant, according to Moroney, that the others on the safety committee at times found themselves depending on Titterton's opinions and inside knowledge.

Titterton himself was questioned at the Australian royal commission about his relationship with other members of the safety committee. Peter McClellan, the counsel assisting the royal commission, asked: 'Were you careful always to tell them everything which you knew?' Titterton replied: 'You are near to being libellous now . . . '

'Perhaps I am, Sir Ernest, but would you deal with the question,' McClellan insisted, 'that you always disclosed everything you knew to your colleagues on the safety committee?'

'Of course not', said Titterton. 'I was subject to American control on information I had in the USA. I was subject to the Official Secrets Act in relation to weapons in the United Kingdom and it was agreed and completely understood by everybody involved that there were certain matters which could not be discussed . . . A great deal of this operation was involved with what I would call a gentleman's agreement and I am very pleased to be able to say that all the people I was involved with both on the Australian side and on the British side come in the classification of genelemen, in this sense'.

Titterton had a propensity for dismissing critics of nuclear weapons and nuclear programs – an attitude encompassed by his view that what matters most in atomic weapons trials is not the copious bundle of pre-trial documents predicting where the fallout will go, or the post trial documents analysing where the fallout went, but the actual scientific result of how the weapon behaved. This attitude, argued by a man, to use the judge's term, of somewhat vigorous personality, had significant ramifications. As the public grew more concerned about nuclear weapons tests, and as doubts began to set in among some Australian officials, including Titterton's colleague, Leslie Martin, about the wisdom of experiments that would leave further radioactive bomb clouds drifting across the continent and plutonium scattered on Australian soil, it was Titterton who pushed most strongly in Australia for the tests, particularly the minor trials, to continue. But, as we shall see further in Chapter Six, the Menzies government by the early sixties had become beset by worries about the political implications of allowing the minor trials to continue; and the British, by then, had detected that Titterton had 'probably overplayed his hand' on the political side, and was having little influence other than on questions of safety.

Judge McClelland asked Titterton at the Australian royal commission if he saw himself fulfilling a political role at the tests, if he played politics. Titterton replied: 'I was doing a job. I was not playing politics. I merely informed my minister. If you take the view his actions were politics, well, I have no comment'.

The question of the political suitability of the Australians chosen to attend the atomic tests was highlighted by the non inclusion of perhaps Australia's most eminent authority on atomic energy, Sir Mark Oliphant. Professor Oliphant, as he then was, had returned to his native Australia in 1950 to become a founder of the new national university in Canberra and the director of its research school of physical sciences. He later became governor, the monarch's representative, in his home state of South Australia. At the age of 48, Oliphant brought back to Australia in 1950 the knowledge and experience of a distinguished career. He had been a pupil of the famous physicist, Ernest (later Lord) Rutherford, at Cambridge and a member of the wartime Maud committee. He was among the first group of scientists from Britain to arrive in the US in 1943 after the Quebec Agreement was signed, signalling the merging of the American and British wartime atomic projects. Instead of joining the team at Los Alamos, he went to work with his old friend and colleague, Ernest Lawrence, at Berkeley, California, where they developed the electromagnetic method of separating uranium 235. Oliphant was Lawrence's second in command and, in effect, the most senior scientist after James Chadwick in the entire British team attached to the Manhattan Project.

The dropping of the atomic bombs on Hiroshima and Nagasaki had a devastating impact on Oliphant. He was among those scientists who argued strongly, before the event and afterwards, that the Americans should have used the bomb as a show of strength to the Japanese, demonstrating its horrific power with a detonation over an uninhabited area, instead of dropping it, without warning, on civilian populations. After the war he devoted his efforts to the peaceful uses of atomic energy: he helped set up the UK atomic energy research establishment at Harwell, campaigned for the international control of atomic weapons and advocated that Australia launch its own atomic energy program, with British help, to develop its vast open spaces, as a hedge against the day when, as Oliphant believed, conventional fuels like coal and oil would run out.

He had been in his post at the Australian National University in Canberra for two years when the first British atomic test, Hurricane, happened in October 1952. But he was not asked to attend as an Australian observer, nor was his invitation sought by the Australian government. Menzies welcomed Oliphant's role as a founder at the national university, but he did not nominate the distinguished nuclear physicist as an observer at the early tests or as a member of the Australian safety committee set up to monitor safeguards at the later trials. Menzies was questioned in parliament about Oliphant's absence from the Hurricane test. His reply was unrevealing:

'The Monte Bello test was a United Kingdom operation to which the Australian government gave every assistance which it could. The test was conducted essentially as a naval operation. Apart from service personnel, only scientists working directly on the test were present'.

Menzies knew, but did not say, that the British really wanted Oliphant kept away from the tests because the Americans considered him a security risk, and they were worried about the effect on their atomic relations with the United States if Oliphant was involved. When the Commonwealth Relations Office in London had briefed the UK high commission in Canberra in a top secret telegram in April, 1952, about Australian scientific observers at the forthcoming Hurricane trial, it addressed just this question. The officials in London saw Oliphant as 'a difficulty'. They told the high commission:

'It is certain that if he took part in the test, the Americans (who regard him as a doubtful security risk) would react very unfavourably. This would make it more difficult to use the test as a means of securing better cooperation from the Americans in future. Oliphant is unquestionably talkative and would give the impression (whether true or not) that he was in possession of all the secrets. It is therefore in the general interest that he should be kept away'.

To overcome this delicate situation, the high commission was instructed to explain the British difficulties frankly to Menzies and to enlist his help.

Whether he was working in Cambridge, Birmingham, Berkeley or Washington, Oliphant's loyalty was never in question. But, in contrast to some of his colleagues, he had developed a reputation for flamboyance and openness which unnerved some people in high places. He distrusted secrecy as a shackle to true scientific endeavour, and he had little respect for politicians. Oliphant had willingly accepted an invitation in 1946 to work as personal adviser to Evatt, then Australian external affairs minister and leader of the Australian delegation at the United Nations debate on nuclear arms control. He got on with Evatt personally, but left the job in frustration after only a few weeks after being appalled at the high handed way Evatt treated his staff.

He had been particularly impatient with the secrecy which prevailed at all levels of the Manhattan Project – forbidding, for example, scientists in one section discussing their work with scientists in another. He believed it had been taken to ridiculous levels, and he said so. At a time when the Americans were particularly nervous over the growing number of British spy scandals, Oliphant's somewhat iconoclastic views about secrecy may have contributed to their wariness of Australian security as well. Oliphant certainly knew that Australia had come to occupy a low spot in the security stakes. In May 1948, he wrote from England to his friend, Sir David Rivett, chairman of the Council for Scientific and Industrial Research (later to become the Commonwealth Scientific and Industrial Research Organisation):

'I find a growing atmosphere of mistrust of Australian security which is likely to prevent any participation by Australia in atomic energy or similar undertakings for some time to come . . . I was told by one critic that 'no

Australian, from the prime minister down, can be trusted not to be careless or worse, and I include you (MLO) in that statement!' [23]

Rivett himself shared Oliphant's impatience on this score. When Australia was exploring the prospect of a postwar atomic energy project with assistance from Britain, John Cockroft, head of the Harwell research establishment, wrote back seeking guarantees of Australian security. Rivett replied to Cockroft in blunt tones:

'As to all this business about classified information, security, secrecy and the rest of it I just loathe it. Of course we shall be prepared to give whatever guarantees may be required if that is the only way we can engage in research work of any value. I have however the utmost distrust of secrecy practices particularly when they are influenced by military people'.

Margaret Gowing, the official historian of the early British atomic project, cites this 'heartfelt outburst' as one that could hardly be taken by the British as an assurance of security.

Oliphant's views on this point certainly had repercussions because, in 1951, the Americans refused to give him a visa from Australia to attend a nuclear physics conference in Chicago. Oliphant, the great scientist the Americans had welcomed to Berkeley during the Second World War and who had made such a significant contribution to atomic research, was now kept out. He was labelled a fellow traveller. With other scientists who had questioned the morality of atomic weapons after the war, and had associated themselves with arms control and disarmament causes. He was not alone. Two other distinguished scientists, and both Nobel prizewinners, the French communist nuclear-research pioneer, Frederic Joliot-Curie, and Oliphant's former Cambridge colleague, the leftwing Patrick Blackett, were not even invited to the Chicago conference because the organisers feared they would strike visa problems.

At the Australian royal commission in 1985, Penney and Titterton were both asked their views about Oliphant's suitability to attend the British atomic tests and the accusations of him as a security risk. Oliphant and Penny had been good colleagues, and had once collaborated in writing the official obituary of Cockroft for the Royal Society in London. Penney replied: 'I got to admire the man, and I'm a Dutchman if he was a security risk. What he was, I am sure, was a vigorous young Australian, and he made his views known'.

Titterton said: 'He had a great skill communicating to people, but . . . I do not think that he did understand people. If I had to make a criticism of Mark Oliphant . . . it would be that he is not a good judge of human beings. He can be taken in very easily, and was on occasions'.

Oliphant himself has since said that if he had been invited to become an Australian observer at the tests, and later to join the Australian safety committee, he would have declined. 'I had become utterly against nuclear weapons and I felt more as time went by that they were something I wanted to dissociate myself from completely'. [24] Perhaps the most significant point is that Penney and his team never even asked him to join in the first place. So the tests went ahead with little, if any, internal dissension. The Australian scientists who were chosen contributed their presence and authority, but not necessarily their skills because the vital scientific information remained in British hands and brains. The British were unencumbered by a plethora of demands on safety from the Australian side, and the Australian government was not to be embarrassed by its own representatives in its bid to support the British bomb. It was a situation full of irony, the type which Oliphant himself truly understood:

'I'd learned by the bitter path that to touch the pitch of secrecy was to be contaminated for a very long time, that governments and politicians wanted not men who believed in the integrity of natural knowledge but men who would tell them what they wanted to hear, and that truth has no meaning for a Churchill, a Morrison, a Menzies or a Casey, if it is politically inconvenient . . . In the end, if we peg away, truth will out. Let's not jump to the lions, but gird up our loins!' [25]

The official British and Australian case over the Australian scientific representation at the atomic tests has always rested on two propositions: that Australia, through its representatives at the tests, had full access to information relevant to the safe firing of the bombs; and that no Australians, white or Aboriginal, suffered from dangerous radiation exposure because their interests were taken care of through these scientific representatives. Much the same official arguments were employed towards the British and Australian service personnel working at the tests.

There is not room here for a detailed examination of the safety committee's performance at each of the atomic tests. However a number of general observations can be made. The 12 bomb tests did expose Australians, and British personnel working on site, to the risk of radioactive contamination because fallout clouds from most of the bombs drifted across the continent towards areas of large population, and in some cases went directly over Aboriginal communities and small townships in South Australia.

There was an essential conflict of interest in the task of the Australian observers and safety committee in coming to grips with the question of just how great this risk was. The Australians, by Titterton's own account, were 'members of a team', with no sense of antagonism between British and Australians. In that sense, they must have shared an interest with the British in completing the tests as quickly, efficiently successfully – and secretly – as possible. There were several points of urgency for Britain to develop and test its nuclear weapons: the fear of the Cold War with the Russians erupting into nuclear war; Britain's pursuit of its own independent deterrent as a means of restoring atomic collaboration with the Americans; and the knowledge at the back of the minds in the government and military that growing worldwide outrage over radioactive fallout could soon lead, as it eventually did, to a ban on atmospheric tests. It was vital, therefore, that no delays or hindrances be encountered in testing the bombs.

But the Australian scientists were charged primarily with looking after the safety of Australians, a task which required a degree of independent judgment and which was hardly compatible with the sort of professional intimacy which Titterton described. Clearly, Titterton himself was a dominant figure among the Australians and, as the British documents reveal, his concern was to allay the fears on safety among officials in Canberra in the interests of allowing the tests to continue. As an important figure in the international nuclear establishment, the need to demonstrate the fruits of nuclear research, through such things as weapons tests, had always taken precedence in his thinking over public fears about radioactivity. Titterton, indeed, consistently played down those fears. In 1985, in the face of considerable evidence to the contrary that had built up over the preceding 30 years, Titterton could state: 'We know positively that the fallout over Australia of all the British weapon tests can have had no effect on the Australian population'.[26]

Several other points are worth noting. The Australian safety committee did not come into being until after three of the 12 bombs had been fired. At the first two trials, Hurricane and Totem, the Australians had merely observer status, with no written brief and no exercise of veto. A condition of Leslie Martin's late inclusion among the observers at the Hurricane trial was that he be given full details of all weapon effects and the layout of the test site. But a year later, the British had still not provided these details. When the Prime Minister's Department in Canberra finally wrote to ask for them, the British high commission furnished a noncommittal reply.[27]

The Australian scientific observers' role at the Totem trials at Emu Field was also curious. It was the first of these, Totem One, which Penney in 1985 conceded, with hindsight, should not have been fired because of the meteorological conditions prevailing at the time. But the Australian observers appear to have raised no objections on this crucial point. At the Totem Two blast, 12 days later, Titterton was the only one of the three Australian observers to attend. Martin had returned to Melbourne University after Totem One and Butement had gone south to look over the proposed Maralinga site before going on to Woomera.[28] The Australians, then, were hardly in a position to conduct a rigorous analysis of safe firing conditions for this bomb. The safety committee, in turn, took no action to stop the firing of the first of the Buffalo series of bombs at Maralinga in 1956, in which the town of Coober Pedy, the centre of Australia's opal mining industry, and several outback stations were in the predicted fallout path.

Moreover, when the Australian safety committee did come into being, it saw its role being confined to assessing safety only from the bomb trials, or major trials. It had no brief, still less control, over the minor trials whose conduct has left the most damaging legacy in terms of contamination of the range.[29] Indeed, no Australian representatives attended the minor trials. Britain kept the details of the minor trials a close secret, much to the growing frustration of the Australian authorities in Canberra who came to believe Australia had gained nothing from letting the minor trials go ahead. The principle operating on the communication of information at all levels during the British nuclear tests was that information should be passed on only if it could be established that the proposed recipient had a 'need to know'; this applied no less to the members of the Australian safety committee than to anyone else.

It would be wrong to assume that the atomic tests were conducted with complete disregard for safety, by either Britain or Australia. But for the Australian government, the presence of Australian scientists at the tests, and the formation of the safety committee, served more of a public relations exercise than any other purpose. The backgrounds of the Australians chosen ensured that they would be acceptable to the British, while their involvement, however compromised by conflicting interests, lent weight to the Menzies government's claims that safety was the primary consideration. The authority of the safety committee's scientists was constantly invoked whenever Menzies, Beale or any other minister faced challenges in parliament or the press. No government spokesman, however, was as fulsome as Beale when he announced to the public the plans for setting up the Maralinga range in May, 1955, soon before the safety committee was formed:

'It is a challenge to Australian men to show that the pioneering spirit of their forefathers who developed our country is still the driving force of achievement. The whole project is a striking example of inter Commonwealth cooperation on the grand scale. England has the bomb and the knowhow; we have the open spaces, much technical skill and a great willingness to help the Motherland. Between us, we shall help to build the defences of the free world and make historic advances in harnessing the forces of nature'.

Thirty years later, Penney observed that that was not a statement which any member of the Australian safety committee would have made.[30]

Chapter Four

EDIE AND DARLENE:
THE STORY OF THE
ABORIGINES

'He is apparently placing the affairs of a handful of natives above those of the British Commonwealth of Nations' – Alan Butement, chief scientist to the Australian government, on Walter MacDougall, native patrol officer for the atomic tests, 1956.

For the first four years of the British atomic tests, just one man had the job of searching for Aborigines through the prohibited range in central Australia, an area of 800 000 square kilometres, or five times the size of the United Kingdom. This remarkable person was Walter MacDougall, a man who became so close to the Aborigines during a lifetime of trekking through the outback that they allowed him the rare privilege, for a white man, of taking part in their initiation ceremonies, and called him *kuta*: brother. For more than 30 years after the tests, the British and Australian governments maintained the fiction that no Aborigines strayed into this vast zone, and that no Aborigines suffered from the tests. The truth, we now know, was otherwise. The Aborigines were the people least equipped to know about the dangers of radioactive fallout from atomic weapons, and they were probably more susceptible to it than anyone else. More than that, the building of bomb sites and weather stations, and the arrival of thousands of British and Australian servicemen to run them, had a terrible impact on the Aborigines' way of life – and it was MacDougall who gnashed his teeth loudly, and with futility, against it.

MacDougall knew more about the Aborigines than anyone who was actually conducting the tests. When the British went to Australia in 1952 for the first trial at Monte Bello, their only source of information about the Aborigines was the *Encyclopaedia Britannica*, according to evidence revealed at the Australian royal commission in 1985. A British official who drew up a pre-firing report on the population of northwest Australia was unable to find any information about the number of Aborigines living there, precisely because Australia at that time still did not include Aborigines in the census, a practice that was not changed until 1967. The British official was able to include in his report, from official Australian information, exact numbers of ducks, hens, cows, beef cattle, horses and sheep, but nothing for Aborigines. Penney told the Australian royal commission that, to his knowledge, no-one considered the prospect of Aborigines living on the northwest coast of Australia, adjacent to the Monte Bello Islands, before the bombs were ignited there. 'Would we not have looked to the Australians for advice?' he asked.

Penney's question was not merely rhetorical. The fact that the Aborigines were not included in the census in the fifties was only one measure of the contemptible way they were still treated in Australia at that time. They had no vote, their claims to their traditional tribal lands were not recognised by any government, state or federal, and the health conditions among many Aboriginal communities was a national, if not an international, disgrace. For most white Australians in the fifties, the Aborigines simply did not count.

The attitude of white Australians towards traditional Aboriginal land was captured in the following submission to Menzies' cabinet in March, 1952. It came from Paul Hasluck, then Menzies' minister for territories, who went on to become governor general of Australia, the Queen's representative. Hasluck told cabinet:

As more and more natives come into touch with mission stations or settlements and adopt European ways the need for large reserves as hunting grounds will decrease, and as the process of detribalisation continues the protection of their tribal grounds and ceremonial areas will become less important.

The fact that the Australian authorities so readily allowed the British to conduct the nuclear tests, without taking any account of the tests' impact on the Aborigines, or insisting on rigorous safeguards for them, was all too typical of the times.

In spite of the Aborigines' sorry history since the arrival of European settlers in Australia less than 200 years earlier, a number of Aboriginal communities had survived reasonably intact to live on tribal lands in Western Australia, near the Monte Bellos, and in South Australia where the Emu Field and Maralinga testing grounds were later established. At that time, many still lived in tribal and semi-tribal conditions – half naked, sleeping in the open and going on walkabout through the mulga and spinifex in search of water holes and food which consisted of kangaroos, goannas and wild plants, all of which were equally exposed to radioactive contamination from the tests. Some of the Aborigines had not come into contact with white people before, let alone experienced the impact of an atomic bomb. According to estimates by MacDougall and others, some 1000 to 1500 Aborigines lived in the Central Reserve of South Australia up to 1955, the year before the Maralinga test site opened for business – in missions, on cattle stations or, in some cases, in tribal groups in the desert. And, due to some exceptionally good seasons, the population was increasing.

Walter MacDougall was born near Melbourne in 1907, the son of a Presbyterian minister, and he died in Melbourne 69 years later after spending an extraordinary life among the Aborigines of central Australia. It was in the Kimberley region of northwest Australia that MacDougall began working with Aborigines as a lay Presbyterian missionary in the 1930s. He married a schoolteacher deaconess and they spent their honeymoon riding on camels through the Kimberleys. Later the MacDougalls moved to another mission, Ernabella, in the Musgrave Ranges of South Australia, about 200 kilometres north of Emu Field. Britain already had a military interest in South Australia dating from 1947, when the Woomera rocket range was set up to test British guided missiles. Two anthropologists, Charles Duguid and Donald Thomson, had argued strongly that movement of whites into the proposed Woomera range would have disastrous consequences for the black inhabitants, and in response to such representations the Australian authorities had decided somewhat reluctantly to appoint a native patrol officer. MacDougall, with his unique experience from the Kimberleys and Ernabella, where he had learned some Aboriginal dialects, got the job.

From the start, MacDougall had to fight with the authorities even to get his own vehicle to patrol the huge range. Later, he was reprimanded when he attended to sick Aborigines living on cattle stations just outside the Woomera prohibted zone. His superiors told him somewhat loftily that he should confine his work to the blacks within the range area. MacDougall replied tersely: 'I consider it part of my duty to defend them wherever the need arises'.

He was a tall, extremely thin man with ginger hair and the sort of snow-white skin totally unsuitable for exposure to the cruel sun of the Australian outback. He would often spend weeks on end travelling between settlements with only his silky terrier dog for company. A loner by nature, he appeared shy and retiring to many who knew and worked with him. But MacDougall was never more at home than when he was spending time on some remote settlement with the Aborigines whose interests he considered almost his own personal property, and his blue eyes would flash with anger whenever some ignorant official back in Woomera or Canberra disagreed with his advice.

It was while he was working in the Kimberleys that he accidentally shot the thumb and forefinger off his right hand with a Winchester rifle. This earned him another name from the Aborigines – *mara pika*: sick hand. MacDougall adapted to writing by learning to hold a pen between his remaining fingers, and he would spend his evenings writing long, detailed and learned reports about how the Aborigines lived and warning of the threat to their future posed by the incursion of white miners, soldiers, scientists, weathermen and others involved with such projects as mineral prospecting and the atomic bomb tests – reports which, for the most part, were ignored in Canberra and never seen in London. Here is MacDougall writing in 1950 in one of those reports about the significance of tribal lands to the Aborigines:

The country that each tribal Aborigine looks upon as peculiar to his family is important to both his domestic and secret life. It is his birth place – his spirit's home. He believes that ceremonies within its boundaries and certain places are necessary for his existence, to ensure the continued supply of game and foodstuffs on which his life depends. If deprived of this by force, he is likely to die of homesickness. If he leaves it voluntarily, he quickly degenerates into the useless outcast seen, among other places, along the east-west line [the railway linking eastern and western Australia]. In fact, he becomes detribalised. Because the law as we know it gives him nothing to take the place of tribal law and culture, he becomes useless to himself or to anyone else.

There were two places, in particular, where Aborigines lived on which the impact of the atomic bomb tests was profound and lasting. The first was Ooldea, a settlement on the east-west railway line about 40 kilometres south of Maralinga itself. This was where William Tietkens, the explorer, had first encountered Aborigines in the 1870s near what was to become the Maralinga test site and had witnessed their colourful tribal corroborees. By the early 1950s, Ooldea had become a very different place. The United Aborigines' Mission, a Christian fundamentalist group, had set up a settlement there in the 1930s in a bid to evangelise the local Aborigines. Daisy Bates, the eccentric Irish writer and adventurer, had gone earlier to live among the Ooldea Aborigines and provided them with clothes and food, although she refused to have anything to do with the missionaries. The attraction of food brought Aborigines in large numbers into Ooldea from traditional tribal grounds to the north. It became a harsh place, plagued by sandstorms and water shortages. By the early 1950s, many of the Aborigines had lost their confidence or incentive to return to their old hunting grounds and were reduced to begging along the railway line or to selling curios to travellers whenever the transcontinental trains stopped briefly at Ooldea to take on water.

In June 1952, the United Aborigines' Mission, as a result of a dispute within their own ranks, decided to close down their mission at Ooldea. In the meantime the state government of South Australia had bought some land on a former sheep station at Yalata, about 120 kilometres south of Ooldea, and it now asked the Lutheran Church to take over Yalata as a mission station for the Aborigines from Ooldea. Yalata was to become a disaster for the Aborigines in every respect. It was just off the Eyre Highway, the main road linking east and west Australia, and much closer to the corrupting influences of white society along the South Australian coast. The ravages of alcohol at Yalata were to become appalling. It was also outside the tribal lands of the Pitjantjatjara people, who comprised the majority of the Aborigines at Ooldea when it closed. Most of them wanted to go north, into the 'red sand' of the Pitjantjatjara land around Maralinga which many of them had known as children, not south into the 'grey sand' of a place like Yalata with which they had no affinity.

This was in June 1952, four months before the first atomic test at Monte Bello, when the British were already secretly discussing the need for a permanent land test site in central Australia. Ooldea's closure was the result of other events: the missionaries' dispute and the government's belief for some time that the Aborigines should be moved away from the harsh environment and the public gaze along the railway line. But there is little doubt that Ooldea would have had to be closed once the decision was made to set up the test sites at Emu Field and Maralinga and the atomic bomb trials started. One British cable at the time described as a 'hitch' the fact that the proposed prohibited bomb trial zone overlapped the Ooldea Aboriginal reserve. The state government of South Australia quickly acquiesced with a later request from Howard Beale, the Australian minister for supply, to revoke its control over the reserve so the bomb tests could take place.

Two anthroplogists, Maggie Brady and Kingsley Palmer, spent several weeks in early 1985 gathering evidence to be presented at the Australian royal commission from the Aborigines who used to live at Ooldea. Brady and Palmer reported:

The closure of the Ooldea mission came as a shock, as there was virtually no knowledge among Aborigines that an argument was brewing over their future . . . There is no doubt that the sudden closure of Ooldea was a traumatic experience. Aborigines described being split up, cut up into groups, not knowing where to go, wailing and crying.

Some actually got on the train in a bid to go to places north of Maralinga like Ernabella, where they knew there could be work, but MacDougall, for whatever reason, persuaded them to return. A year after the enforced move to Yalata, the distress and unhappiness among the Aborigines there so convinced the new secretary of the Aboriginal Protection Board, a man named Bartlett, of their desire to go back to Ooldea that he planned to return them there. This produced a stern cable from the range superintendent to the authorities at Woomera warning them of Bartlett's plan and asking that it be stopped: 'Return of Abos to Ooldea would be undesirable in their own interests and it could be a serious embarrassment to us'.

But it was MacDougall, in one of his many detailed reports, who captured the resignation, apathy and sense of defeat that had set in among the Aborigines at Yalata by 1954, by which time their tribal lands to the north were about to become a full-scale atomic weapons testing ground:

Secret life significance has ended, mainly due to lack of interest shown by the young people and opposition to it by the missionaries. Owing to the fact that there are many of their relatives buried at Ooldea, and that it is the actual birth place of many of them, also that many of them spent their childhood days at the soak [water hole], there is a strong sentimental attachment . . . They all – young and old – have become dependent upon government rations and easily obtained water supplies, and they consider the difficult conditions north of Ooldea as too hard even to contemplate.

The other place where the bomb tests had a significant impact on Aboriginal life was in the Rawlinson Ranges in Western Australia, near the border with South Australia and the Northern Territory, about 560 kilometres northwest of Maralinga. It was here that, in 1956, the Australian government, after a request from Britain, set up the Giles weather station, named after the famous explorer whom William Tietkens had once accompanied. Penney and his meteorological advisers had decided that a weather station was needed at such a location to improve the accuracy of forecasts for firings at Maralinga, where atomic tests were to begin in late 1956. Alan Butement, the Australian government's chief scientist, argued that Penney's request be acted upon, particularly as the proposed weather station was essential for, as he put it, 'ensuring that no circumstances will arise which might cause a change in the drift of the fallout to the east or south east centres of population'. (As events turned out, the weather predictions did not stop this from happening with some of the bombs.) Britain agreed to pay for the station to be built, and Australia offered to pay for the running and maintenance costs for ten years; this worked out at a one-off outlay of 75 000 pounds by Britain and an annual expenditure for ten years of more than 17 000 pounds by Australia.

The Giles weather station brought with it two important events. First, a road was ploughed through the central Aboriginal reserve, where many blacks had rarely, if ever, seen whites, linking the weather station with the outside world at a place called Finke, on the north-south railway line just south of Alice Springs. And another patrol officer was appointed, with his base at Giles, to help MacDougall in the seemingly impossible task of searching the huge Maralinga range for Aborigines. The man appointed was Robert Macaulay, then aged 23, who had just graduated in anthropology from the University of Sydney.

MacDougall and Macaulay shared a deep concern about minimising the effect on the tribal Aborigines of Giles and the atomic bomb tests in general. But in almost every other respect, the two men were worlds apart. MacDougall was the man with no academic training who had lived with the Aborigines for years, knew their customs and tribal laws intimately and spoke their language. Macaulay was the keen, young university graduate, who had virtually not been outside Sydney before he was sent to Giles, could communicate with the Aborigines only through interpreters when he arrived and was given no briefing on their customs and habits before or after he left for the outback. MacDougall was more than twice Macaulay's age, and the Aborigines at Maralinga today still remember Macaulay as MacDougall's son. Macaulay had studied under A.P. Elkin, the noted anthropology professor at Sydney University. It was Elkin who recommended Macaulay for the job at Giles. Elkin was something of a conservative who had clashed with Charles Duguid and Donald Thomson back in 1947 over the setting up of the Woomera rocket range. Elkin had dismissed their arguments that the range should not go ahead because of its encroachment on Aboriginal reserves. He had advised the government that the range would not upset Aboriginal life, subject to certain safeguards such as the appointment of a patrol officer to regulate contacts between blacks and whites.

The different backgrounds of Macaulay and MacDougall did not always make for harmonious relations between the two men, at least initially. Len Beadell, the flamboyant surveyor and explorer who opened up the Emu Field and Maralinga bomb sites, and the Giles weather station, has described the uneasy relations between them:

To start with, it was a bit like a red hound and a black hound. They did not get on because MacDougall said, 'He doesn't know much because he's straight from school'. And the other bloke says, 'Well, Mac doesn't know much because he's been in the bush'. But eventually they did slowly even out. [1]

Richard Durance, the retired Australian army brigadier, who occupied in the fifties the highly sensitive post of range commander at Maralinga, remembered Macaulay vividly. Durance told the Australian royal commission:

He was young and sulky. I think he rather worried about MacDougall being able so easily and competently to discuss things with the different tribes and to be able to go out where there was any suggested bother and sort it out. Macaulay seemed to glower. It may have been a personality clash. I had a feeling that in ten years time we could have a very fine Macaulay.

Macaulay set about earnestly and zealously fulfilling the brief he had been given for the Giles weather station, which was to preserve the local Aboriginal ceremonial grounds and sacred sites from intrusion by whites and to discourage the Aborigines from contact with the weather station. The staff there were strictly forbidden from giving food to the Aborigines or doing anything else that would make them depend on the weather station as a source of supply.

MacDougall completely opposed the setting up of Giles. He argued that the weather station's presence would be an inevitable step in the breakdown of the Aborigines' way of life, and that once they came to rely on it as an easy source of food, water and transport they would lose their native ability to feed themselves. John Weightman, who worked as a welfare officer with the Aborigines' Department of South Australia at the time of the atomic tests, knew MacDougall well and travelled with him in the Maralinga area. Weightman described MacDougall's fears to the Australian royal commission in London in March 1985:

MacDougall was a good bushman. He related well to the Pitjantjatjara people and . . . felt his role was to articulate the interests of these people. He was cynical about the Department of Supply and was critical of various of its policies towards these people, including the making of roads through and the refusal to limit access to the northwest reserve. He felt unable to convince the Woomera hierarchy that these people had a point of view.

I felt that with the resources we were given we had a hopeless task to guarantee that all Aborigines were kept out of the prohibited area. I am sure that was MacDougall's view. He saw himself pretty much as a lone figure. He said that he used to have to take a lot of officers of the Department of Supply from ministerial level out on bush trips. He thought that was a bit of a joke. [2]

MacDougall alarmed the authorities when he gave a newspaper interview in Adelaide in November 1955, in which he sounded off about the impact on the Aborigines of nickel prospectors in Western Australia and the atomic weapons tests projects such as the building of Giles weather station. He told the newspaper that about 2500 natives from South Australia, Western Australia and the Northern Territory were in potential danger:

Whenever the white man finds something of value to him in any Aboriginal area the Aborigines are pushed aside. I believe that what is happening to these natives is contrary to the spirit of the declaration of human rights in the United Nations charter. If no check is possible they seem doomed to increase the number of displaced persons in the work world – to become prideless, homeless vagabonds living by begging, stealing and government handouts. Their only crime, of course, is that they are descendants of a strong, dignified, stone age race not capable of adjusting themselves easily to our civilisation without special help.

This infuriated the Woomera authorities, who tried to have the article suppressed before it was published. MacDougall was given a dressing down, and told to be careful what he said to the newspapers. But MacDougall's life, living in the wide, open spaces with his concerns about the stupidities and inconsistencies of policy towards the Aborigines pent up during weeks of worry and reflection, was anathema to the world of his superiors, with their air-conditioned offices, daily routine and paranoia about civil service rules. Barely four months later, in March 1956, these same superiors were disturbed once again that MacDougall may be about to embark on actions beyond their control. H.J. Brown, the controller of the Salisbury headquarters of the Woomera rocket range in South Australia, wrote a long memorandum to Alan Butement, the Australian government's chief scientist, alerting him to the fact that MacDougall was 'far from satisfied' about several aspects of the Maralinga bomb tests project. In particular, MacDougall was against the Giles weather station being built in the West Australian Aboriginal reserve, and the access road being built to it. MacDougall believed, said Brown, that both these things were a breach of promise on the undertakings the Australian government gave when Woomera was set up, and that the public should be told what was happening. 'It is likely that, in his present frame of mind, he will take some extreme step to draw public attention to what he regards as a breach of promise', Brown warned darkly.

Butement, who, with Titterton and Leslie Martin, was one of the three Australian scientific observers at the Hurricane and Totem tests, and an original member of the Australian safety committee for the later bomb trials, was angered by what he learned, and was apparently determined that MacDougall should be put in his place. Butement shot off a stinging reply:

Your memorandum discloses a lamentable lack of balance in Mr McDougall's [sic] outlook, in that he is apparently placing the affairs of a handful of natives above those of the British Commonwealth of Nations . . . The mere fact that Mr McDougall's views conflict so strongly with those of the Native Affairs Departments of both South and Western

Australia indicates how much he is out of step with current opinion, and the sooner he realises his loyalty is to the department which employs him ... the sooner his state of mind will be clarified ... Mr McDougall might be instructed to get on with the job within his sphere of activity, and leave policy matters to those whose responsibility they are.

This, then, was the view of MacDougall thousands of kilometres away back at headquarters. It did not deter him, and he continued to argue his case copiously in reports and memoranda. MacDougall's views were not as clear cut as one might expect. The official policy towards tribal Aborigines had been segregation on reserves, rather than assimilation with white Australia. Inevitably, this had broken down, but MacDougall believed broken government promises – such as allowing roads to be built into the reserves – were largely responsible. He believed segregation was doomed as a means of preserving the tribal Aborigines' customs and self respect. He advocated a different path, such as training the Aborigines to work the land in European ways so they could take their place alongside twentieth-century whites. The present policy of keeping the tribal Aborigines segregated, but allowing growing incursions on their land by whites, was certain to result, MacDougall wrote, in 'a degeneration from self-respecting tribal communities to pathetic and useless parasites – it has happened so often before that surely we Australians must have learnt our lesson'. He continued: 'There is an ethical aspect in that the country under discussion belongs to the tribe and is recognised as such by other tribes. However we propose to take it away from them and give nothing in return – we might as well declare war on them and make a job of it. We are morally bound to take some action to fit them for detribalised life.'

MacDougall saw the Aboriginal question as 'dynamite', with huge national and international ramifications. Because of the nature of his work, he was often, literally, a voice in the wilderness. But, as we shall see, by the time the atomic bomb trials were over, his unhappy predictions about their effects on Aboriginal life would have come true at both Giles and Yalata.

At the Australian royal commission in 1985, Geoff Eames, one of the two barristers appearing for the Aborigines, suggested that precautions taken to ensure there were no Aborigines on the range during the firing of atomic bombs were not just inadequate: 'They were an absolute farce, a total shambles'. This, said Eames, was no reflection on the efforts of MacDougall and Macaulay. It was a comment directed at the people planning the tests because of the few resources they gave to ensure Aboriginal safety. Certainly, two of the leading scientists at the atomic tests, Penney and Titterton, revealed at the royal commission their almost complete ignorance about the problems of the Aboriginal patrols. 'I did not know how it worked', Penney said in London. 'It was a very empty area. If there had been any Aboriginals I thought he [MacDougall] would know about them and that sort of thing . . . If he was satisfied and he told me it was okay, then that was the best that could be done'. [3] Penney said that, to his recollection, he never called for the reports of the patrols by MacDougall and Macaulay.

Titterton disclosed an even greater ignorance on this question than did Penney. He told the royal commission he had always thought there were six people, not two, patrolling the bomb range for Aborigines. The evidence of Penney and Titterton reinforced the impression that the appointment of MacDougall and Macaulay was more of a public relations exercise than a serious bid to keep the Aborigines out of harm's way. Indeed, a secret Woomera cable in early 1956 frankly described MacDougall's job this way: 'He is an insurance policy ensuring that the Department [of Supply] does not come under public criticism for interfering with tribal natives, and that the government's original promises are not inadvertently broken'.

Yet, until Macaulay was sent to Giles weather station in August 1956, MacDougall was the only man patrolling a range that stretched almost from Ayers Rock in the north to the transcontinental railway in the south. By this time, the two Totem bomb trials at Emu Field were over. Macaulay arrived at Giles to discover he did not even have his own vehicle, and was obliged to borrow one to conduct his patrols during the four Buffalo bomb tests at Maralinga a month later. This, his first patrol in a desert he had never visited before, took Macaulay through the Tomkinson, Mann and Musgrave Ranges along the northern border of South

Australia. But it was hardly the most efficient job, in spite of the young Macaulay's keenness. For part of the journey Macaulay did not have a radio, so that even if he had discovered Aborigines heading south into the testing zone there was no way he could have alerted Maralinga, via Woomera.

Astonishingly, there was never an Aboriginal patrol officer stationed at either the Emu Field or Maralinga grounds during the entire bomb test period from 1953 to 1957. When Macaulay came on the scene, he and MacDougall operated from bases, at Giles and Woomera, hundreds of kilometres apart and often with inadequate communications. Macaulay was able effectively to join MacDougall only for the final round of bomb trials, Antler, in September and October 1957. But this patrol turned out to be stillborn. Macaulay himself explained why when he appeared before the Australian royal commission in Sydney in October 1984:

[My instructions] certainly would have involved me going relatively close to the Maralinga prohibited zone, but the reason I find it difficult to recall exactly what the instructions were is that I never got there. I never became involved because the area through which I had to pass became impassable because of heavy rains and I sat through that [Antler] test period, not bogged, but sitting on a little rocky outcrop, literally unable to move. I was unable to move for at least three or four days, but I estimate my chances of having got through would not have been good for 10 to 12 days. By that stage, it was too late.

MacDougall set out to find Macaulay, but they never met.

While MacDougall and Macaulay were valiantly going about their ground patrols in the inhospitable mulga, spinifex and notorious sandhills around the range, the view from inside headquarters at Emu Field and Maralinga was somewhat more laid back. Alan Flannery was a security officer for the Totem tests at Emu Field in October 1953, and moved to Maralinga as a security officer in October 1956. He told the Australian royal commission that nothing was done at Emu Field to see whether there may have been Aborigines close to the firing zone before the Totem bombs, or to check whether the information on hand, that no Aborigines were in the area, was correct. At Maralinga, workers put up notices near the bomb detonation sites warning people not to come into the prohibited area. But most Aborigines in the area could not read English. Flannery believed that the planning of the tests themselves was meticulous. But he admitted: 'It would have been impossible to prevent anyone entering the area'. Peter McClellan, the counsel assisting the royal commission, asked: 'Do I infer what you are saying to me is that, as far as you were concerned, any attempts to secure the range area – the whole of the range area – was a hopeless task?'

'Impossible', said Flannery.

Macaulay himself frankly explained to the royal commission the limitations of his job. Could he have given an assurance at the time of the Buffalo trials at Maralinga in 1956, he was asked, that no nomadic natives were or would be in the danger zones?

No, of course not. I did not know where the danger area was. I had never been there and I was six or seven hundred miles away from it. All I was pre-pared to do at that time, and I believe I did do, was to indicate to others where people were and what their likely movement patterns would be over the next few weeks or months.

Apart from the ground patrols by MacDougall and Macaulay, there were also at Maralinga air patrols by the Royal Air Force before each bomb trial. These were by no means systematic, but more in the nature of general sweeps. One thing the RAF pilots would look for was smoke from Aborigines' fires. But Aborigines who camped on the range at the time of the bombs told the royal commission when it visited Maralinga in April 1985, that they would smother their fires at the first sound of an approaching aircraft because they were frightened. Richard Durance, the range commander at Maralinga, believed the air patrols were 'extremely valuable', although he admitted in late 1984 that the whole business of security on the range could have been improved if the authorities had provided more patrol officers and facilities.[4]

But Durance's sanguine view of the air patrols was not shared by one man who actually took part in them. John Weightman, the welfare officer who went to Maralinga in 1957, briefed the RAF pilots and went on most of their patrols, sitting up front with the crew. He remembers most of the flights simply following the roads around the range and not going over the bush because he and others thought the country was too vast to cover in a grid pattern.

It was like looking for a needle in a haystack given the vastness of the area and the means at our disposal. There were not many obvious things to look for from an aeroplane 500 feet up and travelling at, say, 200 or 300 miles an hour. The obvious things were smoke by day and fire by night. To look for an Aboriginal person in that sort of country from an aeroplane and to find him would be quite impossible. [5]

Even before the bomb trials began at Maralinga, when the range was still being built, a somewhat happy-go-lucky means of pushing the Aborigines out of the area was hit upon that had all the hallmarks of a scene from the American Wild West. As mentioned earlier, the closure of Ooldea on the edge of the Maralinga range had left the Aboriginal community there destitute. By 1954, the Ooldea water supply had all but dried up after repeated use by the steam trains stopping at Ooldea on the transcontinental railway. Aborigines still wandering around the area would often try to jump on the trains heading east towards Port Augusta or west towards the frontier mining town of Kalgoorlie in Western Australia, 800 kilometres away. Durance explained:

Kalgoorlie seemed to be some sort of star to go to. But they were not wanted, any more than they were in the depression days. It was the Commonwealth Railways guards' job, particularly on the tea and sugar, which was the train that brought provisions through to all settlers and stations along the run to Kalgoorlie, to remove them.

But with the bomb trials imminent, the British authorities hit on an idea: why not let the Aborigines stay on the trains, and the British would pay their fares? As Durance put it:

The Commonwealth Railways could put in a charge for any Aboriginals who climbed aboard that train going east or west, as long as the object was to keep them going for at least 200 to 300 miles . . . Kalgoorlie, I have been told by the MacDougalls of life, was a glittering Las Vegas. If they could only get to Kalgoorlie – I don't know, but I do not think it was the dream when they got there. But that was it . . . I thought it was an excellent way of being quite sure that those who were wandering around the northern edge of the Nullarbor Plain, if it was their desire to go west, that they did so.

Geoff Eames, the counsel for the Aborigines, asked Durance: 'Was there ever any thought given by anyone that the impact on Aboriginal people taken on the train ride to the Las Vegas of the west might be disastrous?' 'Not to my knowledge', said Durance. 'It was far preferable that they were alive and safe than at that stage being concerned with whether it was right or wrong.' [6]

In spite of the train rides to Kalgoorlie, the exhausting and frustrating work of MacDougall and Macaulay and the air patrols, Aborigines remained living in the Maralinga region at the time of the atomic bombs. In July 1959, Macaulay reported encountering on a patrol 34 natives at Shell Lakes and Lake Ell, on the West Australian side of the South Australian border. He concluded that tribal natives from this area had travelled about halfway to the forward area at Maralinga, the actual point where the bombs were fired. The following year, he and MacDougall made a more amazing discovery when they came across an Aboriginal group of two men, four women and eight children, only one of whom had seen whites before. The encounter happened near Lake Wyola and Vokes Hill, barely 160 kilometres northwest of Maralinga. The group had been living there permanently; MacDougall and a police constable tracked them down by following their footprints. The Aborigines appeared to be in good health, and lived on a diet of witchetty grubs, lizards and water which they eked out from mallee roots. Macaulay reported: 'The natives said they heard the atomic bombs at Maralinga a few years ago and were very frightened. They did not see any flashes'. Although they were still living in a totally tribal state, these Aborigines were becoming increasingly interested in the activities of the white man: they had been using empty food tins they found tossed along a nearby track and were looking for discarded pieces of bread.

Macaulay's conclusion after this patrol, in September 1960, was unequivocal: 'Natives have been living well inside the Maralinga prohibited zone continuously from before the establishment of the atomic weapons testing grounds', he wrote in a secret report to the authorities at Woomera. In the light of this, it is interesting to note that another three years were to go by before the Australian safety committee first raised with the Australian government the need to secure the actual sites where the bombs had been detonated: at a meeting in July 1963, the safety committee agreed 'in principle' that fences should be built around the bomb sites, radioactive debris collected and buried and 'appropriate' warning signs erected. Once again, most Aborigines could not understand the signs.

Some of the Aborigines, whom Macaulay reported in 1960 had been left in the Maralinga country when the bomb tests were going on, told their stories to the Australian royal commission when it visited Maralinga in April 1985. One of them was Henry Anderson (his European name), who described through an interpreter how he and his family had lived in the Maralinga lands for years, and were wandering in the bush west of Maralinga living off 'bush tucker'. In those days, the people did not have clothes. They heard an explosion, the ground shook and they got very frightened. Afterwards, Henry saw smoke swirling to the northwest. He thought the smoke was a snake that came from a place called Wantu. It was a dangerous snake, eating people up. His family were worried about what the smoke would do to certain Aboriginal places in the region. It killed a place called Out Well, dead. It hurt Lake Dey Dey, and spoiled Bulgunnia. 'Those places were the old men's places. They are the holders of the sacred things', said Henry. Before the bomb exploded he had seen aeroplanes flying around the country. What did his family do when the aeroplanes came? 'They got up and hid themselves. The people were frightened. They put out the camp fires.'

The most spectacular case of Aborigines straying into the bomb zones involved a tribal family called the Milpuddies. They lived in the north of South Australia, near the Ernabella mission station, and were what the Aborigines themselves called spinifex people – nomadic bush natives. In May 1957, almost midway between the end of the Buffalo bomb trials at Maralinga and the start of the Antler trials the following September, the Milpuddies had gone south on walkabout, following the water holes towards Ooldea where they intended visiting relatives.

They had led such an isolated life in the spinifex that they did not know Ooldea had been closed down five years earlier. The family consisted of Charlie Milpuddie, his wife, Edie, a little boy, Henry, and Rosie, a girl of four. Unknown to them, their trek took them directly into the path of a crater at a site near Maralinga called Marcoo where, seven months earlier, an atomic bomb had been exploded on the ground giving a yield of 1.5 kilotons. The reasons behind this particular bomb test could not have been further from the world of the Milpuddies: this, the only atomic bomb actually set off at ground level in Australia, was designed to observe the radioactive fallout pattern compared with an air burst and the effect of an atomic bomb exploded at ground level, say, in a city like London or Birmingham.

The Milpuddies spent the night of 13 May camped near the Marcoo crater, where they lit a fire and dined on a kangaroo Charlie had killed. At around 9 the next morning, a military officer from Maralinga was stunned to see Charlie Milpuddie wandering towards a nearby site called Pom Pom, where a caravan was stationed for the health physics team, the experts in charge of monitoring radiation exposures and carrying out decontamination. Frank Smith, then a member of the radiation detection unit at Maralinga, got an urgent call to rush to Pom Pom. When he saw what had happened, he persuaded the Milpuddies to go to the health physics caravan but decided not to put on his white protective clothing and head gear because he thought the sight may frighten them. When the Milpuddies were found, their only possessions were a clutch of hunting spears and 12 pelts from dingos, which they were apparently hoping to sell at Ooldea. Charlie Milpuddie and the boy were checked and the boy was found to be contaminated. So the whole family were put under showers in the caravan, then loaded with their four hunting dogs into a Land Rover and driven to Yalata, 200 kilometres south.

When the Australian royal commission visited Maralinga in April 1985, Edie Milpuddie, through an interpreter, told the story she experienced as a young woman almost 30 years earlier. The setting for the hearing was the red dust and green mulga scrub just south of what remains of the Maralinga village, where about 150

Aborigines had set up a makeshift camp after travelling hundreds of kilometres from Lake Dey Dey, in South Australia, and Cundeelee, in Western Australia especially for the event. Edie Milpuddie, surrounded by women from Lake Dey Dey, knelt shyly on the ground, the women whispering and giggling selfconsciously among themselves. Judge McClelland, dressed in designer jeans, an open-necked shirt and dark glasses, and his two fellow royal commissioners, Jill Fitch and Bill Jonas, sat rather awkwardly on camp chairs with a blue tarpaulin strung between mulga bushes behind them as a windbreak. The gallery consisted of an unlikely combination of the Aboriginal womens' menfolk and children, and a brace of newspaper and television reporters from Australia's big cities.

Edie Milpuddie said that her family were naked when the soldiers picked them up at Marcoo. She had never seen a motor car before. She had never seen a shower. When she went to the shower in the caravan, she thought there was another Aboriginal woman there too. Then she realised she was seeing herself in a mirror. After the shower, the soldiers held something near her that made a clicking noise. Later, Edie and a group of women friends retired into the scrub nearby with McClelland and Jill Fitch, where they told him privately about something that happened to Edie soon after the Milpuddie family arrived at Yalata. Geoff Eames, the counsel for the Aborigines, explained publicly to the royal commission: 'The circumstances are such that it is simply too hard for her to say in a formal session'. But, said Eames, the senior Aboriginal women at Lake Dey Dey had agreed that Eames himself should say publicly what fate had befallen Edie Milpuddie after her ordeal.

What was not known then, and I don't think has been known until now, was that at the time that Edie Milpuddie and her family were discovered at the Marcoo crater she was pregnant. When she was relocated at Yalata she gave birth out bush to a child which was dead. She buried that child out bush. She and the women at Lake Dey Dey believe that that fact is related to the [Marcoo] experience and to what they describe as the poison from the range. They believe that, while that matter should be told privately to the commission, it should be more widely known because it is a matter which might help people understand why they have particular concerns to know about the level of safety for Aboriginal people on the Maralinga lands.

Edie Milpuddie's next child, Allan, was born in 1961 and died of a brain tumour two years later. Sarah, the child who followed Allan, was particularly premature and weighed only one or two pounds at birth. Rosie, the daughter discovered with Edie at Marcoo, herself lost a child in 1973. Edie's husband, Charlie, died at Yalata of pneumonia and heart failure in 1974. Eames told the royal commission that the evidence of Edie Milpuddie's story was 'not necessarily conclusive, but certainly suggestive that her family and, indeed, her grandchildren since that time seem to have suffered extraordinary ill health and numerous deaths'.

How badly contaminated were the Milpuddies when they were picked up at Marcoo? Harry Turner, the Australian health physics representative at Maralinga, went to Pom Pom when the Milpuddies were being decontaminated, took photographs of them after their showers and wrote a report of the incident four days later for the authorities at Maralinga. Turner's report said:

The only variation from normal background was found on the right side of the boy's hair and on his buttocks. The counter reading in both cases was about 10 counts per second above background. None of the others had any detectable contamination on their bodies or clothing ... There is no possibility that any of the family could have experienced any radiation injury.

Lawyers for the Aborigines at the royal commission, and McClelland himself, challenged this conclusion. Frank Smith, the radiation officer who took the Milpuddies to the Pom Pom caravan, had supervised their decontamination and showering. Smith told the royal commission in June 1985, that Turner had not been present during the monitoring, and that Turner had prepared his report from information Smith himself had given. As Smith told it, the details of the story were somewhat more complex than Turner's official report conveyed: in fact, neither Edie Milpuddie nor her daugher was ever checked for radiation:

The elderly English pilot officer did not mind us washing the son and the father. But he had some sense of indignity that we would get too close to the female members of the tribe. I do not know why, but he insisted that [there was] no hanky panky, etcetera, and that is why we did not go on with that. I did not monitor the bodies of the mother and the child. I monitored the external hair, but I could not go over other parts of her body.

Smith said that when Edie Milpuddie got under the shower she washed only her hair, arms and legs. No-one helped her to shower, as they had helped the father and son. Was it possible, he was asked, that, if there was any radioactivity on parts of her body other than her head, it was not washed off?

I cannot say what happened as a result of the water going on her hair. We had pressurised water there, and she was in there for about five minutes. I was able to get the boy to put his hand in the foot-hand [radiation] monitor, and the father, and they thought it was great fun. There was no way in the world I would have been able to get the mother and the daughter to do it. They were like a cat on a hot tin roof. They were nervous. They were shy.

Smith likened the Milpuddies' experience at Pom Pom, suddenly surrounded as they were by soldiers in uniforms and being confronted with geiger counters, showers, cameras and jeeps, to that of white people suddenly landing on Mars. 'The whole family were disoriented.'

The Milpuddies' story is remarkable not just for its bizarre impact on the family, but for the light it throws on the paranoia and frenzy which the incident generated among officials in Maralinga and Canberra. Their greatest fear was that if the story leaked out it could threaten the future of the bomb tests. The Milpuddies were secretly and swiftly removed from Maralinga to Yalata with almost indecent haste. Astonishingly, no follow-up medical checks were ever made on the surviving members of the family until 1981, 24 years later, after the bare bones of the incident had finally found their way into the newspapers. Both Penney and Titterton told the royal commission in 1985 that they did not hear of the Marcoo incident at the time, which is, perhaps, a significant admission in itself. But Howard Beale, the Australian minister for supply, did hear about it. According to Durance, the Maralinga range commander, what worried Beale was that the Mulpuddies' hunting dogs were not checked for radiation before the family were spirited down to Yalata. Beale acted quickly. 'Mr Beale got through to his department and told them to tell me to shoot the dogs', said Durance. 'I do not know why the Department of Supply, through the minister, wanted them shot but they wanted them shot and said so. I had it done.' The slaughter of the dogs in front of the Milpuddie family outraged Charlie Milpuddie and he demanded, unsuccessfully, to leave Yalata after it happened.

The men working on the Maralinga range were called together and told to keep quiet about the Milpuddie affair. One of them was John Hutton, a 19-year-old soldier in the Australian army at the time, whose job involved building fences for the scientists to store equipment near the bomb sites. Hutton recalled the men being mustered together and addressed by 'a colonel who wore red braids', who told them they had not seen the Milpuddie incident because the British and Australian governments had poured a lot of money into the atomic tests and if it got out to the newspapers the money would have been wasted. The colonel reminded them, said Hutton, that they were bound by the Official Secrets Act, and they could be shot or sent to jail for 30 years if they were found guilty of transgressing it.

Retired brigadier Richard Durance, the Maralinga range commander at the time, was then a colonel. He came out of retirement to tell the royal commission he was undoubtedly the officer who warned the men:

I would be the only one wearing what is colloquially termed a red hat . . . I have no recollection of this, but it is what I would have done and if I could remember back I am sure that I would have taken the action I have been told occurred.

Why?

The whole range was a very secret affair. The less that was said about it the better. Any knowledge that started to seep out to the public, certainly about an incident of that nature, would, I think, have been very serious. It could have been an embarrassment to both [British and Australian] governments, plus the South Australian state government who were responsible for Aborigines in their state.

Durance also told the royal commission he could not agree with the optimistic conclusion of Harry Turner's official report, that there was no possibility that any members of the Milpuddie family could have experienced radiation injury.

Even for some Aborigines at Maralinga who did not stray into the actual bomb sites, the atomic tests had shocking repercussions. Perhaps the most tragic story of all belongs to Darlene Stevens, who was living in the bush with her family west of Maralinga at the time of the bomb tests. Ever since the late fifties, patrols had gone out from Cundeelee, a mission station on the transcontinental railway in Western Australia, to locate Aborigines in the desert zones adjacent to Maralinga and bring them into Cundeelee. It was both a humanitarian and a missionary exercise. Darlene Stevens' group, however, remained in the desert.

Macaulay reported that he and MacDougall had first encountered Darlene and her family in August 1960, three years after the bomb trials finished, near Nurrari Lakes, about 200 kilometres northwest of Maralinga. Three years later, Macaulay and Tom Murray, a Commonwealth policeman from Maralinga, came across them in the same territory again, this time about 100 kilometres closer to Maralinga. Although the bomb trials were long since over, the 'minor trials' were still going on and the Maralinga region was still a prohibited zone. The group consisted of Darlene's father, his two wives and three children. Darlene – or Tangawunu, by her Aboriginal name – was then aged about 12.

Macaulay reported that the family had never visited any of the main mission stations scattered through Western and South Australia, at Ernabella, Warburton and Cundeelee. Instead, they moved through a region bounded by lakes, most of which were often dry, in the Great Victoria Desert in the northwest of the Maralinga prohibited zone. Macaulay noted that Darlene's family had had an opportunity to leave the desert and move to Cundeelee mission in Western Australia in 1960; but they had elected to stay in the desert around Maralinga. The meeting with Macaulay and Tom Murray happened on 25 July 1963, according to Macaulay's report. The family appeared to him to be in good health. 'They had been waiting for some time to see me, and departed the morning after our meeting, heading to the Serpentine Lakes and points west', he wrote. 'A follow-up patrol to see them again was cancelled when it was learned that they had moved into Western Australia about their normal business.' A hint of concern crept into Macaulay's report when he added: 'It is not known how long they intend staying out there'.

Macaulay's report gave no hint of what happened to Darlene and her family after this encounter, nor did he appear to know at the time he prepared his report back at Woomera. When they met the Aborigines, the patrol officers told them they should go to Cundeelee mission station, 650 kilometres away. As the story was later told to the Australian royal commission, a dispute broke out between the patrol officers over whether the Aborigines should be provided with transport, and the final instructions given to the family were to walk and stay on the road. So they did.

Darlene herself told of the terrible tragedy which followed, during the royal commission's hearings in the bush at Maralinga in 1985. She answered questions, through an interpreter, from Geoff Eames, the Aborigines' counsel. 'What happened when you went walking off with your family after you had seen that white man?' asked Eames.

Interpreter: 'She said the man that was wanting to take them to Cundeelee was told off by another man and told not to take them there, that they should go on foot'.

Eames: 'When the man said that you were not to be taken in the car or taken in the Land Rover, did your family start to walk off?'

Interpreter: 'Darlene said yes'.

Eames: 'Did anyone tell you you had to stay on the road?'

Interpreter: 'Darlene said she was told to stay on the road all the way'.

Eames: 'When you were walking along the road, could you find any water?'

Interpreter: 'She said no to that question'.

Eames: 'And could you find any food?'

Interpreter: 'There was no food'.

Eames: 'And what happened to you and your family when you were walking along that road?'

Interpreter (indicating Darlene and her companions): 'I think it is causing some disturbance there'.

Eames: 'Yes, okay. Perhaps you might check this – if you could ask did a couple of her family perish on that trip?'

Interpreter: 'She said they left her mother towards the Rawlinna road, this side of it, and she left them there and they never came back'.

Eames: 'And eventually did you come to a place where they had helicopters and then some people helped you into Cundeelee?'

Interpreter: 'She said that after she lost her mother . . .'

At this point, the interpreter broke down and sobbed. He was a white man who had worked closely with Darlene and other Aborigines at Cundeelee mission. The judge discreetly adjourned the proceedings. This is how Darlene's story ended: She and her family set off, as instructed, along the road leading west from the Nurrari Lakes region of the Maralinga zone. They kept walking through the desert for almost 450 kilometres until they reached Neale Junction, in Western Australia. There they turned south on the road towards Rawlinna, a settlement on the transcontinental railway another 350 kilometres away. This was the only road leading south that would eventually take them to Cundeelee. But they never got to Rawlinna. Unable to find food or water, the family was in a desperate state. Somewhere along that road, Darlene's mother and father died of thirst and starvation. One of the two little boys in the party, aged about three, wandered off into the desert and was never seen again.

So the group, by now reduced to Darlene, the other woman and another child, retraced their steps back to Neale Junction – the place where the helicopters were, in Darlene's story. The helicopters belonged to an army survey team, who alerted the authorities, and eventually Darlene and her fellow survivors were taken to Cundeelee, where they continued living for many years.

There is a chilling sentence in Macaulay's 1963 report – written from Woomera, almost 1000 kilometres away to the east – which gives no clue to the events that surrounded it: 'A recent message from an army survey team at Neale Junction indicates that a woman and two children have turned up there, and this may indicate that they are seeking a way to Cundeelee mission'. Macaulay himself had reported a year earlier, in August 1962, a food shortage in the Great Victoria Desert, the area through which Darlene and her family had to trek. Aborigines there were having more difficulty finding food than water: the main foods were lizards and grubs, but there were very few rabbits, kangaroos or emus.

At the time of this tragedy, the Department of Supply had laid down strict rules for its employees, including the patrol officers, to follow towards the Aborigines. One instruction was that no Aborigines must be carried in government vehicles except in cases of illness or at the request of employees of those working on stations. Another order stressed that, 'it must be remembered at all times that intended kindnesses may in many cases result in harm to natives'.

In their final submission to the Australian royal commission, the lawyers for the Aboriginal groups affected by the atomic testing said:

Communication with the Aboriginal party was undoubtedly difficult. Macaulay had not understood any Aboriginal language although no doubt had picked up a few words by 1963, and . . . the survivors had 'language difficulties' which made them unable to converse with the army survey party that they stumbled across at Neale Junction.

We do not report these events in order to attribute blame to any of the patrol officers who dealt with this party. But it is clear that range policy (to move people off the range) and range convenience (to have people on the roads where they could be easily located) were factors in the deaths of the three people.

But the more important factors were the general policy of closing the traditional lands, discouraging people from using their lands, opening the lands up to white intruders and generally terrifying and distressing the people by the range activities. To the white patrol officer it no doubt seemed sensible for the Aborigines to be directed to stay on the roads. But to the Aborigines the roads, unlike Aboriginal routes, had no logic as pathways between water and food locations.

This difference in perception is perhaps just one illustration of the lack of comprehension of Aboriginal lifestyle and culture that was a feature of the entire British nuclear test program. In the end it was this gulf in understanding which contributed to the deaths of the three people.

In October 1953, when the first British atomic bombs were exploded on land at Emu Field, in South Australia, Almerta Lander and her husband were living at a place with the improbable name of Never Never, about 200 kilometres away to the northeast. The couple had gone to Never Never, near Welbourn Hill station, so that Almerta's husband could take a job building a windmill and a yard. It was in the heart of the South Australian desert – flat, stony country with a few little hills and low slung scrub, but otherwise, as Almerta remembers it, nothing outstanding.

About ten one morning, the Landers looked up from their chores and noticed a cloud coming towards them from the southwest, the direction of Emu Field. 'It was unusual', Almerta Lander remembered:

Although it was the colour of a rain cloud, darkish, it did not have the compact, rolling look that a rain cloud would have. It was just a sort of mass, and it had at the top of it a banner that stretched upwards. We had been told that they were testing at Emu Plains. That is why we took notice of it, because there were not any other clouds in the sky. None whatsoever.

The base of the dark cloud was in the top of the mulga trees, and as it got closer to where the Landers were working it appeared to stretch from horizon to horizon. It passed directly over the top of the caravan in which they lived, and by lunchtime it had gone. Almerta Lander had lived in this country since 1939, and had seen almost every strange and turbulent weather phenomenon the Australian outback is capable of producing: wind storms, dust storms, rain clouds, the lot. This was nothing like any of those. It appeared to have something she had never seen before – trails of fine dust trickling down from the cloud. 'It was very sticky. It was really very, very fine, very soft and sticky.' It was different from any dust storms they had lived through. 'I would just flick the dust off with a feather duster and then sweep it off the floor. But this could not be flicked off. It had to be wiped off with a damp cloth.'

Almerta Lander always did the cooking outside the caravan in camp ovens, and at the time the cloud passed over it shed its sticky dust into pots and billies which were on the stove with food and water in them. 'Whatever was there, we drank it.' Afterwards, the Landers went to nearby Welbourn Hill station and talked about what they had seen with the station's owners, the Giles family (no connection to the weather station). Mrs Giles told them she had seen the same dark cloud, and that it had left the same sticky dust behind.

The Landers and the Giles had witnessed the notorious Black Mist, one of the most mysterious and controversial legacies of the entire British atomic tests program. The timing of the phenomenon put it squarely as a product of the first of the Emu Field bombs, codenamed Totem One. Aborigines living around Wallatinna and Welbourn Hill stations also witnessed the strange cloud, and many, living as they were in the open or in meagre humpies, were stricken with terrible illnesses soon afterwards. While she was living near Wallatinna in the early 1940s, Almerta Lander had met two Aborigines, Pingkayi and Kanytji, who worked with her husband. When Pingkayi and Kanytji's son was born it was Almerta who suggested the name, Jimmy. Later, Jimmy took on the name, Yami Lester. In 1945, Almerta and her husband began travelling around the stations where her husband took contract jobs erecting windmills and building fences. Yami and his parents went to live at Wallatinna station, and Almerta did not see Yami Lester again for many years. The next time she saw him was after the Totem tests when he was a young man – and blind.

Yami Lester saw the Black Mist as a child from Wallatinna station, where he was born and was living with his family at the time. One morning, when he was up early and playing, he heard an explosion away in the south that sounded like three or four bangs. Everyone in the camp started talking about it, and someone said 'it was the army'. Later that day, he saw a cloud.

It was coming from the south, black – like smoke. I was thinking it might be a dust storm, but it was quiet, just moving through the trees and above the trees. It was just rolling and moving quietly.

Lester remembered the old people in the camp being frightened. 'They reckon it was *mamu* – something that could be a bad spirit or evil spirit.' Some people brandished their woomeras, or spear throwers, to try to make the cloud change direction. Others dug a hole for people to climb into. Yami Lester's parents, Pingkayi and Kanytji, also recalled the awesome sight. Kanytji heard two noises from the southwest just after sunrise. At first he thought it was someone shooting, then he thought it may have been the *Wanambi*, the water serpent of the dreamtime, making a noise as it created water holes. Pingkayi also heard two noises, and remembered the cloud depositing a black, moist substance on the leaves and ground. She was struck by how the cloud had a really strong smell which made her vomit.

These and other first-hand accounts of the Black Mist were given when the Australian royal commission went to Wallatinna and nearby Marla Bore in April 1985, to hear the Aborigines' own stories. The Aborigines also told about what happened to some of their people after the Black Mist had passed. Pingkayi said that within a day, there was a lot of vomiting, diarrhoea and stomach pains. Some people were coughing and had headaches. Pingkayi herself had sore eyes. Asked whether anyone died following the *puyu* (Black Mist), Pingkayi said 'one thousand people died' – although, as the interpreter explained, the figure should be taken not literally but as meaning many people.

Yami Lester also recalled suffering from vomiting, sore eyes, diarrhoea and skin rashes. He thought some people died because he could remember others being upset and crying and the camp was moved twice, a traditional practice when deaths occur. He had good eyesight before the Black Mist, but straight after the event he could not see at all. Eventually the sight came back in his left eye, but his right eye remained blind. The sight in his left eye, however, was impaired and some years later he lost it completely.

Yami Lester has always maintained that his blindness was the eventual result of damage caused by the Black Mist – a claim which scientists close to the atomic tests, and their aftermath, have hotly disputed. He says the connection between his lost eyesight and the nuclear tests has never been properly investigated by doctors or scientists. It was Lester who began the Aborigines' campaign to get a royal commission set up when, as he recalled, in 1980 he heard Sir Ernest Titterton talking about the British atomic tests on a national radio program in Australia.

I was upset about that. I thought that scientist was talking a little bit the wrong way. Nobody knew about the Aboriginal side of the story, so after the program I got out of bed and rang up the Adelaide *Advertiser*.

Thus began a long campaign by the Pitjantjatjara council, a campaign during which Lester and his wife travelled to London, and eventually culminated in the royal commission they had demanded going to Wallatinna and Maralinga itself. What, then, was the story behind the bomb that caused the Black Mist?

The performance of the bomb in question, Totem One, was the subject of some of the most astonishing evidence of the Australian royal commission's inquiry. Totem One and the other bomb in that round, Totem Two, were fired from towers at the Emu Field testing ground in South Australia in October 1953. At 10 and 8 kilotons respectively, each was about a third the strength of the earlier, and first, British atomic test, Hurricane. The Totem trials were scrambled together, as Britain sought to perfect the next stage of its atomic arsenal using cheap plutonium as the weapon fuel, produced from its new, dual-purpose nuclear reactors. Even the test site at Emu Field was something of a stop gap; the two Totem tests were the only ones ever held there, and the place was abandoned soon afterwards because it was geographically unsuitable for any more bomb tests. Penney himself, during a reconnaissance trip to search out a more permanent testing ground further south at Maralinga, told Alan Butement, the Australian government's chief scientist: 'The investment at Emu is part of the price that we have to pay for rushing the Totem trials'. [7]

The behaviour of the cloud carrying the radioactive fallout from the Totem bombs would depend, as it does for all atomic blasts, on the crucial factor of weather conditions. Put at its most simple, the principle centres on the wind patterns: the higher the cloud goes, and the more scattered it becomes, the less concentrated is the radioactive debris falling back to earth. If, on the other hand, there is little wind shear – that is, winds dragging the cloud about in different directions at different levels of the mushroom cloud – then the danger of the fallout staying bunched together and plummeting down in more concentrated volumes is much greater. Titterton and Leslie Martin, who were to be Australian observers at the Totem trials, had sought information from Penney five months before the tests on the question of the likely bomb cloud heights. They were worried about any possibility of fallout on population centres to the southeast of Emu Field, as far away as Melbourne, in the event of local unexpected rain. Penney replied that the UK team did not anticipate the cloud rising above 30 000 feet (about 10 000 metres) and were confident that their meteorological service would give them sufficient knowledge of upper wind conditions to fire with no possible risk of danger to health.

On the basis of this, Titterton and Martin sent Menzies a top secret letter in June 1953, four months before the Totem trials, giving him a guarantee that everything would be all right. The sweeping and self-confident nature of their assurance is remarkable in the light of revelations 30 years later about how the Totem One bomb actually behaved.

We are able to assure you that the isolation of the site of the trials precludes any possible damage to habitation or living beings by the 'shock' wave, thermal radiation, gamma rays and neutrons. It is possible for us to assure you that the time of firing will be chosen so that any risk to health due to radioactive contamination to our cities, or in fact of any human beings, is impossible. To sum up, on the basis of information before us, we are able to assure you, Sir, that no habitations or living beings will suffer injury to health from the effects of the atomic explosions proposed for the trials.

Penney arrived at Emu Field for the Totem One test on 28 September 1953. Two days later, Lord Cherwell, Churchill's atomic adviser who was then on an official mission to Australia, arrived at Emu Field with other top officials amid great secrecy. But Penney and his team faced growing frustration. Their first attempt to ignite the bomb, on 7 October, had to be called off because of bad weather. Rain over the next few days meant that standby could not be ordered again for another week.

Totem One was finally exploded at 7 in the morning on 15 October. The top of the cloud went to 15 000 feet (about 5000 metres). It dispersed slowly and drifted northeast, across Wallatinna, producing a narrow band of contamination on the ground. The cloud was so concentrated that Australian air force crews sent to monitor it several hours later reported being able to locate it visually even at night. American air force pilots, well experienced in monitoring US atomic bombs, and who had arrived secretly to conduct their own analysis of the Totem tests for the Pentagon, later told the Australians that the radioactivity from Totem One was the most intense they had ever encountered. The Americans' sensitive measuring equipment became saturated, and they were unable to use it until some of the radioactivity had decayed.

The key to what happened was contained in a document prepared for the British Ministry of Supply five months before the Totem trials, and unearthed at the Australian royal commission in London in early 1985. The document had the innocuous title, 'High Explosives Research Report No. A32', and was a bid by a group of leading Aldermaston scientists to describe the likely impact of airborne contamination from Totem One. The A32 document became, in effect, the 'smoking gun' of the Totem trials.

It was a crucial document, sensational for what it revealed, because the British scientists were still, in effect, feeling their way in calculating such things as the size of fallout particles, the way they are carried about by the cloud and the rate at which contaminated particles of different sizes and volumes fall back to earth. A great deal of fallout from nuclear weapons consists of earth and other bits of material pulverised by the blast which, depending on how high above the ground the weapon is exploded, are then sucked up into the fireball where they become instantly contaminated with the 'fission products', before drifting off into the atmosphere. Depending on their size and density they fall back to earth either very quickly or stay aloft for weeks, months or even years.

Totem One was only the second atomic bomb the British had exploded, and the first they had detonated on land. They still had no inside information on these questions from American scientists about the 37 atomic bombs the Americans had tested in Nevada and the Pacific Ocean over the previous two years. The British scientists, like everyone else, could only go on what was published in US atomic energy commission official reports.

A32, then, began with an explanation of how the fallout particles to a large extent would be carried by the wind currents, both vertically and horizontally. The contamination on the ground would steadily decrease as the distance downwind from the blast decreased. So the further the particles could be carried before falling to the ground, the less dangerous the contamination would be – and this would depend on the behaviour of the wind. The document admitted that very stable atmospheric conditions often prevailed at the Emu Field site, in which case diffusion of the cloud would be slight. It concluded that the least favourable conditions for firing a bomb would be a steady wind blowing in the same direction at all heights of the bomb cloud – in other words, an absence of wind shear – because this would concentrate the contamination in a narrow band, rather than scatter it about. If these conditions did prevail, the document warned, then there should be no population centres in the area over which this narrow band would travel for a distance of 190 kilometres. Wallatinna station was 195 kilometres north east of Emu Field, the precise direction the Totem One cloud took.

The A32 document's calculations assumed the bomb would yield about 5 kilotons of energy. In fact, it turned out to be twice that strength. And another secret document, prepared after the Totem trials, reported that the climatic conditions at the time of the bomb's detonation were precisely those which A32 had warned would produce a maximum danger from fallout. On the strength of this, both Penney and Ronald Siddons, one of the scientific authors of the A32 document, made the astonishing admission when questioned by the Australian royal commision in London in early 1985 that, with hindsight, the Totem One bomb should not have been fired.

Penney agreed with the suggestion that the way the Totem One cloud stayed together was exceptional compared with each of the 11 other atomic bombs exploded in Australia. Penney's admission on the Totem One bomb came reluctantly and dramatically, on the very last day of the royal commission's hearings in London that had gone on for ten exhaustive weeks. Peter McClellan, the counsel assisting the royal commission, had taken Penney through the documentation step by step for more than an hour before putting to him an unequivocal proposition: 'You did not know what was precisely going to happen after the event, on the information available to you at the time. It should not have been fired – with hindsight, would you agree?' Penney replied: 'With hindsight I would agree. That is a very different statement.' Then, explaining the difficulties of calculating risks then, compared with now, he added: 'The attitude in those days was different'.

Ronald Siddons's revised thinking on Totem One proved to be far more startling than Penney's. Siddons was no peripheral figure to the event. He was a mathematical scientist involved in measuring gamma radiation doses from the Totem trials and, as we saw, a co-author of the A32 document. He played a key role in fallout forecasting at the Antler trials at Maralinga four years later, and by the time he appeared before the royal commission in 1985 he had risen to become a deputy director of the atomic weapons research establishment at Aldermaston, the centre which Penney inaugurated in 1950 where the British atomic bombs were designed and built.

Siddons helped to re-evaluate the A32 document for the royal commission, and disclosed that some of its calculations were wrong. It actually underestimated by three times the contamination from the bomb. His own calculations had shown that Penney's statement about the amount of contamination observed 130 kilometres from the blast was an underestimation of the real levels by six or seven times. And, because the Totem One bomb turned out to be twice as powerful as the predictions had assumed, the risk level would have extended not 190 kilometres from the blast but at least 270 kilometres. That would put Wallatinna squarely in the risk zone.

Siddons said that Penney, and his colleagues, who made the decision to fire Totem One, had the basis of these modified estimates and calculations before them at the time. 'They were in possession of the information which is available to us now . . . I believe that it was unduly risky to proceed with Totem One at the time it was fired. If I had been asked at the time, my advice would have been not to run the risk.'

Penney has said he had never heard anything about a Black Mist from the Totem One bomb until 30 years after the tests. Titterton has always treated the affair contemptuously. At a secret meeting with members of the Australian Ionising Radiation Advisory Council as late as 1981, Titterton said:

This story is laughable from the physical, meteorological and medical points of view. I am not denying that there may have been a black cloud; what I am denying is that it's physically possible for a black cloud travelling at ground level to have emanated from a nuclear explosion. [8]

Yet the story was not new. It certainly pre-dated the controversy over the conduct of the British atomic tests that erupted in the early 1980s. Tom Murray, the Australian Commonwealth policeman who travelled extensively between cattle stations and missions in the central desert between 1953 and 1967, first heard of the Black Mist at Emu Field or Maralinga in the mid-fifties, when the bomb tests were still going on. He told the royal commission the story he heard then: 'That the natives went blind and all sorts of things, and were really ill. This was only something I took no notice of whatsoever. It was just a sort of gossip thing.'

When the Black Mist affair first surfaced in the British press in 1983, the Ministry of Defence in London denied any connection with the Totem One bomb. But the atomic weapons research establishment at Aldermaston secretly commissioned William Roach, a meteorologist, and Derek Vallis, a scientist working in radiological protection, to investigate the allegations. Roach and Vallis examined such things as the size of the mushroom shaped cloud from Totem One, the amount of radioactivity produced in the explosion, the volume of soil swept up into the cloud and the size of the radioactive particles which composed the cloud. But, Vallis later told the royal commission, this information was not obtained from measurements made at the time, but from theorectical calculations based on the known explosive yield of the bomb. There was no doubt a good reason for this: no-one had bothered to take ground readings of Totem One's fallout around Wallatinna. As a result of this serious scientific omission, no reliable on-site data exists about the level or extent of contamination or about the wind conditions at Wallatinna at the time.

Roach and Vallis reported in August 1984, that the Black Mist phenomenon could well have occurred. As Roach told the royal commission a year later: 'The fallout cloud would have been seen from the affected site [Wallatinna] about mid-morning, possibly as an extended black curtain'. But they refused to link the existence of the black cloud with illness among the Aborigines, saying that the highest possible radiation doses they could calculate for Wallatinna could not have resulted in short-term adverse health effects. Even so, Vallis told the royal commission that their estimates of the radiation doses were bound to carry large uncertainties, and could not be calculated more accurately than to a factor of ten either way.

Geoff Eames, one of the counsel for the Aborigines, acknowledged the difficulties of relating the Black Mist to health effects when the royal commission travelled to Wallatinna and Marla Bore. The biggest problem was the sheer lack of medical records. In 1981, the state government of South Australia commissioned an epidemiological study of Aborigines to look at, among other things, long-term effects of the bomb testing on cancer rates. But the study discovered that there were virtually no medical records for the northwest of South Australia for the period of the bomb trials, and certainly no records at all for Wallatinna on health, sickness, disease and other medical problems. What records did exist were sparse, and some had been lost in a fire at Ernabella. There were other problems to do with Aboriginal custom and lore. Aborigines in that part of South Australia adhere strongly to the practice of not mentioning the names of dead people. Nor do they have the same concept of time and numbers as whites. Those things, alone, made it particularly difficult to relate Aboriginal deaths to certain dates or people.

For these reasons, Eames explained, the Aborigines had agreed that the royal commission would not be in a position to make a positive finding on the relationship between the deaths and sickness after the Black Mist and the Totem test. But, the Aborigines' lawyers argued, the state of knowledge about medicine and the effects of doses with low-level radiation was such that the whole question should be left open. 'The scientific evidence now discloses that, at the dose levels which could have occurred at Wallatinna, the adverse health effects which the lay witnesses described may have resulted'.

One expert who gave extensive evidence to the royal commission about a possible connection between the illnesses at Wallatinna and the Totem bomb was Sir Edward Pochin, a member of the scientific staff of the British Medical Research Council for 33 years until his retirement in 1974. Pochin was a former chairman of the International Commission on Radiological Protection, the body whose recommendations on radiation exposure rates were followed by the British at the bomb tests. Pochin flew from Britain to Australia to give evidence, during which he highlighted a whole host of scientific unknowns about the effects of low-level radiation. For instance there was, and remains, little information about the effects on a group of people such as the tribal Aborigines at Wallattina compared with white people living town or city lifestyles.

The Wallattina Aborigines had already lived through epidemics from diseases such as measles in the fifties, and many suffered from poor nutrition. Some scientists argue that if such a group's immune system was suppressed from conditions of this sort, then the radiation dose required to produce immediate health effects could be lower than that for other people. Pochin agreed that the state of knowledge did not enable anyone to assert that Aborigines would not have a significantly greater sensitivity to the effects of radiation than non-Aborigines. He drew attention to a vast array of factors which can affect a person's response to radiation exposure – and he believed they had the potential to apply at Wallatinna. They included the rate of human cell proliferation, age at the time of irradiation, body temperature, blood flow, genetic background, physiological condition, hormone balance, stress, trauma and other forms of injury.

Pochin had something of an open view about Yami Lester's eye injuries. The royal commission had heard earlier that Lester suffered from trachoma, an eye disease with a high incidence among Aborigines, and had probably had measles. Pochin was questioned about the possible effect of measles and trachoma, through cell damage and cell regeneration, on the way a person may respond to radiation doses at low levels. He was asked: 'So the situation with Mr Lester is this, is it not: that you are unable to say that if each of those events occurred – radiation at low dose, trachoma, measles or any two of the three – they can exclude radiation as being an accelerating or aggravating factor in his condition?'

'That is correct', replied Pochin.

The whole question of just how dangerous exposure to low-level radiation is for human health is one which has split the scientific and medical communities for many years. (It is discussed further in Chapter Seven.) When the British atomic tests began, most scientists still accepted that there was a threshold of radiation exposure below which a person's longterm health would not be affected. That notion has since been discredited. But the scientists at the British tests made no special allowance at all for the Aborigines. David Barnes, the British health physicist who, with Penney, helped devise the standards for radiological protection at the beginning of the tests in 1952, told the Australian royal commission in London in January 1985: 'I think, as we are speaking now, we might very well have taken more account of the Aborigine population'. Just how ignorant the British scientists were about the way the Aborigines actually lived – and how far the Australian authorities failed to inform them – came out in this exchange at the royal commission between Barnes and Andrew Collett, one of the Australian lawyers appearing for the Aborigines:

Collett: 'You were not aware that the Aborigines had different cooking and preparation techniques for their food, were you?'

Barnes: 'No'.

Collett: 'Neither were you aware at that stage that Aborigines in that area [Wallatinna] slept on the ground rather than in beds – is that not the case?'

Barnes: 'Yes, we took no different account of Aborigines than we did of the white population. We treated them the same way. I have made this admission a number of times.'

Collett: 'Would you agree now that, had you known about what I have just told you about the state of the Aborigines in the region, it would have been desirable in 1952 and 1953 to have had a separate standard of exposure then?'

Barnes: 'Had this been brought to our notice – by anybody – I feel sure we would have taken that into account'.

It was only after the first five of the 12 atomic bombs had been fired that the authorities belatedly recognised that the Aborigines could be exposed to more danger because of their migratory lifestyle, open-air living and lack of conventional clothing. In 1956, the Australian safety committee recommended that an exposure level be set for Aborigines for the final two rounds of trials, Buffalo and Antler, which was lower than that which the experts considered acceptable for the white population. 'This will impose a further restriction on the choices of suitable firing conditions, beyond those already agreed with the UK', the safety committee warned in a secret report to Menzies. The government agreed to the measure. But the new regulations still accepted the notion of a threshold, a level below which exposure to radiation would be safe. Even by then, this idea was beginning to come under vigorous challenge among scientists around the world. By 1956, the International Commission on Radiological Protection, whose recommendations formed the basis for the radiation exposure policy at the British tests, had already tightened its recommended 'safe' levels from those which applied at the time of the Hurricane and Totem tests. The ICRP continued to revise its standards during the fifties to the extent that, according to calculations done by Ronald Siddons, the tighter contamination standards set by 1959, and adopted by the British, would have been exceeded by 60 times in the fallout from the Totem One bomb experienced by the people at Wallatinna.

Notwithstanding the enormous research problems struck by the epidemiological study of Aborigines mentioned earlier, which the South Australian health commission embarked upon in 1981, the royal commission asked that the study be continued, and a report was finally produced in early 1985. The South Australian study identified 30 cases of cancer among Aborigines between 1969 and

1980, most of them in the zone north of the bomb sites; 27 of the cancer victims had died. Of the 30 cancers, two were thyroid and two leukaemias. The report pointed out that the quality of the data was inadequate for epidemiological research of good quality, and concluded that, on balance, there was no clear evidence of a developing trend of diseases among Aborigines in South Australia which could be related to radiation exposure.

During its hearings in London, the Australian royal commission asked Dr Alice Stewart, a noted radiation expert from Birmingham, to comment on the findings. During the 1950s, Stewart became the first person to document the effect of low-level radiation on the human foetus, thus opening up a whole new debate about the wisdom of using X-rays for diagnostic purposes, particularly on pregnant women.

Alice Stewart agreed with the suggestion that the South Australian study was 'an epidemiologist's nightmare'. She said:

It does not even get into being reasonable to think you could do anything even if you had the very early records available for 1200 people. You could come to no conclusion for a very low-dose effect in the time you have allowed. I think the whole thing sounds hopeless from start to finish.

But some findings did strike her as significant. She believed the total number of cancers among the Aborigines was 'far too high', and of the two thyroid cancers and two leukaemias she said:

That, to me, is the only distinctive finding of the whole study and I think that should have been mentioned in the conclusion. It is a very odd figure. First of all, thyroid cancer is rather famous for not killing, and certainly very rare. In the whole of the Hanford study [involving about 25 000 radiation workers in the US – see Chapter Seven] we never had a case. And leukaemia is normally only 5 per cent of cancer deaths.

Stewart agreed that thyroid cancer was regarded as a particularly good marker of radiation:

It is known to be associated with one of the biggest products which tends to get lost because of its content of iodine – it is a good marker because iodine has associations with radioactivity and fission products and with the thyroid gland.

In December 1984, a group of Pitjantjatjara Aborigines made a triumphant journey to Maralinga to celebrate the return of ownership over the Maralinga lands to their people. After a long battle, the state government of South Australia, headed by John Bannon, had recognised their traditional rights to this land in a special act of parliament. But this was by no means the end of the Aborigines' story.

At the time of the atomic tests 30 years earlier, the Aborigines had not been consulted or informed about the use of their tribal lands as a testing ground. Most of the Aborigines living in the paths of the radioactive clouds were barefooted and wore little or no clothes. They lived in the open and gathered their food and water from sources open to the elements. They were not given an opportunity to protect themselves: indeed the precautions taken for the British and Australian personnel at Emu Field and Maralinga, even though they were not always enforced, stand in stark contrast to the completely dismissive treatment of the Aborigines who lived there permanently.

The actual bomb sites at Emu Field and Maralinga were not included in the land returned to the Aborigines in 1985 because the South Australian government believed the question of the contamination remaining there should be resolved first. Several sites at Maralinga are still contaminated with plutonium, which remains radioactive for thousands of years and is capable of causing cancer in humans if inhaled or injested. (The story of how it got there, during the minor trials of 1959-63, is discussed more fully in Chapter Six). The Aborigines have built up a deep fear of what they call this 'poison', and its potential to scatter beyond the fenced zones to contaminate their water holes and food sources.

Even before the historic land rights legislation of 1984, many Aborigines who had been living at Yalata for the past 30 years had begun to reject it as a place to live, with all its problems of social stress and dislocation. In 1982, about 80 Yalata people and their children travelled about 280 kilometres north to establish the first camp, or outstation, on the Maralinga lands at Lake Dey Dey, northwest of the Maralinga range. Making Lake Dey Dey their base, they waited patiently over the next two years as the negotiations went on for the legislation which finally gave them the right to return to their country for good.

The Australian royal commission finally recommended at the end of 1985 that Britain should pay for a clean-up of the plutonium contamination at Maralinga, to make the land safe again, and that Australia should compensate the Aborigines for the loss of their lands. It appeared to be an attempt to reach an evenhanded solution, even though Australia years earlier had absolved Britain of any further responsibilities in this regard. Both tasks will be hugely expensive, and will not be achieved quickly, probably not for many more years while the governments negotiate between them the best deal possible – and the Aborigines go on waiting.

All the worst fears which Walter MacDougall held about the impact of weather stations, roads and contact with the whites on the tribal Aborigines came to pass. The Giles weather station, built to assist forecasting for the Maralinga bombs, proved to be a total disaster for the Aborigines who lived nearby in the Rawlinson ranges. MacDougall and Macaulay sought to enforce rigidly a policy which was aimed at not allowing the Aborigines to seek out easy food and water from Giles, and thereby lose their traditional hunting methods. But the inevitable breakdown gradually happened, in spite of their efforts.

By 1959, Macaulay reported that the continual contact of workers at Giles with the Aborigines through trading and game shooting had made the Aborigines part parasites on the weather station. He had an incinerator installed to burn all edible refuse to stop the Aborigines fossicking in rubbish tins. In January 1962, Macaulay reported that about 50 Aborigines were camped about 1 kilometre from Giles.

They are in poor condition and deteriorating as the season worsens. Food is becoming very scarce and the kangaroos are dying out. There are reports from Giles of children eating grass and leaves. The staff at Giles is worried.

Five months later, Macaulay reported that one family was persistently living on scraps recovered at night from the incinerator. He decided to move this family to the Warburton mission.

For the most part, the response of government officials was to try to stop this sort of thing from coming to public notice. In May 1957, an Australian government film unit travelled to Giles to make a film about the weather station. The director of meteorology in Melbourne wrote to inform the Department of Supply about the film crew, and certain instructions they had been given:

The unit has been briefed carefully on the necessity for discretion in filming the natives and that any film sequences taken by them are to avoid any impression that the natives are starving or that the establishment of Giles has interfered with their tribal way of life.

But nowhere, perhaps, was the legacy of the atomic tests on the Maralinga Aborigines captured more starkly than in this description of the degeneration of conditions at Yalata, the mission settlement set up near the transcontinental highway in 1952 to take the Aborigines who were moved away from the Maralinga lands around Ooldea. It came from Hans Gaden, who helped to bring the Aborigines out of the Maralinga lands and who worked for many years at the Lutheran missions near where Yalata was situated. Gaden here was giving evidence in July 1983, to a select committee of the South Australian state parliament on the land rights legislation which eventually returned the Maralinga lands to the Aboriginal owners:

We brought out 67 Kokothas and 401 Pitjantjatjaras. They were nice people, what I consider to be some of the nicest people I have met. But they were scrub people. They should never have been brought out from there. They should have been taken the other way rather than south.

I am afraid that it is all 31 years too late. These people have lived at Yalata for 31 years. During that time they have come into contact with plenty of alcohol, plenty of dirty white men and everything that oppresses them. When I look back at what they were like 31 years ago and what they are like now it is disgraceful.

The situation at Yalata should never have occurred. It came about because of the atomic bomb. Although we did not blow them up, we ruined them. Aborigines are not like white people. There are some fine Aborigines and some of them are better than the whites. Full-blooded Aborigines go to pieces after drinking alcohol. What kind of work will they have? They want to earn money. The first thing they told me when I brought them out [of Ooldea] was that they wanted work. On Friday nights, before they were legally permitted to drink, a taxi driver would bring them alcohol. On one occasion, I heard them the following morning. You had to see it to believe it. I dosed them up with coffee to sober them up. They drank 34 flagons of wine from Friday night until Sunday morning.

If I could have found that white man I probably would have shot him.

That is what had become of the Aborigines from Maralinga. It almost makes me cry when I see them today. They are not the same people.

Chapter Five

1956: 'SHE SHOOK THEM'

'Atomic weapons . . . take precedence over every other activity in the UK'
– Australian government document of the mid-1950s.

The Hurricane test at Monte Bello in 1952 had put Britain in the nuclear power league and had demonstrated to the Americans that British scientists were capable of building atomic bombs themselves without access to American nuclear secrets. But there was considerable confusion about what the next stage should be. Churchill, to begin with at least, was unenthusiastic about the enormous expenditure which an ongoing atomic weapons program for Britain implied. He still held out hopes for some sort of shared package deal with the US, in which the Americans would supply their junior partner with atomic weapons in return for access to British scientific and technological expertise. But Britain's military chiefs of staff were keen to build up a stockpile of atomic weapons which could be carried by the RAF's new generation of V-bombers, whose production by then had been given the go-ahead. As we saw earlier, the military chiefs had decided that Britain should work towards a target of producing 200 atomic bombs by the late fifties as its contribution to a combined Anglo-American stockpile. In this, they had the support of Lord Cherwell, the prime minister's atomic affairs adviser.

So the next two tests, the Totem series at Emu Field in South Australia, were ordered to be got ready for the target date of October 1953. Australia agreed to the holding of the Totem trials with as much alacrity as it had agreed to the original request for the Hurricane test at Monte Bello. Around the middle of 1952, even before the Hurricane trial had happened, the British were thinking about the need for a land site for future tests. Len Beadell, the Australian surveyor and explorer, had been instructed by Australian officials in great secrecy to scan the Great Victoria Desert region of South Australia for a suitable area. Beadell eventually found a site in what was completely unexplored country about 220 kilometres northwest of Mabel Creek station, within the prohibited area of the Woomera rocket range. It consisted of a vast claypan, which made an excellent natural airstrip, and a promising test site nearby to the south; Beadell called them Dingo and Emu claypans respectively (Beadell himself has given an excellent account of this arduous discovery in his book, *Blast the Bush* – see Bibliography).

Penney visited this site, again in total secrecy, in September 1952, on his way to the Monte Bello Islands for the Hurricane trial. Earlier the same month, Sir John Cockcroft, head of the atomic energy research establishment at Harwell, was having talks with Menzies on several atomic energy topics, including British help in uranium exploration in Australia and a possible Australian domestic atomic energy program. Cockcroft raised with Menzies Britain's wish for a feasibility study on a new site in Australia for future atomic tests, and Menzies immediately agreed 'in principle' on behalf of the Ausralian government. As Cockcroft reported back to London:

I saw the Prime Minister today and asked him whether we might have facilities on Woomera Range for further tests if desired. He is agreeable in principle and to Penney making reconnaissance for possible sites.

Penney was satisfied with the Emu Field site, although there were obvious problems with its physical isolation and poor access given the tight schedule he envisaged for holding the trials there. Back in London in November, after the successful completion of the Hurricane trial, Penney impressed upon the British authorities the urgency of testing the performance of the latest atomic weapons then being developed. By December, Churchill had agreed to a new round of trials, to be called Totem.

Menzies himself was in London at this time, and when Churchill approached him to seek agreement in principle for the Totem trials at Emu Field in October 1953, Menzies was reported as replying he felt certain the Australian government would agree to the suggestion. The formal British request came in an *aide-memoire* handed by Lord Cherwell, Churchill's adviser, to Menzies on 12 December 1952. 'The test has become necessary in order not to delay the rapid development of the United Kingdom atomic energy programme', the *aide-memoire* explained.

It was a Friday when Menzies received it. Menzies' staff were instructed to cable the text of the British request urgently to Canberra, where it would need to be seen by the acting prime minister, Sir Arthur Fadden, and to have a reply back in London by Monday. The telegram arrived in Australia at midnight on Saturday, with the following message from the head of the Prime Minister's Department, Allan Brown, who was travelling with Menzies in Britain:

EMERGENCY. My immediately following message contains the text of an aide memoire handed to the Prime Minister by Lord Cherwell. Please convey it urgently to the Acting Prime Minister. Mr Menzies feels that the Australian government will certainly agree to the suggestion and hopes to inform Mr Churchill of this agreement on Monday morning before he leaves. He would appreciate receiving confirmation before then if this is possible.

When he received this cable in Canberra, Fadden conferred with the defence minister, Philip McBride, then authorised a telegram confirming that the Australian government would agree in principle to the British request. The reply arrived in London, as Menzies had requested, on the Monday morning. From then until the end of July 1953, when the Totem trials were publicly announced, a cover plan was devised to respond to any questions about work at the Emu Field site by associating it with ordinary rocket range activities at Woomera.

The controversial nature of the Totem tests, involving the Black Mist and the unsuitable weather conditions in which the first Totem weapon was fired, were described in the previous chapter. The Totem bombs were experimental devices similar to the warheads being built for the Blue Danube weapons system, whose delivery to the RAF took place soon after the Totem tests were over. But one problem for the atomic weapons program after that was that plutonium production in Britain was insufficient to meet the targets set for the output of weapons. Following the Totem tests, therefore, the government authorised the building of further atomic reactors in order to achieve a substantial rise in the production of fissile material by the end of the decade. At the same time, the scientists at Aldermaston began work on the Red Beard variety of strategic atomic weapon, with the aim of producing bombs that were lighter and smaller than the earlier, Blue Danube version, but with the same explosive yield. But just as these developments were getting under way, the strategic outlook changed dramatically.

In November 1952, the Americans had exploded the world's first thermonuclear device, codenamed Mike, at Eniwetok in the Pacific Ocean. This was more of an experimental device than a usable hydrogen bomb. Less than a year later, in August 1953, the Russians stunned the Pentagon when they tested their first thermonuclear device in Sibera. From all accounts, this was a proper, deliverable bomb. If so, it meant that the Russians had beaten the Americans in the race for the super bomb. Seven months after that, the Americans exploded their first deliverable hydrogen bomb, codenamed Bravo, at their Pacific Ocean testing ground in the Marshall Islands. At 15 megatons, Bravo was 750 times more powerful than Hiroshima. It was also the biggest hydrogen bomb the US has ever tested – and, we now know, it was the 'dirtiest' in terms of fallout. This was the bomb that really alerted the world to the dangers of radioactivity.

The hydrogen bomb, also called thermonuclear or fusion bomb, added an entirely new and awesome dimension to the arms race. Its operating principle was the reverse of the atomic bomb which derived its energy from the splitting, or fission, of atoms of heavy elements like uranium and plutonium. The H-bomb was based on fusion, or the joining together of isotopes of the lightest element, hydrogen. Massive temperatures were needed for the fusion reaction to occur, hence the term thermonuclear. The only way known so far to produce the high temperatures needed for fusion is by an atomic bomb. Every hydrogen bomb therefore consists of at least two stages: a fission, or atomic bomb, which acts as the trigger, and the fusion mixture which is ignited in the heat created by the trigger.[1]

Two points are worth noting about the hydrogen bomb. First, if the required high temperatures and pressures are achieved there is, in principle, no limit to an H-bomb's explosive power. In 1961, the Soviet Union made the largest single test explosion of an H-bomb, with an explosive power of about 60 megatons, or 60 million tons of TNT – about 3000 times more powerful than the Hiroshima bomb. There would be nothing stopping the Russians or the Americans achieving even higher yields if they wanted – except the practical question that with such bombs of really big megaton yields, much of the energy would be wasted: it is considered today that it would take a bomb of only 10 megatons to destroy even the largest population centre. Second, because the fusion process produces no radioactive isotopes, a fusion bomb does not leave much radioactive fallout. What radioactivity there is comes from the fission trigger, but it represents only a very small fraction of the total energy released by the bomb. A two stage fission-fusion thermonuclear bomb, then, is considered relatively 'clean'.

That is why many scientists were puzzled by the huge amount of radioactive fallout that came from the Americans' first proper hydrogen bomb, Bravo, exploded in the Marshall Islands in 1954. Among the scientists who did their own independent calculations of the effects was Professor Joseph Rotblat, a Pole who began working in Britain before the Second World War and who joined the British team on the Manhattan Project. Rotblat later disowned nuclear weapons and helped found Pugwash, a peace movement among atomic scientists. He correctly solved the mystery about Bravo: it was, he discovered, a fission-fusion-fission bomb – a three-stage device. To the fission trigger and the main fusion bomb core the American weaponeers had added a third stage by wrapping a large amount of natural uranium around the fusion bomb. The effect of this third stage was to make Bravo a much dirtier bomb, with more radioactive products in the debris which composed the fallout. In fact, as well as producing enormous quantities of radioactive substances, this third stage also had the effect of increasing the hydrogen bomb's explosive power. Since then, most of the thermonuclear weapons held in the arsenals of the superpowers have been assumed to be of the three stage fission-fusion-fission variety – very 'dirty' bombs, in which about half the energy released is due to fission and half to fusion.

The Americans had secretly begun development work on the hydrogen bomb as early as 1950, two years before Britain had even tested its first atomic device. The Soviet atomic explosion of 1949, the Korean War and the steady worsening of relations between East and West had convinced Washington of the political need to maintain a visible military superiority over the Soviet Union by building bigger and better weapons. Although British scientists had been aware of the scientific principles surrounding the hydrogen bomb for some years, the appearance of these super bombs presented Britain with a dilemma. Was she to take part in the thermonuclear arms race or opt out of it? Could she afford to join in? Dare she, with national prestige involved, stand aside?

There were typical fears in the British bureaucracy of too much information about the hydrogen bomb leaking out to the public. In July 1953, a few months after the first American thermonuclear test at Eniwetok, the British embassy in Washington sent a secret memorandum to the Foreign Office in London, noting that President Eisenhower, who had succeeded Truman after the 1952 Presidential election, had recently expressed himself against secretiveness in atomic matters, and that in this he was supported by a growing section of American public opinion. Eisenhower at this time was busy formulating his 'Atoms for Peace' plan which he announced five months later, a much trumpeted public relations exercise in which the President proposed the setting up of an 'atomic pool' of fissile material from East and West which could then be used for peaceful atomic energy development projects around the world. The British memorandum addressed the unpleasant prospect of what the President's purported new stand on public frankness could mean:

Startling revelations by the President may well therefore throw public opinion into great disarray and touch off one of those 'great debates' which we find so dangerous and disconcerting. The fact remains, however, that this is a problem which has still to be faced and in a typical American manner it will not be solved without the participation of the whole nation in

• NO CONCEIVABLE INJURY

the discussion. We had therefore better be prepared for it.

The debate within Churchill's cabinet over whether Britain should build hydrogen bombs was in stark contrast to the complete secrecy with which Attlee hid from his ministers seven years earlier the decision to manufacture atomic weapons. By 1954, the growing public concern over nuclear weapons and their effects obliged Churchill not just to inform his ministers about what was going on but to allow them to discuss it before any decisions were taken. But the impression of cabinet government on this issue should not be taken too far. From the somewhat dry official records of the discussion recorded by the cabinet secretary, Sir Norman Brook, it is clear that the subject was sprung upon ministers without warning. Again, Churchill, by then 80 years old, was not leaving the final decision up to his cabinet; he was merely 'suggesting' that they formally approve a decision which had already been taken secretly by the defence policy committee. Nevertheless, the cabinet debate took place over three days in July 1954, with Churchill himself opening by saying that Britain could not expect to maintain its influence as a world power unless it possessed the most up-to-date weapons. The primary aim of British policy was to prevent war, and he had no doubt that the best hope lay in making it clear to potential aggressors – by which he meant the Soviet Union – that they had no hope of shielding themselves from a crushing retaliatory use of atomic power.

The ministers then thrashed out several aspects of embarking on a hydrogen bomb program – financial, moral and political. To every doubt, there was always a pragmatic answer. For instance, the cabinet minutes reveal a considerable distrust among Churchill's ministers towards American actions and motives with the newly acquired super bomb – and a feeling, similar to that which existed in some quarters after the Second World War, that Britain needed to act as a restraining force on its Atlantic partner by being able to match it in nuclear capability. Some British ministers felt the greatest risk to peace was that the United States might plunge the world into war, either through a misjudged intervention in Asia or in order to forestall an attack by Russia. The cabinet minutes continued:

Our best chance of preventing this was to maintain our influence with the United States government; and they would certainly feel more respect for our views if we continued to play an effective part in building up the strength necessary to deter aggression than if we left it entirely to them to match and counter Russia's strength in thermonuclear weapons.

How much would it cost to build the hydrogen bomb? The cabinet was never told.

The only information it received was that the capital cost should not exceed 10 million pounds, and that thermonuclear bombs would be made in lieu of atomic bombs at a relatively small additional production cost. In any case, the official argument went, 'in terms of explosive power the thermonuclear bomb would be more economical than the atomic bomb'. Another question was asked: was it morally right that Britain should manufacture weapons with this vast destructive power? Several ministers were already anticipating a public backlash, as the minutes record: 'There was no doubt that a decision to make hydrogen bombs would offend the conscience of substantial numbers of people in this country'. Again, the doubters were confronted by two countervailing arguments: insofar as any moral principle was involved, it had already been breached by the Labour government's decision back in 1947 to make the atomic bomb. In any case, the moral issue was not really one of possession but of use. And if Britain was prepared to accept the protection offered by the United States' use of thermonuclear weapons, no greater moral wrong was involved in Britain making them herself.

But, in the end, the arguments boiled down to one overriding proposition, the same one which had governed so much of the original decision to manufacture atomic weapons back in 1947. As the cabinet records put it:

No country could claim to be a leading military Power unless it possessed the most up to date weapons; and the fact must be faced that, unless we possessed thermonuclear weapons, we should lose our influence and standing in world affairs.

Although Churchill's cabinet formally approved the hydrogen bomb program in July 1954, the decision was not made public until the defence white paper the following year. At that stage, the military chiefs had scheduled a new round of atomic bomb trials for Australia towards the end of 1956. But the hydrogen bomb program now dictated that proving trials for the new weapon be pushed ahead as rapidly as possible. It was against this background that the decision was taken to hold another set of trials, codenamed Mosaic, in Australia even earlier in 1956. The Mosaic trials were always presented to the Australian public as tests of atomic weapons. In fact, as Penney admitted to the Australian royal commission 30 years later, they were tests of triggering devices for the full-scale hydrogen weapons which Britain began testing in 1957. One of the two Mosaic bombs actually contained the components of a fission-fusion device.

Mounting public concern over the enormous explosive power of thermonuclear weapons meant that the British H-bomb trials themselves could not be held in Australia. They were held instead at Christmas and Malden Islands, in the Pacific Ocean, between May 1957 and September 1958. Unlike the atomic bombs tested in Australia, no details have ever been released about the explosive yields of the Pacific Ocean tests, although all are assumed to have been in the megaton or high kiloton range.

As well as rescheduling its military program to include the manufacture of thermonuclear warheads, Britain also pushed ahead with tests to refine its atomic weapons. There were two reasons for this. Atomic devices with increased efficiency were needed as triggers for the hydrogen weapons, and an atomic weapon stockpile capable of rapid deployment would be an insurance against any possible interruption to the development of the hydrogen bomb. The most immediate threat of such an interruption came from mounting international pressure for an end to nuclear weapons tests. Should the Americans and the Russians come to such an agreement, the British would be unable to ignore it. The American Bravo hydrogen bomb test of 1954 had produced a motion in the House of Commons from a large group of Labour party MPs calling for an end to such tests, and this was soon followed by the formation of the Campaign for Nuclear

Disarmament. With the great philosopher and mathematician, Bertrand Russell, at its helm and several notable scientists like Linus Pauling, Joseph Rotblat and Frederic Joliot-Curie among its supporters, CND began waging a strong and effective campaign whose actions and messages quickly spread beyond the shores of Britain.

So a further series of three atomic weapons tests, codenamed Buffalo, was hurriedly set up for the new permanent testing ground at Maralinga for September and October 1956, followed by a final series of three bombs, codenamed Antler, for the same months of 1957. The Buffalo trials were designed as refinements to the Blue Danube weapon, and comprised tests of four weapons exploded at various heights above the ground and on the ground itself. One of them involved the first full-scale release of an atomic weapon from an aircraft; this was both an operational exercise for the RAF and a political demonstration that Britain could not just build and explode atomic weapons but was able to deliver them to an enemy target. The Antler trials, like Mosaic, were publicly presented as atomic tests but in fact involved testing triggering mechanisms for the thermonuclear weapon.

Speed was now a crucial factor in both the atomic and thermonuclear tests. The fact that Britain was prepared to pour enormous financial and technological resources into both programs, and into the setting up of two testing grounds on the other side of the world, in Australia and Christmas Island, showed the extent to which the government was determined to push ahead with Britain's independent nuclear deterrent before vital testing time ran out. Between May 1956, and September 1957, Britain tested 18 atomic and thermonuclear weapons in Australia and the Pacific. In October 1957, one month after the last of these tests, the United States, the Soviet Union and Britain agreed to a moratorium on all nuclear testing. It was to last for just three years.

The thorny old question of Britain's atomic relations with the United States had resurfaced at the time of the first of the land-based atomic trials in Australia, Totem, in 1953. By then, the Americans had conducted 41 postwar nuclear weapons tests in Nevada and the Marshall Islands. They were obviously more experienced than the British in monitoring fallout from atomic clouds and measuring such things as weapon yields. Now they were keen to monitor the British tests as well – not just to see what the British were up to, but to gain further practice in their techniques for the long-range monitoring of Soviet nuclear explosions.

This presented Whitehall with a quandary. The British understandably were irritated that the Americans had frozen them out of atomic collaboration, but now were bold enough to turn around and ask for landing rights in Australia so they could monitor the Totem trials. A secret document prepared for the British government posed the dilemma succinctly:

It appears that they intend to take samples of the cloud with aircraft based on Guam, whether we agree or not, but that it would be more convenient for them to have these landing facilities. Washington embassy urge that if we do not meet this request for facilities we shall lose US goodwill to no purpose, since the Americans intend to take the cloud samples anyway.

In going ahead with the Totem and later trials, the British had never lost sight of the ultimate aim of renewing the atomic collaboration with the Americans which had been snatched from them after the war. They were therefore very keen to impress the Americans at every stage of their weapons-testing program. Even as the Totem trials were being planned, in July 1953, a public relations officer from the British Ministry of Supply arrived in Washington with a copy of the official film of the Hurricane explosion at Monte Bello the previous October packed in his suitcase. He set up a screening at the State Department, but the event was something of a disaster. Sir Roger Makins, the British ambassador in Washington and later chairman of the UK Atomic Energy Authority, drafted a terse letter to the Foreign Office in London describing what happened and suggesting how the British should make use of the film.

Purely by chance, a member of my staff heard about it [the film] and went to the showing. The film was very badly wound on unsuitable spools and came to pieces in the middle of the performance. The B.I.S. [British Information Service] then took charge of the film, had it properly wound and arranged, with my approval, to have it shown . . . to a select group of representatives of the atomic energy commission, the joint congressional committee on atomic energy, the State Department and the United States armed services. I was present and spoke a few words by way of introduction.

Makins, who clearly had not been informed that the film was being brought to Washington, continued:

In the meantime, the B.I.S. are trying to clear up, through the information policy department of the Foreign Office, why this propaganda asset, by far the most effective (after the Coronation) we have had in our hands in recent months, has been handled in this incredibly amateurish manner.

He urged that arrangements be made for the film to be shown commercially throughout the USA. 'It is far too good an opportunity to be thrown away.'

It was against this background of trying to tread a fine line on atomic public relations with the US that the British reluctantly gave in to the American request to monitor the Totem trials in Australia the following October. The Australian authorities granted landing rights for two US air force B29 superfortress and two transport support aircraft at the Australian air force base at Richmond, near Sydney. The American aircraft agreed not to fly closer than 640 kilometres downwind of the Totem explosions, and the British asked to be given cloud samples of their own bomb picked up by the B29s. The Australians sought to cover up the true nature of the B29s' mission by issuing a press statement through the Australian air force announcing that the American aircraft were 'flying meteorological laboratories' and were there to give meteorological help. The press statement failed to mention that the planes were also equipped with sophisticated radiation detection equipment, and that the crews were well experienced in locating and sampling the radioactive content of clouds from atomic explosions.[2]

The Americans also knew a 'hot' aircraft when they saw one – and in this, their presence turned out to be a bonus because of the extraordinarily lax radiation protection procedures for the Australian air crews who took part in the Totem trials. Three sets of aircraft were involved in monitoring the radioactive cloud from Totem One – British, American and Australian. In each case, different arrangements were made, or, in the Australian case, not made, for the protection of the air crews and for decontamination of the crews and the aircraft after they landed.

The British service chiefs had decided that a Royal Air Force crew should fly a Canberra aircraft through the atomic cloud as soon as possible after the Totem One explosion to assess the aircraft's behaviour under such conditions of atomic warfare and the risk to air crews from radioactivity. The Canberra was also to be fitted with canisters to pick up samples of the radioactive cloud. London asked Australia to provide the Canberra, but Australia was unable to spare one so the British supplied their own. Australia did, however, agree to a British request to provide ten Lincoln aircraft and crew to monitor the direction and radioactive intensity of the cloud as it drifted across the continent. The Lincolns were divided for the exercise between bases at Woomera, in South Australia, and Richmond, near Sydney.

According to Penney, these cloud-sampling exercises were not necessarily to diagnose the behaviour of the bomb. They had more to do with intelligence, and, in particular, enhancing Britain's ability to monitor Russian and American tests. As Penney somewhat coyly told the Australian royal commission: 'The Americans wanted cloud samples for the same purposes as we did'.

Operation Hotbox, as the Canberra flight was aptly called, went off flawlessly. Six minutes after Totem One exploded, the RAF crew of three, flying at 3000 metres, took the aircraft through the cloud at a tangent then turned around and made another run straight through the centre. Inside the cloud, their ship shook from the turbulence and they had to turn the lights on in the cockpit because it was so dark. Before takeoff, the Canberra had been completely sealed with tape in a bid to stop radioactive dust getting inside, and the crew were told to wear oxygen masks during the entire flight. When they landed at Woomera, they taxied to a special position where filters, which had been attached to the Canberra to catch samples of the cloud, were released into a pile of sand. Then they took the aircraft to the end of the runway where it remained for four hours until tests showed enough radioactivity had decayed to make it safe to be towed away. Finally, an Australian air force crew, specially decked out in protective overalls and masks, decontaminated the Canberra by thoroughly washing it down at least four times, after being briefed on this by the British radiation hazards group at Emu Field. Meanwhile, The Canberra's crew underwent decontamination showers of their own after their clothing and gear had been carefully taken away and monitored for radiation.

No such precautions were set up for the Australian Lincolns and their crews. They had the job of following the cloud across Australia to see where it actually went. The two American B29s also did this independently of the Australians, although they kept in close liaison with the air force base at Richmond. Five of the Lincolns took off from Woomera at intervals several hours after the early morning Totem blast and headed for northeastern Australia where the cloud appeared to be going. The Australians later reported seeing a big cloud, still intact, which they thought was swinging towards Darwin. The Americans, by contrast, maintained that the cloud had broken up into small patches which appeared to be moving towards Brisbane. The American air crews also signalled that the radioactivity was the most sensitive they had ever encountered – so much that their radiation detection equipment had reached its full-scale reading; it stayed there for several hours until some of the contamination on the B29s had decayed. In a bid to reconcile the conflicting reports, the controller at Richmond air force base sent up another Lincoln with orders to reconnoitre both alleged paths to see if two separate clouds had developed. The Lincoln's crew of seven flew around central Queensland for several hours and announced they had sighted the cloud west of the outback town of Charleville. This turned out to be dubious information because the Lincoln's navigation system had broken down and the aircraft, in fact, was lost.

So the Lincoln was ordered back to base at Richmond. But because the crew had been in the air for almost 12 hours they looked like running out of fuel before they got there, so they landed at Williamtown, a base 120 kilometres northeast of Richmond. Even then it was a split-second landing: one engine cut out as they touched the tarmac and the other died as they taxied in, leaving the plane stranded in the middle of the runway. The flight tower radioed to the crew to stay in the aircraft, which they did for half an hour. No ground crew came near the aircraft. Eventually they were allowed out, but had to wait on the tarmac near the aircraft for two hours until another aircraft arrived to take them back to their Richmond base. 'Bud' Puxty, one of the Lincoln's crew members, later recalled: 'This was highly unusual, particularly after such a long flight, and has never happened to me. Guards were placed around the aircraft at about 100 yards distance.'

Next morning, Puxty and the rest of the crew flew back from Richmond to Williamtown to pick up the Lincoln. They took with them one of the American airmen from the B29s, who had heard about the strange flight and offered to check the Lincoln for radioactive contamination. The American walked around the aircraft with his geiger counter, checking the fuselage, the wheels and then the interior from the rear turret right up to the nose, muttering grimly as he went: 'Oh, shit . . . oh, shit'. As they left the plane by the front ladder, the Australians asked the American if he wanted to catch a lift with them back to Richmond. 'Christ no!' he exclaimed. 'That bloody machine is hot. I'm not going anywhere near it.' So the American left the Australians to fly the contaminated Lincoln and caught the train instead.

The American air crews, like the British 'Hotbox' crew in the Canberra, had made their own special radiation protection arrangements. The four American crew members in each B29 carried film badges and dosimeters to check their exposure levels, they used oxygen from the time they made contact with the bomb cloud until they landed at Richmond and they were forbidden to eat or smoke from the time they made contact with the cloud until after they had washed and changed at Richmond. Their aircraft were well sealed during flight, and were isolated and checked after their return. The Australian crews in the Lincolns, less experienced than either the Americans or British in this regard, received no protection at all. Bruce Stein, one of 'Bud' Puxty's fellow crew members in the Lincoln which had so horrified the American, remembered just how casual the arrangements for the Australians had been:

When flying the Lincoln through the mushroom cloud, and at all times, we wore only normal air force flying gear. We had no respirators or protective clothing and, as the flight level was below that at which oxygen masks were required, we did not use those either. During the flight, even when we were in the mushroom cloud, we ate in the normal way and it is quite likely that I could have ingested radioactive particles. The plane was again used and I flew in it on three subsequent occasions. [3]

The British, in fact, had told the Australian air force chiefs in charge of the Lincolns before the Totem One operation that there was little chance of contamination to either the Australian aircraft or their crews. So no decontamination procedures were set up at either Woomera or Richmond. It was left to the Americans, through incidents such as those at Williamtown, to alert the Australians to the fact that contamination posed a bigger danger than they had been led to believe. A secret report prepared by the Australian air force soon after the Totem operation disclosed just how significant this advice was: 'It was only through seeking assistance of the US air force specialists and equipment that it was at all possible to ascertain that Lincoln aircraft and personnel had obtained any degree of contamination'.

Even though the British had told the Australians there would be nothing to worry about, the captain of the first Lincoln which returned to Woomera after tracking the Totem One cloud radioed ahead that he was worried about the excessive readings on his aircraft's radiation detection equipment. So Herbert Gale, a British scientist in charge of the technical aspects of the air sampling operations, met the aircraft. He, too, became worried by the contamination level, and ordered the cloud filter samples the Lincoln had collected to be left for another nine hours before anyone handled them. As the rest of the Lincolns returned, impromptu decontamination methods were set up. Two of the five Lincolns dispatched from Woomera had spent ten minutes in the Totem One cloud, and the other aircraft 30, 45 and 55 minutes respectively. At the distances the Lincolns tracked it, hundreds of kilometres from ground zero, the cloud was far more dispersed than it had been for the Canberra's Operation Hotbox. Another British expert was called in, Group Captain Denis Wilson, a radiologist who had been in the Canberra crew for Operation

Hotbox. Wilson checked the first Lincoln with his equipment, and later concluded: 'It appeared that the Lincoln constituted something of a dust trap and was unsuitable for use in cloud tracking. Not unexpectedly, the engines and radiators were the most contaminated area.' [4] Wilson recommended that all five Woomera Lincolns be isolated for 12 hours, and he instructed their crews to wash immediately. Afterwards, the men were checked for contamination and found to be clear.

Two days later, David Stevenson, another British scientist, arrived at Woomera from the test site at Emu Field. Stevenson was one of the UK Atomic Energy Authority's experts on decontamination, and was deputy leader in the radiation hazards group team responsible for decontamination at the Totem trials. He had gone to Woomera to help check the decontamination of the Canberra from Operation Hotbox; but he found a group of Australian air force officers simmering with anger over the way nothing had been planned to decontaminate the Lincolns and their crews. 'I was metaphorically roasted', Stevenson later recalled. 'They were clearly somewhat upset.' Astonishingly, Stevenson – one of the key British decontamination people – knew nothing about the role which the Lincolns had played: 'This was the first intimation I had that Lincoln bombers were involved in the exercise at all'. [5]

Although Stevenson had gone to Woomera to check the laundry measures for the clothing worn by the air and ground crew responsible for the RAF Canberra, he decided to examine the Lincolns in view of the unexpected fracas. He found the leading edges of the wings and tailplanes and the engines of most of the Lincolns were contaminated. The levels were below those permitted by the radiation hazards group for vehicles, but there was still a risk from ingestion of radioactive particles; all ground crew were told to wash before smoking or eating after they had worked on the aircraft.

In the meantime, ground control had still not determined the precise location of the Totem One cloud. So the remaining five Lincolns from Richmond were sent to monitor the skies around north Queensland, where they eventually determined that the centre of the cloud passed across the coast at Townsville before moving out to sea. All ten Lincolns, from Woomera and Richmond, later returned to their home base at Amberley, in Queensland, for more decontamination.

The Totem affair had been a rude shock to Australian air force officers. Some of the Lincolns used in the Totem One cloud tracking had also flown at Operation Hurricane in the Monte Bellos a year before, and it now seemed likely that they had never been decontaminated in the meantime. So the Australians insisted that two members of the British radiation hazards team from Emu Field go to Amberley to advise on proper decontamination of aircraft, equipment and men. Most of the Lincolns were flown back from the Totem operation still contaminated: an inspection on arrival at Amberley revealed that nine of them were either heavily contaminated or slightly contaminated with 'hot spots'; the worst one was the plane that made the unscheduled visit at Williamtown and so horrified the American airman.

In March 1954, five months after the Totem operation, the Lincolns were stripped down, their engines removed and airframes opened up in a major inspection. David Thomas, a scientific adviser to the Australian air force, visited Amberley with a group of senior officers for the inspection. They found the interiors of 24 and possibly 32 engines were still contaminated. Thomas recommended that a full-scale decontamination centre with steam-cleaning facilities be built at Amberley. This was eventually done, but it was not entirely foolproof. The new centre did not start operating for another year, too late for the Totem Lincolns. The procedure involved towing contaminated aircraft into a bay and blasting them with high pressure steam and hot water hoses until their radioactivity level was down to a nil reading. The crews doing this were supplied with ordinary overalls, cotton gloves, rubber boots and berets, but as they climbed over and under the aircraft with their high pressure hoses they invariably ended up soaked with contaminated waste water dripping over their faces and down their necks.

It may have been the Lincolns which needed proper cleaning but, as Thomas later explained, it was the fate of the men who flew them which worried him:

• NO CONCEIVABLE INJURY

When the Lincolns came up for major inspection and the heads were taken off engines and turbo superchargers were dismantled, we found a lot of radioactive dust inside those engines, those Rolls Royce engines. And therefore you would say to yourself, 'Well, if all this stuff has got inside the engines, inside the superchargers and inside the cylinder heads, what about the hapless crews? What would they get on board when they are flying?'

The fiasco over the Australian Lincoln aircraft at the Totem trials was a classic example of the British scientists failing to warn the Australians of possible dangers from the bombs and of the Australians failing to ask the right questions – or, in this case, enough questions. It should have occurred to both sides that aircraft and their crew flying through a radioactive bomb cloud, even a diluted one hundreds of kilometres from ground zero, would end up contaminated and would need protection. But the attitude, before and after the event, was remarkably casual. David Colquhoun, then the Australian air force group captain who was commander of the Lincoln task force, recorded the events a few weeks later with a mixture of concern and reassurance. In a secret report to the Australian air force home command soon after the Totem operation, Colquhoun wrote:

The contamination of the aircraft was, of course, completely unforeseen and caused considerable inconvenience. Had the information on the possibility of contamination been available, suitable provisions could have been made to meet the case.

Colquhoun also wrote a letter from Woomera to the senior air staff officer at home command:

All the scientists are somewhat nonplussed with the amount of radioactivity registered in Totem One and are most apologetic that the matter was not fully covered by briefings, and the issuing of equipment before Totem One. They are cooperating fully now . . . I would like to stress that there is no risk or undue concern over this radiation business. I am assured that the risk to aircrew is negligible but there is a possibility that the ground crew could, by swallowing radioactive particles, suffer some discomfort in later years. The latter is the reason for our precautionary measures.

Because the Australian crews flying the Lincolns at Totem One were given no personal radiation monitoring devices – unlike the British and American air crews – their levels of contamination were difficult to assess and, indeed, will never be fully known. A report by the UK atomic weapons research establishment a year later attempted to estimate the contamination of the crews based on readings of the radiation monitoring equipment inside their aircraft and the activity of the bomb cloud samples trapped by the filters installed outside the planes. According to these estimates, the crew of one Lincoln received a slightly higher gamma ray dose than that set down by the safety orders as the lowest permissible dose, while the rest of the crews received gamma ray doses within the limits. But these estimates took no account of possibly inhaled or ingested radioactivity: the Lincoln crews – again unlike their British and American counterparts – wore no masks at Totem One, and freely ate their rations during their long flights. As for the Australian air force ground crews working on decontamination of the Lincolns at Amberley, no medical records of their dose levels have ever been found.

Soon after the magnitude of the contaminated Lincolns at Totem One was realised, Colquhoun flew from Woomera to the operation headquarters at Emu Field and called for extra members of the British radiation hazards team to help with their cleaning. The Totem Two bomb was exploded at Emu 12 days after Totem One. It yielded about 8 kilotons, slightly less than the earlier bomb. Because the wind conditions were more turbulent and unstable than for Totem One, the Totem Two cloud spread more widely and the fallout was less heavily concentrated.

The RAF Canberra did not fly through the second Totem cloud because the British scientists decided they had had enough cloud samples from Totem One, and, in any case, the three RAF crew members had received more than their permissible radiation doses during Operation Hotbox. Penney told the Australian royal commission that although Hotbox was an operational exercise ordered by the military chiefs, he vetoed it being repeated at Totem Two because of the radiation hazards. 'The men were themselves prepared to do it again. I said, "No, enough is enough". ' Only four Australian Lincolns were sent to track the Totem Two cloud; this time, their crews were instructed to wear oxygen masks inside the cloud and were given film badges and dosimeters to measure their personal radiation exposures.

The lack of communication between the British scientists and the Australian air force involved in the same operation seems remarkable. It was Whitehall who asked the Australian government to loan the Lincolns, and once Canberra agreed the whole business disappeared into a chasm of secrecy. James Austin, a senior scientist from Aldermaston who was head of the decontamination team for the Totem trials, told the Australian royal commission in London in February 1985:

We did not know about the participation in particular of the Australian air force before we left England.

Why? he was asked: was there a communication or a 'need to know' problem? Austin replied:

I would have thought it was very much a result of the secrecy attached to certain parts of the operation. But I have never understood why the Australian air force did not seek advice in matters of decontamination before their operation . . . I am sure if it was known that we were planning a decontamination team with several people specialising in that field well ahead – many, many months ahead – of the operation, I cannot understand why the information did not get to the Australians.

Another two and a half years went by after the Totem trials in October 1953, before Britain tested its next nuclear weapons in Australia. The delay was very much a strategic and practical one: the military planners needed time not only to develop different types of atomic weapons, but also to find a suitable new place to test them. In the earlier years of the atomic program, no one had given much thought to what sort of atomic weapons Britain should be planning for the future, or how they should be deployed. In 1951, the Defence Research Policy Committee, a body set up to advise the minister of defence and the chiefs of staff in Britain, had begun to confront this question. Apart from blasting and burning cities, it was clear these weapons could be deployed in other ways if the designs were modified: for example, tactical weapons to be used against troops and artillery had to be considered as well as strategic weapons.[6] Penney's knowledge about the effects of atomic weapons, and the discussions of how strategy, tactics and hardware needed to accommodate them, led to the decision to pursue physically smaller atomic weapons with lower explosive yields. But the lead time to develop these new types was up to three years. The Buffalo series of tests in 1956 were to prove that Britain had this capability. At the same time, as we saw, the Soviet and American hydrogen bomb tests sparked off a parallel bid in British planning for high yield thermonuclear weapons, with a similar development timespan.

A top secret report by the Defence Research Policy Committee in May 1953, spelt out the large list of questions which the military and civil service departments in Britain wanted answered from future atomic trials. This document caused a press sensation in Britain and Australia when it was declassified in 1984 over what some newspapers interpreted as its apparently blunt demands for experiments involving human guinea pigs. The Royal Navy, it said, wanted information about the effects of different types of atomic explosions on ships. The Royal Air Force wanted to know about the effects of atomic bombs used against airfields. 'The army must discover the detailed effects of various types of explosion on equipment, stores and men with and without various types of protection.'

Did this involve stationing groups of men in the forward area at the tests, without protective clothing? Certainly, this happened at some of the American atomic trials in Nevada in the early fifties, where thousands of soldiers were positioned a few thousand metres from the blasts and then ordered to move even closer in after the detonation. One aim of such experiments was to study the psychological impact of atomic warfare on troops in the field. At two of the British tests, in the Buffalo series, a special 'indoctrinee' force of officers was chosen to witness the blasts for similar reaction studies, but there were no close-in manoeuvres; and there appears to be no evidence of unprotected troops being deliberately stationed close to any British atomic blasts.

Questioned at the royal commission in London in 1985, Penney denied that unprotected troops were used in experiments during the tests: 'Looking at this [document] now, I would say that drafting was pretty dreadful because it can lead to misunderstandings. To me, that was not what was meant.' The experiments certainly happened, but Penney insisted they were all done with dummies, propped up in jeeps or laid out on the ground. With some dressed in ordinary British and Australian army uniforms and others in protective clothing, the models joined a vast collection of other 'target response' items at Emu Field and Maralinga spaced out around the ground zeros – Centurion tanks, jet aircraft, aircraft frames, concrete shelters, specially built girder bridges and railway tracks, mines, food, glass, drugs, jerry cans filled with water, sacks filled with earth, and even live animals. All were there, as the newsreel commentaries of the fifties echoed the official line, 'in the interests of science' – to test the effects of heat, blast and radiation from the bomb.

Apart from the time needed to develop the new weapons, Britain now also needed a new testing ground. Emu Field had been good enough for the Totem trials, but it would not be suitable as a permanent testing ground for the trials which Penney and his team now envisaged would last for the next ten years. Emu Field had been chosen partly with secrecy in mind: it was about as remote as you could get and everything had to be brought in by cargo aircraft, which made it enormously expensive to maintain.

Ministry of Defence officials in London had already drawn up an extensive list of possible sites all over the world, but all of them had been rejected for one reason or another. The secret list contained eight places in the Indian Ocean alone, including the Seychelles – 'too populated and-or too hilly'; Rodriguez – 'too populated; mountainous'; Diego Garcia – 'land area not suitable'; and Addu Atoll – 'belongs to Ceylon. Over populated'; and three sites in Africa, including British Somaliland – 'Nomadic population. Doubtful whether climatic conditions are suitable for dispersing cloud.' (As events turned out, much the same could have been said for Maralinga and Emu Field in Australia.)

The Ministry of Defence had also considered, and rejected, four places in the Atlantic, one of which, the Falkland Islands, was 'too far away. Too difficult of access', and another, the Bahamas, was turned down because 'wind direction unsuitable. American guided weapon range a complication.' The Pacific islands were rejected because they were even further in time from the UK than Australia; they were 'relatively densely populated' and air access was difficult. This view changed when Britain went to Christmas and Malden Islands in the Pacific to conduct its hydrogen bomb tests in 1957. But, for the moment, it seemed to be stuck with Australia.

The task of initiating the search for a new site fell to Air Marshal Sir Thomas Elmhirst, who was chairman of the UK Totem executive, the Whitehall body charged with planning the Totem tests. Elmhirst first approached the Australian authorities in July 1953, only four months before he was due to leave to take up his new job as governor of the Channel island of Guernsey. Thus began a flow of correspondence which was remarkable for the gulf of knowledge between the two countries which it revealed.

Already, British officials had held behind-the-scenes talks in London with their Australian counterparts, who had given them the nod to pursue the possible opening up of a permanent test site in Australia. 'I am surveying the world', Elmhirst wrote to Major General Jack Stevens, of the Australian Department of Supply. 'But more particularly, at the moment, Australia.' Elmhirst explained that Penney wanted the permanent site for air bursts over land and ground bursts as well; if possible, Penney wanted a 160 kilometre radius free of human habitation. From his 'preliminary study' of Australia – by which, no doubt, he meant a map – Elmhirst had concluded there were only two possible sites: somewhere on the Woomera rocket range in South Australia, or Groote Eylandt, off the coast of the Northern Territory in the Gulf of Carpentaria.

Stevens' reply must have left Elmhirst particularly dispirited:

The specifications set out in your paragraph 4 are very drastic and few, if any, places in the world could meet all of them'. 'I think you can wash out the latter [Groote Eylandt] as it is most unsuitable – barren rock and densely wooded flats, 35 miles by 15 miles and only 22 miles from Arnhem Land in which there are many natives, a Church of England Mission and an Island population of seven Europeans and 400 to 600 natives. A timber company is seeking and may have obtained a timber concession. There are no port facilities. It has a wet season from November to February.

As for the Woomera rocket range, Stevens pointed out that its water supply was uncertain and limited, and a permanent atomic bomb site on the axis of the range could, in time, be 'an embarrassment'.

Undaunted, Elmhirst in London presented a report to the chiefs of staff, and wrote again to Stevens in Sydney the following August:

In discussing my report with my master, Lord Cherwell, he was very much in favour of a big island if one could be found and he spotted on the map a Cape Barren Island off the north shore of Tasmania. I suggested to him that the island was probably a big sheep station? His answer was that to pay for the removal and setting up again of a few people and animals would be far cheaper than building say a hundred miles of railway!

This new suggestion impressed Stevens as little as Elmhirst's earlier letter; in a slight tone of despair, Stevens wrote to Frank O'Connor, the head of the Australian Department of Supply, that the British suggestion of Cape Barren Island scarcely seemed wise in view of the island's winds and settlement. 'All told, we don't seem to have a suitable island', Stevens told O'Connor. 'I do not propose to make any further inquiries unless I am asked to. It's all yours!'

While the bureaucrats were exchanging letters, Penney was holding secret talks with Australian officials about his needs for an alternative site to Emu Field. The main requirement was a place with Emu Field's isolation, but closer to the transcontinental railway so that supplies and equipment could be brought in by train rather than by air. So while Penney was in Australia for the Totem trials in October 1953, a secret expedition led by Len Beadell, the discoverer of Emu Field, set out from there and headed south.

Beadell, again, has given a firsthand account of this expedition in his book, *Blast the Bush*, in which he describes how the party came across some remarkable Aboriginal relics from the 'dreamtime'. These were undoubtedly the first white men to stumble upon the sites, even as late as 1953, and their discovery was a sombre sign of just how significant these lands must have been to the Aborigines. The first, a few kilometres south of Emu Field, consisted of a large collection of stone posts standing upright in the ground and placed apart at regular intervals. There were also about six smaller clusters of stones, each one consisting of an upright slab with several smaller stones leaning inwards against it. Beadell and his companions gave this ancient Aboriginal ceremonial ground the name of Aboriginal Stonehenge. The other discovery came near Tietkens Well, the area eventually chosen for the new weapons testing ground. It was a more pathetic sight: two mounds of earth, clearly the graves of an Aboriginal adult and child. A hunting spear and woomera, the spear launcher, had been carefully laid out on top of the large mound, while a tiny spear which the child must have used as a toy rested on the smaller grave.

The site Beadell and his party settled for, about 200 kilometres south of Emu Field, became the Maralinga testing ground, and it appeared to have everything Penney wanted. It was only 35 kilometres north of the railway line, near Ooldea, which meant it could easily be serviced from the siding at Watson. It had a beautiful setting of dense mulga and salt bush scrubland and trees in an undulating plain, which would be a perfect site for the large village that had to be built for the servicemen; and about 30 kilometres further north of that was a flat, featureless and open desert where the bombs themselves could be ignited. On 17 October, two days after he had directed the firing of the Totem One bomb at Emu Field, Penney secretly flew in a Bristol freighter to the new site, which was then referred to simply as A. He landed on a makeshift runway which Beadell and his companions had hastily cleared from the bush by dragging pieces of railway lines behind their Land Rovers. Alan Butement, chief scientist to the Australian government, was also in the party, and as they stood under the hot sun surveying the scene, Penney pronounced himself satisfied. He told Butement:

The area A is, in my opnion, a first class site. It would give us all that we wanted for many years to come and I see no difficulty in testing 20 or more weapons here. The site, I should say, should be considered to extend at least as far south as Tietkens Well.

Penney then asked about Aborigines in the area, and Butement told him:

I am given to understand that this area is no longer used for Aborigines. There was a track from Ooldea up to the north through the area roughly where Emu now is. But here again I understand that this is now not used, except by one or two elderly blacks and then on rare occasions, and that there is no need whatever for Aborigines to use any part of this country around the proposed area.

'That sounds very satisfactory', Penney replied.

After a short stay in the bush camp, which included a haircut administered by the versatile Beadell, Penney flew back to direct the firing of Totem Two at Emu Field. He concluded: 'I do not think there will be any quarrels with our decision to move to A provided that the cost of A doesn't run into too high a figure'. [7]

The cost of A, or Maralinga as it was soon called, turned out to appear far cheaper than Emu Field. After the Totem trials, Penney saw Menzies and Beale to discuss planning for future tests, and, following his return to Britain, the Australian government commissioned a report to compare the cost of setting up Maralinga with keeping Emu. It concluded that the cost for Maralinga would be about 1.9 million pounds against about 3.6 million pounds for Emu Field. The total cost of the Totem trials at Emu – excluding the equipment and the building of the bombs – had been 828 000 pounds. Australia's share of this was 134 000 pounds, the bulk of it spent on pay to Australian servicemen, and Britain's contribution 694 000 pounds. [8] Beale informed the Australian cabinet almost a year after the Totem trials that Britain had initially 'intimated' that she was prepared to pay for the lot; but Australia offered to pay the cost of its own servicemen who had prepared the Emu site, and Britain agreed to this. (In fact, the British *aide-mémoire* mentioned earlier, requesting Australian permission to hold the Totem trials at Emu Field, had been quite direct in its offer to pay Australia's share. It said: 'The United Kingdom government would be very happy to make suitable arrangements to reimburse [the Australian] Government for the special costs which it incurs'.)

Britain was now keen to get Australia's agreement for Maralinga as soon as possible, as it wanted to hold the next round of trials during the first half of 1956. But several conflicting strands in the story made their unwelcome appearance again. Clearly conscious of the mounting public concern about nuclear weapons tests, British officials were anxious that the new venture should have all the appearances of a joint Anglo-Australian undertaking rather than simply another British project on Australian soil. The Australian public, they discerned, would be unwilling for too much longer to accept the latter. To this end, they wanted Australia to contribute to the cost of the project. But the British were still completely unprepared to share any scientific and technological secrets from the bomb trials with Australia for fear of upsetting the United States.

They no doubt had a convenient excuse here in the form of assurances from Menzies himself. Lord Cherwell had talked with Menzies during a visit to Australia in late 1953 to discuss, among other things, future British access to Australian uranium. This was yet another ironic element in the delicate Anglo-Australian atomic relationship at this time, and it is worth digressing slightly to explain it.

After the Second World War, the British and the Americans had sought to locate and secure the world's known accessible uranium supplies in a bid to deny them to other countries, particularly the Soviet Union. The machinery they created to do this was the Combined Development Agency (CDA), essentially a uranium-procuring body whose costs were shared by both countries. The arrangement had actually begun during the war, when it was agreed that all uranium should go to the United States. In the postwar years, the machinery came under pressure because both countries now had atomic projects of their own which were hungry for uranium. The picture was further complicated by the opening up of new uranium sources, including South Africa and Australia, new types of ore, new mining techniques and new pricing policies. Very soon, the British and the Americans found themselves de facto competitors for this uranium, despite the continued existence of the CDA with its overtones of purchasing collaboration.

In March 1952, the Americans sent a team acting for the CDA to Australia to hold talks about buying uranium and the possible building of an ore-processing plant under CDA auspices. The negotiations were to centre particularly on South Australia and its premier, Thomas (later Sir Thomas) Playford, a skilful and enduring politician who was keen to give his state's mainly rural-based economy a more solid industrial and manufacturing base. Playford was a strong states rights man in this and almost every other sense, and he did not want the federal, or Commonwealth, government in Canberra dictating the terms under which South Australia might do a deal with the rest of the world over its uranium deposits.

Even though British officials were attached to the American visit to South Australia, the British were clearly worried that South Australia may be about to enter into an arrangement with the United States that would leave Britain disadvantaged. One of the British visitors, Cedric Cliffe, wrote a long, informal account of the proceedings to a Foreign Office mandarin in London, asking that, before the official reports of the tour arrived via the British high commissioner's office in Australia, his personal impressions be passed on to Sir Roger Makins, a senior Foreign Office official who specialised in atomic energy policy and who was about to become British ambassador in Washington. Cedric Cliffe's frank letter of March 1952, gives some flavour of the currents operating at various levels.

You will remember that some concern was caused at home by the South Australians starting off to try and deal with the Americans on their own, but that later on we were reassured by the news that the Commonwealth government had got on to this and were prepared to exercise any necessary control. To understand the whole business, you must know a little about Tom Playford, the premier of South Australia, who is the moving spirit of the whole thing, at any rate as far as South Australia is concerned.

He is quite an extraordinary character with something in him of the late

J.H. Thomas, something of Arnold Bennett's 'The Card' and a good deal of Bottom the Weaver. He has enormous energy, a very shrewd political sense and (by our standards) no dignity at all. He loves horseplay and wants to do everything himself, down to driving the jeep or handling the geiger counter. He is nominally a 'Liberal' (roughly equivalent to our Conservative), but is much more what we should think of as a Labour type. Anyhow, he has got the Labour people in South Australia so well in hand that he has managed to remain in office for fourteen years on end! Despite his buffooneries, he has done a very great deal for South Australia, in the promotion of local industries &c; he is first and last a South Australian, and has very little time for the Commonwealth or for Menzies.

Playford himself had initiated the American visit by travelling to the US to drum up interest in Washington in his state's uranium. The main deposit was at Radium Hill, about 300 kilometres northeast of Adelaide. But there was a second promising field, which interested the Americans equally, at Rum Jungle near Darwin, in the Northern Territory, which came under federal government control. Cedric Cliffe wrote:

Of course there is no real question of any 'rivalry' between Radium Hill and Rum Jungle, except insofar as it may prove beyond Australia's unaided power to develop both fields. Nevertheless Playford, that unscrupulous fellow, was trying to crab Rum Jungle with Jesse Johnson [leader of the American team] as a corollary to boosting his own goods.

He concluded his letter to London on a note of concern for the British position:

The Australian Press has naturally been very interested in the whole visit. Unfortunately it has throughout spoken of the mission as if it was purely American; but Davidson [a British geological consultant] tells me that Jesse Johnson himself has always been most scrupulous in stressing the fact that the potential buyers are an Anglo-American agency. It is a good thing (though purely a matter of luck) that Davidson was about the place to show the UK flag a bit.

In June 1952, three months after the Americans' visit, the US

Atomic Energy Commission invited Menzies, then making his annual visit to Britain, to stop over in Washington so he could discuss the possibility of developing the Rum Jungle deposit quickly and making the uranium available to the CDA. The meeting was also attended by Sir Percy Spender, the Australian ambassador in Washington, and Sir Christopher Steel, of the British embassy. Gordon Dean, the chairman of the US Atomic Energy Commission, told them the US needed access to more uranium to meet its planned expansion of fissile material production:

The entire expansion program is predicated on the notion that we need so many bombs as to be reasonably sure that, in the event of an all out conflagration, the Western world could smash the Russians. In other words, uranium ore from whatever origin – the Congo, Canada, South Africa or Australia – is for the common defence program.

Menzies agreed that the best immediate use should be made of uranium for weapons production, but he demurred with the American proposal of handing over the Rum Jungle deposits completely for two reasons. He was worried about the price, and particularly about not being seen to sell the Rum Jungle uranium more cheaply than uranium from Radium Hill in South Australia; and, because Australia still harboured ill-defined notions of developing atomic energy for its own industrial needs, he wanted Australia to retain some reserves of its own instead of being left by the Americans with nothing but a worked-out mine. The Americans made it quite clear to Menzies that they saw no prospect of using atomic energy for their own domestic power system for at least another ten years. Instead, their position was, as Sir Christopher Steel, the British representative at the meeting, later reported to London, that 'every scrap of metal [uranium] they received was either put into bombs or used in research programmed for use in bombs'.

The British, who were planning a domestic atomic power program side-by-side with a weapons program, were worried that they might be about to miss the bus in Australia, particularly as Rum Jungle then looked like one of the most promising new uranium finds in the world. They rightly feared that the Americans were engaged in building up an enormous uranium stockpile, using as an excuse the argument that uranium needed to be utilised solely for defence purposes. Although uranium procurement, through the CDA, was at this time the only area of atomic co-operation between Britain and the US, neither country clearly trusted the other even in this regard, and each was prepared to explore its own ways of dealing with supplier countries such as Australia to meet its own needs.

Steel, who had attended as Britain's representative at the Washington meeting between Menzies and the Americans, later reported to London that – on the principle of showing as much sympathy to the Australians as possible – he had supported Menzies' arguments that Australia wanted to keep some uranium as a hedge for its own industrial development. 'I hope that the modicum of support which I gave the Australians was not mistaken', Steel wrote to the Foreign Office. 'I considered that while they might be asking for something the Americans did not want to give them, it was better to help them a little and keep our foot in the door.'

The Menzies government appointed a special cabinet committee to examine the American proposals over the next few months, and by early the following year, 1953, Australia had signed contracts with the CDA for the sale of uranium from both Radium Hill and Rum Jungle, uranium which, under CDA, and therefore American, rules was reserved for military use. The Menzies government had agreed to sell the whole of the Rum Jungle deposits to the CDA over a period of ten years, and it had done so without striking a hard bargain over price. The Americans had refused to tell Australia what price the CDA was paying to other supplier countries such as Belgium, South Africa and Canada; they had offered simply the same price as that paid for the deposits at Radium Hill. Menzies' cabinet agreed, according to the record of its discussion, that, in spite of the scantiness of the information available to it, the modest price for a commodity in such keen demand represented a real contribution by Australia to the common defence effort, and it believed Australia should, therefore, receive some credit for this in other negotiations with the US and the UK.

By early 1953, more promising uranium discoveries were beginning to appear in Australia, just as the Cold War between East and West was intensifying. Fearing that the Americans would try to snap these up for their military stockpile as well, Britain made a deliberate bid to secure any further Australian uranium on an exclusive basis. In June that year, Menzies met Lord Cherwell, the paymaster general and Churchill's adviser on atomic matters, at Christ Church, Oxford, where Cherwell lived. Cherwell wanted to sew the question up quickly by getting an agreement in principle between the British and Australian governments: Australian uranium in return for British know-how on the industrial uses of atomic energy. He knew he was handicapped somewhat in being able to fulfil this because of the *modus vivendi* arrangement with the Americans which restricted the amount of atomic information Britain could pass on to third countries, even members of the Commonwealth like Australia. Cherwell promised Menzies to approach the Americans about having this arrangement altered, but in the meantime it was important to get a working agreement going with Australia over uranium supplies. Menzies demurred once again, saying that before any government-to-government agreement was arranged the whole question of uranium supplies should be investigated by experts.

Five days later Cherwell and Menzies met again, this time with Thomas Playford, the premier of South Australia, to discuss further the prospect of Anglo-Australian collaboration on the industrial uses of atomic energy. They agreed that nothing should be said to the Americans about their talks, and Menzies pressed Cherwell to visit Australia so he could see what was happening on the spot.

In September 1953, Lord Cherwell flew to Australia in a bid to offer the Australians a knowledge-for-uranium deal, and in characteristic fashion he tried to shroud his visit in complete secrecy. On both counts, the visit failed. London had cabled ahead to the British high commissioner in Canberra that Cherwell hoped contacts with the Australian press could be kept to an absolute minimum and would much prefer, if possible, to escape their attentions altogether, particularly those of photographers. Unless the high commission or the Australian authorities regarded it as essential for him to attend press conferences, he hoped even this might be avoided. The British, moreover, were to take a strict line on what was said publicly about the purpose of Cherwell's visit. They were to emphasise that he was there to arrange for technical assistance to Australia in the development of its atomic energy program, but there was to be no mention of uranium sales.

Cherwell began his visit with a secret flight to Emu Field where that curiously parallel strand of Anglo-Australian atomic relations, the Totem bomb tests, were about to be held. Then he met Menzies and an inner group of ministers over three days in early October. The agreement he had hoped to extract from them would have given Britain an option for up to 30 years over two thirds of the Australian uranium not committed to the CDA, which Britain would use for its expanding atomic energy industrial program. The remaining third was for Australia to keep for any domestic atomic program of its own. In return, Britain would seek from the Americans a reinterpretation of the *modus vivendi* arrangement, which would permit Britain to give the Australian government classified technical information without having to obtain US consent.

There was, of course, no guarantee and little likelihood that the Americans would ever agree to such a relaxation, particularly in view of the continuing American distrust of Australian security. In any case, Menzies and his ministers rejected Cherwell's proposition. They were unwilling to commit themselves to offering Britain a fixed percentage of uranium ore, arguing that they had no idea how much would be discovered or what Australia's own requirements were likely to be. All they proposed was to throw open the mining of uranium to private companies and to treat the UK as a preferred customer to whom they would give first offer of any surplus uranium at current prices.

The collapse of the talks understandably displeased Cherwell, who proposed to his own government that Britain should henceforward remain noncommittal on the question of giving Australia atomic technical information. If Britain was to secure its industrial requirements of uranium in some way other than through Australia, it would be unwise to risk American goodwill by raising the question of reinterpreting the *modus vivendi*. Britain would have to inform Menzies in due course that, for the moment, Australian requests for technical assistance would have to be dealt with on an ad hoc basis.

Apart from the degree of retribution implicit in Cherwell's reaction, it was also, perhaps, an implicit acknowledgement that, even if Australia had agreed to the British scheme, the probability of Britain securing Amerian approval for exchanging sensitive information with Australia was always very slim. After Cherwell's departure for home, the *Daily Mirror* newspaper, of Sydney, commented:

Government publicity merchants have been working overtime trying to create the impression that all was sweetness and light during the recent discussions on Australian uranium with Lord Cherwell. They have an uphill fight. This newspaper and most Australian people are satisfied that his Lordship left this country in a huff after having failed to pull what the Americans would call a 'very fast deal'.

It is clear Lord Cherwell came to Australia with the idea of making a 30 year contract for Australia to supply uranium to Britain on the cheap. His proposition was so one sided that not even the Menzies-Fadden government would fall for it. The result was his Lordship flew back to England in a very angry mood.

The haggles over uranium supplies were a significant episode in Anglo-Australian atomic relations of the fifties which, by sheer good luck for the British, managed to remain divorced from the bomb-testing program. Australia never sought to make its generous provision of bomb testing sites an extra lever to its uranium supplies in its requests for technical information from the British about atomic energy, although it was in a perfect position to do so. It did, however, stand up to Britain on the uranium question and appeared to be prepared to play the British and the Americans off against each other. This was the one area in Anglo-Australian atomic relations where Australia drove any sort of bargain with Britain, and it stood in stark contrast to Australia's compliance over the conduct of the British atomic tests. Too much should not be made of this, however. A British memorandum prepared after Cherwell's uranium talks in Australia noted:

Mr Menzies was himself more in favour of our proposals than most of the other members of his cabinet, and a direct reply to him might single him out in a manner which would prejudice our ultimate object.

The ultimate object, of course, was uranium, and before too long the British returned with a less stringent proposition which stipulated no fixed proportion of Australia's uncommitted uranium supplies, but merely a wish to buy as much uranium as it could in return for technical information. This was accepted by the Australians. Britain had taken a fairly cynical stand throughout, dangling the prospect of collaboration before Australia, knowing that it might never be able to deliver on this promise because of its overriding commitment to restoring full-scale atomic collaboration with the United States.

To return to the negotiations over the establishment of the Maralinga testing site: Cherwell had gone back to Britain after his abortive uranium talks in Australia with a firm impression on one thing, at least. He reported that Menzies had told him Australian ministers had made it quite clear they had no interest in atomic weapons. They did not wish to receive any information specifically related to the design and production of atomic weapons as they would, on no account, embark on any expenditure for such a program. Cherwell believed, nevertheless, it would be reasonable to expect that Australia would want to be informed on the effects of atomic weapons on people and the environment.[9]

In spite of Menzies' private assurance to Cherwell, the British were concerned that they may not be able to keep Australia at bay on this question of sensitive technical information forever. Nine months later, in July 1954, when the time came for Britain to approach Australia with a formal request for the Maralinga site, the Whitehall insiders planning the exercise had become slightly nervous. The Commonwealth Relations Office warned the British high commission in Canberra of its view that the Australians were unlikely to be content indefinitely with limited information given to them in the past, and may insist on being given fuller information on the form and manufacture of weapons. As things stood, that would certainly create difficulties with the United States, London warned, adding: 'In the meantime you should be cautious about any approach from the Australians on this question since we do not wish to prejudice closer collaboration with Americans in this field'.

A few days later, the high commission in Canberra wrote to Menzies with a formal request for provision of a permanent testing ground and for Australian co-operation with the atomic weapons tests that were likely to continue for the next ten years. The letter said the UK would depend on Australia for help with the provision of works and services, and it hoped, therefore, that the provision of the required facilities could be undertaken as a joint project – in other words, that Australia should share the cost. The UK would leave the final choice of site to Australia, but UK experts believed that under suitable meteorological conditions Maralinga would provide an adequate safety margin for atomic weapons of somewhat higher power than those at the previous trials. There would be no question of testing hydrogen weapons.

This letter was largely window dressing to provide public formality for a situation which had already been decided in secret. Penney, as we saw, had already nominated the Maralinga site nine months earlier and Menzies had indicated to the British his willingness for the future tests to proceed. Indeed, for a time Menzies appears to have been terrified that Britain might choose a permanent site in Canada rather than Australia. The British, however, were able to reassure thim that they did not regard Canada as a suitable site owing to climatic conditions in uninhabited areas – an ironic situation in view of the patently unsuitable climatic conditions that prevailed at some of the tests in Australia. Even before the British request for the permanent test site had been presented to Menzies' cabinet, a senior diplomat from the British high commission in Canberra was able to cable to London that he had seen Menzies.

I think that he is personally favourably disposed to the idea and would welcome the prospect of continued collaboration between the United Kingdom and Australia. I felt it best to use discretion and scotch any suggestion that we had been thinking of Canada as an alternative.

Three weeks later, on 26 August, Beale submitted the British request to a special, inner committee of Australian cabinet ministers handpicked by Menzies, whose role is discussed further below. They agreed in principle to the establishment of a permanent testing ground and Australian co-operation in the new series of atomic tests. Menzies himself had received some interesting advice in a note from one of his senior advisers in the Prime Minister's Department, supporting the argument that Australia should agree to the British request. The note to Menzies said:

It is part of the United Kingdom grand strategy to possess a stock of nuclear bombs because otherwise the United Kingdom considers it will have no control over the way in which these weapons are used by the United States strategic airforce.

The United Kingdom Chiefs of Staff also contemplate that in the event of global war, the United Kingdom might transfer its manufacturing potential for nuclear bombs to Australia as an area remote from attack. The argument against consenting to the establishment of the testing ground in Australia is a political one, mainly the peculiar public revulsion at, and fear of, atomic weapons. But this could probably be handled in accordance with the principles which you enunciated in your statement on the hydrogen bomb.

This last remark was a reference to Menzies' statement to parliament in Canberra the previous April, after the explosion of the American hydrogen bomb, Bravo, in the Pacific. Menzies had argued that the hydrogen bomb's development was justified to meet the challenge of the Soviet arms build up, and that Australia should be thankful that 'our great friends and allies of the United States' had been willing to accept the burden to maintain a clear world leadership:

It follows that Australia will not put pressure upon the United States to desist any more than would any of the other nations with whom Australia is honourably and vitally associated . . . In common with the British people all over the world, the Americans desire peace.

Although Menzies' committee of ministers now agreed in principle to Britain's request for a new permanent test site, they directed an interdepartmental committee to examine the question of Australia's contribution and participation. This committee went away and questioned various government departments about their ability to provide men and money for the project. Its conclusion was glum: the Australian defence services could not provide men for construction work due to other commitments, and it was doubtful if the job could be done satisfactorily by civilian labour.

The interdepartmental committee also made a significant observation. It pointed out that Australia had still not been informed of the results of the Hurricane and Totem tests, and it considered that, as atomic weapons would be vital to Australia's defence, a firm request should be made to the UK for information on the results of future tests for strategic planning purposes. It suggested that Menzies raise this question in his reply to the UK high commissioner's letter. Leslie Martin, the scientific adviser to the Australian Department of Defence, and one of the three Australian scientific observers at Hurricane and Totem, had already indicated in Melbourne that the UK made available no information of any value after the last test.

Menzies had confined discussion of the Maralinga project to an inner sanctum of ministers known as the Maralinga committee of cabinet (not to be confused with the Maralinga Committee, a body later set up by Beale to be responsible for organising the planning and construction work at Maralinga, and composed of civil servants as well as people from Australia's domestic security organisation, ASIO, and the Australian Atomic Energy Commission). The Maralinga committee of cabinet consisted of Menzies, Beale, Sir Arthur Fadden, the treasurer, or finance minister, and Sir Philip McBride, the minister for defence. After the cabinet's Maralinga committee had considered the interdepartmental committee's report, Menzies wrote to the British high commissioner on 25 October confirming Australia's agreement to make Maralinga available as the permanent testing ground. He added that, because of pressure on Australia's service and civil resources, it was unlikely that Australia could make little more than a token contribution towards construction and preparation of the ground.

Menzies did not raise in his letter the question of Britain supplying information to Australia about the results of future atomic tests.

Menzies visited Britain again in early 1955, and on his return he told the cabinet's Maralinga committee that Australia, after all, should be able to provide forces for the construction of the test site and for care and maintenance of the ground between tests, and that Australia should bear the cost of any service personnel it provided. The cabinet committee later agreed to this. Meanwhile, British and Australian officials had begun negotiating the memorandum of arrangements covering the operation of the Maralinga ground, and had become bogged down over the wording of a key clause – the clause covering compensation claims for death or injury due to the atomic tests. Australia took the view that since it was the tests themselves that created the hazard, the UK should foot the bill for all claims, British or Australian. Britain's view was that it would indemnify Australia for all valid claims, except those from Australian personnel contributing to the conduct of the tests; they should be Australia's responsibility. After almost 10 months of bickering between London and Canberra on this question, Australia caved in to the British proposal and the memorandum was eventually finalised in March 1956. As the Whitehall officials apparently suspected, the compensation clause was to become a flashpoint of attention 30 years later.

There was now great pressure on Australia to have the Maralinga ground built and ready for the next round of weapons trials in the Australian spring of 1956. It was a remarkable year in many ways. The Soviet occupation of Hungary and the build up to the Suez crisis helped fan the flames of international tension which the government and military chiefs had perceived all along as the justification for the development of the independent nuclear deterrent. There could be no delay in testing the weapons once they were ready. A secret Australian document of March 1955, stressing the need to get Maralinga ready by the target date, even offered as one reason the fact that the tests could not be held much beyond September the following year was because UK scientists were unused to the exceedingly hot conditions of the Australian summer from October to March, when temperatures in the outback frequently approached 50°C; even many instruments used in the trials would have to be redesigned to operate in such hot conditions. The Australian document claimed: 'Atomic weapons have been accorded "super priority" by the UK government and take precedence over every other activity in the UK'.

In June 1956, Howard Beale, the Australian minister for supply, flew to Woomera and Maralinga with a party of journalists for a public relations exercise to show off the testing ground as it was nearing completion. As the DC3 carrying the journalists approached Maralinga, the air hostess on board, Nan Witcomb, was ordered to draw the curtains on the starboard side so none of the passengers could see what was happening below or get a feeling for the layout of the test site, such was the paranoia about security. But Witcomb could not resist taking a peek as she closed the curtains – 'being a woman', as she explained years later.

The settlement she saw was far more sophisticated than the one built and then abandoned at Emu Field for the Totem tests three years earlier. In the space of 12 months, the desert around Tietkens' plain had been transformed into a township of shining, prefabricated living quarters for almost 1000 men, with its own power generators, tennis courts, gymnasiums, hospital and cinema which showed pictures three times a week. William Tietkens had been right: the underground water was all salt, but the builders of Maralinga had installed special distillation equipment to produce 60 000 gallons of fresh water from the 120 000 gallons of salt water pumped up from the bores each day. Later, huge underground tanks were built to catch the rainwater that flowed off the airstrip and this became Maralinga's main water supply. The airstrip itself, built between the village and the bomb sites, cost 1 million pounds and was then the longest runway in Australia. The town, the airport and the bomb sites were all connected by a network of 130 kilometres of sealed roads. The whole of Maralinga cost 5 million pounds to build, a considerable sum of money in 1956.

Beale's press visit was big on style but short on hard information. The journalists were told almost nothing about the forthcoming weapons tests at Maralinga and, in frustration, were reduced to writing human interest stories about how some of the workers there could save up to 40 pounds a week through overtime payments, again big money in those days. The Australian safety committee, the body of scientists which, as we saw, was set up in 1955 to monitor future tests, had been asked to provide background information on such things as weather conditions and physiological effects of atomic weapons, in anticipation of the reporters' questions. But the safety committee, continuing the tradition of secrecy, loftily declined to co-operate. It considered the request at its meeting in Melbourne a month earlier, but concluded, according to the record of the meeting, 'that it had nothing to convey to the Press in these matters'.

So many of the stories from the Beale visit inevitably focused on the unexpected arrival of an attractive air hostess in a secret desert town of men. Strangely enough the press visit to Maralinga coincided with the detonation of the second of the Mosaic bombs in the Monte Bello Islands, which will be discussed shortly; it deflected attention from the Mosaic tests only briefly. In a display which smacked of an intoxicating Hollywood film poster of the 1950s, the *Sun* newspaper, of Sydney, splashed a huge picture of Nan Witcomb above a smaller picture of the Monte Bello blast, with the headline: 'She shook them . . . more than this explosion'. The story went on to describe 'beautiful, green-eyed air hostess Nan Witcomb' who stepped out of a plane at an atom outpost in front of 1700 men who had not seen a woman for a year. 'Bronzed, bearded and lonely labourers stopped, stared and then ran to tell their mates. Maralinga range commander, Colonel R. Durance, was worried about Nan's effect on his women-starved men.'

Some newspapers tried valiantly to produce serious stories from the visit about cheaper types of atomic bombs with 'simpler mechanisms' to be tested shortly at Maralinga, but the information available was insufficient to give the public any meaningful idea of what was going on. Many newspapers dramatically described Maralinga as the Los Alamos of the Commonwealth, highlighting the Anglo-Australian joint venture side of things, a line which had been carefully nurtured in the on-site briefings. Most reports, in the end, resorted to the tone of this article from the *Daily Telegraph*, of Sydney:

Out in the great Australian loneliness 900 miles north west of Adelaide today I sat in an air conditioned hut and ate a lunch of lobster and iced asparagus washed down with cold beer. Across the road which a year ago was a dingo pad (wild dog run) a group of bearded men stared in stunned silence at the first woman most of them had seen in six months. She was Nan Witcomb, of Adelaide, air hostess on the plane which brought me to this outpost. Small wonder the men stared for this is the only womanless township in the world.

In spite of the growing public and press interest in nuclear testing, the official obsession with secrecy over the British atomic project had not changed much, if at all, since the early days of the Hurricane test in 1952. Initially, the authorities in Whitehall had decided to ban all press representation at the Totem trials at Emu Field the following year. But this produced such a clamour of protest, particularly from the Australian press, that they were obliged to change their minds at the last minute and allow nine journalists each from Britain and Australia to attend the Totem One trial. The reporters, however, were not to be permitted any closer than 25 kilometres from ground zero and were to be kept completely segregated from the scientists. Lord Cherwell was nervous even about these tight conditions, and suggested that if the press were to attend Totem One there should be a further advance public announcement to the effect that the bomb was a tactical weapon – 'otherwise an acute observer might start a story that the test had been partially unsuccessful'. Cherwell wanted no announcment at all, however, about the nature of the Totem Two bomb: 'On this, rumour should be given free rein'.

The policy of allowing rumour to be given free rein had begun to rebound on the authorities in Britain and Australia as the press, left as they were to speculate before and after each trial, published stories which were often inaccurate and sometimes fantastic. Thus, breaking the news of the Totem tests, in June 1953, before they were announced officially, the *Daily Express* in London asserted they would include the world's biggest ever atom bomb. In fact, the Totem bombs were only one third the yield of Britain's first atom bomb, Hurricane, and a fraction of the yield of the world's biggest known atom bomb to date which had been exploded by the Americans in the Pacific back in 1948. Australian newspapers picked up the story, and suggested that the Totem tests would involve pilotless planes carrying atomic bombs, and the testing of a cobalt bomb. Menzies and Beale accused the press of scaremongering over many of these stories, but they failed to acknowledge that the blame lay more often than not with the blanket of secrecy imposed in the name of security. Menzies dismissed suggestions that the tests should not be held in Australia as 'awful and silly nonsense'. He said: 'What is being done is to save life, not imperil it'. And, after the Totem trials were over: 'We have greatly improved our capacity for defence as a genuine effort on behalf of the British family'.

Throughout the test period in the fifties, most Australian newspapers accepted the government's argument that the tests were a vital British, Australian and Commonwealth contribution to the Western world's defence. They made no attempt to analyse the separate issues of radiation exposure and health, the fate of the Aborigines, Australia's sovereignty or even whether Britain's independent nuclear deterrent was really necessary. The serious British newspapers made a bigger effort than their Australian counterparts to describe and analyse the nature of the bombs Britain was testing, but they disclosed little information beyond that contained in the meagre and limited official statements from Whitehall. The contrast with the press in the United States at this time could not have been greater. There, reporters were given frank briefings on technical aspects of atomic weapons, which managed to circumvent obvious security breaches, and were even encouraged to embark upon analytical articles probing America's nuclear weapons program.

In 1956, as Britain's and America's separate testing programs stepped up (there was virtually no information about Soviet nuclear tests at the time), other world events overshadowed what was happening at Maralinga, Bikini and Nevada. In July, President Nasser of Egypt announced that he had nationalised the Suez Canal, and Britain and France responded by sending troops into Egypt after British bombers had attacked Egyptian airfields. The Suez crisis dragged on for the rest of the year, until Britain and France responded to a United Nations call to withdraw their forces after what had become a fairly catastrophic exercise in gunboat diplomacy by both countries. In November, the Soviet Union invaded Hungary in a bid to put down growing dissidence in one of its East European satellites.

To the mainstream press at the time, these events tended to reinforce the portents in many quarters of an unstable world drifting inexorably towards full-scale war. And in Australia, the glamour and excitement of the Olympic Games held in Melbourne at the end of 1956 helped to push the events at Maralinga even further on to the inside pages of the newspapers. Among the newspapers in Australia, the *Sydney Morning Herald* was one of the most consistent supporters of the British atomic tests, with a series of editorials that spanned the decade. The *Herald*, like the Menzies government, took the view that by contributing the test sites Australia gained a special advantage in the defence umbrella of the big powers – an argument that was to resurface in the sixties in support of Australia's contribution of troops to the Vietnam war and in the seventies and eighties over Australia's agreement to the operation by the United States of secret defence communications bases on Australian soil.

The *Herald*, however, did not accept meekly the secrecy with which Britain surrounded the tests or the Menzies' government's acquiescence in it. In August 1953, the newspaper joined the chorus of press dissent over the initial decision to keep journalists away from the Totem trials, albeit in restrained and loyal tones:

The Briton's traditional reluctance to blow his own trumpet, while it has gained him a certain reputation, puts him at a sad disadvantage when it comes to publicising his achievements in a competitive world. It must be hoped that this racial inhibition will not operate to prevent – as it did in the case of the Montebello tests – the proper reporting of the forthcoming experiments at Woomera.

A fortnight after that editorial, however, the *Herald* slammed Menzies over the secrecy business: 'It is not too much to say that the arrangements for preliminary publicity for the experiments have been grossly bungled', it thundered.

Ministers, it seems, are too easily frightened by the latter day Word of

Power: Security. They would do well to remember that the public which foots the bill and stands the consequences has rights which cannot be overridden by such convenient formulae. Security has its place, and is all very well in its place, but when it seeks to cast its cloak over governmental activities and expenditures which are of urgent public interest, then its exponents should be bluntly told they have exceeded their functions . . . Australians, moreover, whether taxpayers or not, are equally entitled to know what is being done inside their borders . . . It is absurd that the most the Prime Minister of Australia can find to say on a matter of such vital public interest is that 'none of these experiments will endanger the people of Australia'.

By 1956, the *Herald* had stopped attacking the government on the secrecy score and had turned its guns on the emerging body of dissenters who were calling for a ban on further atomic tests in Australia.

An artificially stimulated nervousness in this country has tended to discredit the Government's policy of assisting Britain in her atomic tests. Australians should accept these Maralinga tests with at least as much calm as the people of Nevada have regarded the 44 explosions in their desert.

In Melbourne, the *Age* welcomed the Hurricane test in October 1952, for bringing Britain into the nuclear club: 'The whole British Commonwealth – and not least Australia, on whose soil this epoch-making event took place – rejoices at the achievement'. The *Age* at that stage was prepared to condone the whole secrecy business:

It is better that we should know too little than run the danger of putting information into the hands of those who, at this moment, are, no doubt, seeking to discover the scope and potentialities of the Monte Bello experiments.

Two years later, in December 1954, the *Age* was beginning to have second thoughts on this score. It detected growing anxiety over plans for future atomic tests in Australia, and genuine apprehension in many quarters:

No-one seeks the abandonment of all security measures. But in a loosely informed nation uncertainty and conjecture provide a breeding ground for fear. The people should be taken into the Government's confidence as far as possible ... In this respect something more than vague official statements and the varying opinions of individual scientists are required.

Almost alone among the Australian press to oppose the British tests consistently was the *Daily Mirror* of Sydney. The *Mirror* was a lone voice of scepticism towards Menzies' repeated assurances of safety, and a fortnight before the Totem trials in October 1953, it asked in headlines: 'Is there no real danger Mr Menzies?' The *Mirror* declared: 'There is plenty of scope in the Antarctic for such an explosion – not in Australia. Mr Menzies' responsibility is, indeed, a fearful one.' In 1956, the *Mirror* cited the repeated delays in firing the first of the Buffalo bombs at Maralinga, due to unfavourable weather conditions, as evidence of the unpredictability of winds which could blow the radioactive clouds over population centres to the northeast. It announced in huge headlines: 'Penney's Got the Wind Up!' The *Mirror* in July that year called for the cancellation of all new atomic tests on Australian territory: 'Australia simply cannot afford to take the risk of inflicting irreparable damage on the health of her people – in spite of all the assurances of the experts of adequate precautions'.

Ever since the early 1950s there had been a small coterie of anti-bomb activists in Australia composed mainly of trade unionists, academics, and leftwing intellectuals. But in the hysterical anti-communist atmosphere that prevailed at the time, any pronouncements they made were branded as red propaganda and they were forced to hold their meetings almost in the fashion of a clandestine underground cell. Menzies unsuccessfully held a referendum in 1951 in which he asked Australians to vote for banning the Communist Party, and three years later he dramatically plunged the nation into a political crisis over the defection of a KGB agent from the Soviet embassy in Canberra amid allegations of communist sympathisers in the opposition Labor party. Menzies used the Petrov affair, named after the defecting Soviet diplomat, to appoint a royal commission into Australia's security, a move which certainly assisted his victory in the general election of 1954. In the aftermath the Labor party split, with a right wing, staunchly anti-communist faction hiving off to form the new Democratic Labor Party. In this frenetic domestic political climate, Australia's own version of McCarthyism, any sustained opposition to nuclear testing was swiftly discredited as a disloyal campaign by fellow travellers of communism.

But by 1956, as we have seen, things were changing under the international reaction to the Soviet and American hydrogen bomb tests. Trade unionists in Adelaide and Brisbane held protests that year against further British tests in Australia, and nine scientists in Adelaide wrote to the *Advertiser* newspaper in that city challenging statements by Titterton that the tests held no risk to the public. Even so, the reaction in Australia to nuclear testing – a place where tests were actually going on – was more subdued and less flamboyant than in Britain where the Campaign for Nuclear Disarmament got under way with a manifesto drafted by Bertrand Russell. Albert Einstein signed the manifesto two days before his death in April 1955, a move widely seen as a dramatic act of penance for his letter to President Roosevelt years earlier that had helped spark the Manhattan Project. The international attention which flowed from CND led, in 1957, to the formation of the Pugwash movement, when 24 noted scientists from both sides of the Iron Curtain met at Pugwash, Nova Scotia, to discuss the risks of nuclear war and to commit themselves to a campaign against nuclear weapons.

Beale's visit with the press to Maralinga in June 1956, took place against a background of mounting international opposition to continuing tests by all three nuclear powers: America, Russia and Britain. Less than two weeks before the Maralinga visit, Sir Anthony Eden, the British prime minister, had come under sustained questioning in the House of Commons about Britain's forthcoming hydrogen bomb tests at Christmas Island in the Pacific, and their contribution to the radioactive products which had concentrated in the upper atmosphere from all the other nuclear tests up to then. At the end of 1955, Eden had proposed that the nuclear powers explore ways of regulating and limiting test explosions as a means of controlling the growing radioactive contamination of the atmosphere. This British proposal was abandoned later by Harold Macmillan, Eden's successor as prime minister, under pressure from the Americans. Nevertheless, it did act as a starting point for the discussions which eventually resulted in the Americans, Russians and British agreeing in October 1958 to a suspension of nuclear testing. France, which became the world's fourth nuclear power when it exploded an atomic bomb in the Sahara in 1960, ignored the test moratorium.

In the weeks leading up to Britain's hydrogen bomb tests at Christmas Island in May 1957, both Japan and India called on Britain to abandon the tests. Japan was already worried about fallout from Soviet tests in Siberia drifting over its territory, and the Pacific tests presented an added hazard. India's prime minister, Jawaharlal Nehru, took a broader, Third-World view and condemned all three nuclear powers. He obliquely, but unmistakably, criticised Menzies, as well, who had said it would be a triumph if the conference to be held in Canberra by the now defunct South East Asia Treaty Organisation (Seato), an American sponsored alliance, 'ushered in 1000 years of peace'. Nehru commented: 'I suppose that means a continuation of the Cold War for 1000 years'. He condemned the arms race and alliances like Seato and the Warsaw pact, saying that if they persisted they would lead to final catastrophe. Seventeen years later, in May 1974, India, under the leadership of Nehru's daughter, Indira Gandhi, stunned the world when it exploded an atomic bomb of its own.

The growing fear of war in the mid-fifties was not accompanied by a corresponding acceptance of nuclear weapons as a means of deterring or fighting that war. An opinion poll taken in Australia in June 1957, found 49 per cent of those questioned were against testing atomic bombs in central Australia, with 37 per cent in favour; the rest were undecided. Opinion had swung dramatically since 1952, the year of the first British atomic test, when a poll found 58 per cent in favour of the tests and only 29 per cent against. By 1957, the poll found, women were two-to-one against atomic testing, with men about equally divided. Another opinion poll taken in Australia in February that year found that 66 per cent of those questioned wanted all atomic bomb tests stopped by international agreement.

Faced with this growing challenge to the British and other tests from public opinion, Beale set out to counter it with a propaganda war. He told the Australian cabinet in September 1956, that he had given a great deal of consideration 'to the question of educating public opinion on this matter'. The campaign which resulted involved an assault on the way the media were reporting the atomic tests – it could hardly be described as critical, but there were apparently enough negative points emerging to convince Beale that a change was needed. In an uncharacteristically open gesture, he made Penney available for a press conference in Sydney before the Buffalo trials which began at Maralinga in September. He also arranged for Penney to give a national radio talk on the Australian Broadcasting Commission in a Sunday night program called 'Guest of Honour', during which Penney emphasised the progress made in Britain's development of atomic energy for peaceful purposes and said atomic energy would play a vital part in developing Australia.

Both Beale and Titterton joined this media political counterattack by preparing articles under their names extolling the virtues of the tests, which were then sent to the major city newspapers, some of which published them. A series of three articles by Titterton appeared, for example, in the *Courier Mail*, of Brisbane, in late 1955. The headline on the final instalment said: 'Our A bomb tests are a MUST. They can't harm us'. Another article by Titterton, with a less fulsome headline, appeared in the *Age* in July 1956, after the Mosaic trials at Monte Bello, assuring readers that reports of radioactive rain had 'caused quite unnecessary concern in the public mind'.

An article by Beale headed, 'Why Australia Provides the Site for Atomic Tests', appeared in the *Sydney Morning Herald*. Beale, as we have seen, enjoyed issuing long and dramatic statements, although their overenthusiastic tones did not always please others in Canberra and London. Beale's undoubted touch for hyperbole and his keenness for being at the forefront of public reassurance surfaced at several points during the atomic tests. But his biggest trial of all in this regard came in June 1956, shattering the solemnity and tranquility of his visit with the press to Woomera and Maralinga.

The two tests codenamed Mosaic were held in May and June 1956, and culminated during Beale's visit to the outback. Britain's decision to develop thermonuclear, or hydrogen, weapons, taken, as we saw, by Churchill's government in 1954, had put enormous pressure on Aldermaston to perfect these weapons as soon as possible. As Penney explained, the Russians' explosion of a hydrogen bomb in 1953 had had a dramatic effect on the military in Britain. By April 1955, Britain's thermonuclear work had proceeded at a faster pace than expected. The scientists at Aldermaston calculated that, if they were to meet their target of testing a full-scale hydrogen bomb by early 1957, they would first need to conduct other weapons tests aimed at giving them vital data on the H-bomb's design. But Maralinga would not be ready as a test site until September 1956. So Britain approached Australia once again to ask if it could hold these other trials in their original testing ground, the Monte Bello Islands.

The Mosaic trials were to be, in effect, preliminary tests for the thermonuclear trials in Christmas Island. But the Australian people were never told by their own government or by Britain the real purpose or nature of them. Hydrogen bomb tests by the mid-fifties had aroused a growing groundswell of public opposition because of the sheer magnitude of the weapons and their perceived potential for spreading radioactivity. Menzies and Beale had always insisted when challenged in parliament that there would be no hydrogen bombs exploded in Australia. The events that followed were a particularly vivid encapsulation of the key strands of the 1950s story: the unwillingness of Britain to take Australia fully into its confidence and the consequent communication gulf between the two countries; Australia's dilemmas over trying to please Britain and safeguarding its own national interests at the same time; the indifference towards the Aborigines; the public fear over radioactivity – and, most of all, the obsession with secrecy among scientists and civil servants at all levels.

Sir Anthony Eden, who had succeeded Churchill as prime minister, sent a personal message to Menzies in May 1955, asking for Australia's agreement to two firings at Monte Bello early the following year. The message avoided precise details, but it made it quite clear that the proposed trials were to be connected to thermonuclear tests:

You know well importance we attach to speediest development of efficient nuclear weapons and of great part they can play in interests of Commonwealth strategy. Our research and development work is going so well that we hope to carry out certain experiments early in 1956 and to have a full scale test of thermonuclear weapons in 1957.

Eden explained that if the 'experiments' could be done at Monte Bello in April 1956, Britain would save six months of valuable time in its weapon development program, and get better value from a further round of tests that were scheduled anyway for Maralinga the following September and October. He then described the nature of the proposed Monte Bello program:

Experiments would consist of atomic explosions with inclusion of light elements as a boost. It would, of course, be made clear in any public announcement that explosions were atomic and not thermonuclear.

The smaller of the two shots would be fired first. If this was successful the second 'and slightly larger' shot would not be fired. Neither blast would be more than two and a half times more powerful than the Hurricane bomb of 1952. They would be exploded on towers to reduce the contamination, and the fallout would be less than one fifth of that of Hurricane. Australian scientists would have the same facilities for checking safety measures as they had at previous trials and would have at Maralinga. Finally, Eden said Britain would be prepared to pay for the operation but asked that Australia provide logistic support such as refuelling, stores and facilities for aircraft.

Several points are worth noting about Eden's message. First, this appears to be the only information Australia was given about the nature of the Mosaic bombs right up to the time of their firing. Eden's description of Mosaic as 'atomic explosions with inclusion of light elements as a boost' was an interesting choice of words. As we saw, the difference between atomic and thermonuclear explosions is one between fission and fusion. Thermonuclear explosions are achieved by the fusion of isotopes of the light element, hydrogen, using an atomic bomb as the trigger. Or, as Penney explained it in disarmingly straightforward language to the Australian royal commission: 'The atomic bit produces the great heat and so on that ignites the rest and then you have this great big explosion'.

The Mosaic tests, then, were clearly to be in the nature of a thermonuclear explosion. They were, as Penney described them 30 years later, 'experiments [that] would later lead to our knowledge enabling us to make a thermonuclear explosion'. But at the time, this caused paroxysms of agony among the planners in Britain about the likely reaction in Australia. One interdepartmental cable in June 1955, warned: 'Any mention of thermonuclear is political dynamite and must be avoided in announcements of trials'. Another secret message to the British Ministry of Defence stated bluntly:

The greatest difficulty relates to the reason we give for the decision. We cannot avoid telling the Australians that the bombs fired will contain small quantities of thermonuclear material. In the statement attached, the reason for the trials is linked with the development of small atomic bombs, the yields of which are boosted by using small quanities of thermonuclear material . . . The correct reason is to obtain early information on the likelihood of success of the one megaton weapon as conceived at present.

The power, or yield, of thermonuclear weapons is usually measured in megatons, or millions of tons of TNT, rather than kilotons.

Second, Eden's remark to Menzies relating the proposed yield and fallout of the Mosaic blasts to those of the Hurricane bomb was rather curious. Neither the estimated nor the actual yield of Hurricane, three years earlier, had yet been disclosed officially to Australia.[10] Third, the British prime minister's assurance that Australian scientists would have the same facilities for checking safety as they had at earlier trials was also strange. At those trials, Hurricane and Totem, the three Australian scientists, Titterton, Leslie Martin and Alan Butement, were observers only with no authority to take part fully as safety advisers. In fact, their power to insist on certain safety standards at those trials had been almost zero. As a result of that glaring gap in Australia's role, the Australian safety committee had been formed only in 1955, with all three as inaugural members, for the precise purpose of safeguarding the safety of Australians; the Mosaic trial was to be the first they would attend in that capacity, the first test of the safety committee in operation.

Five weeks after Eden's request arrived, Menzies replied that Australia agreed in principle to the proposed tests; but he warned that Australia may not be able to provide all the logistical help Britain would like because Australia's military commitments were already stretched – in Malaya, where Australia was contributing with Britain to a Commonwealth strategic reserve force which had been fighting against communist guerrillas, at Woomera and at the preparations for Maralinga itself.

In September, Britain and Australia made a joint announcement that the trials would take place in the Monte Bello Islands, giving the target date of April 1956, and that another series of tests would happen at Maralinga later that year. None of the tests, it said, would exceed 'a few tens of kilotons in yield'. As we shall see, this was a misleading statement as far as the Mosaic bombs were concerned. But true to the spirit of Eden's message to Menzies, every effort was made to stop the thermonuclear connection of Mosaic from getting out. The Australian government, partly out of ignorance about the true nature of Mosaic but also out of unwillingness to push the British too far on this, went along.

Anticipating further questions from the press following the bland and unrevealing announcement of Mosaic, the British authorities drew up a list of likely questions that could arise and the answers that should be given to them. They sent the list to the Prime Minister's Department in Canberra, which, in turn, sent it to Beale with a prudent note, 'They hope, of course, that we would take a similar line'. The list amounted, in effect, to Beale's promptings. The first hypothetical press question on the list, and the answer given for it, was a wonderful example of clever, if deceptive, official wording.

Q: Have any of these tests any connection with an H-bomb? A: There will be no explosion of an H-bomb, nor any explosion of the character or magnitude of that bomb, but all atomic tests contribute information of value to the development of H-bombs.

Another example clearly anticipated journalists probing deeper:

Q: Are these actual weapons or are they test equipment which may be used in various types of weapons? A: No statement can be made.

Professor Mark Oliphant, the Australian nuclear physicist who had been frozen out of any role in the British tests, was quoted in one newspaper as predicting, correctly as it turned out, that the tests could be of a trigger mechanism for an H-bomb. But the British were keen that there should be no room for disagreement or independence from Australia on the conduct of these or any other trials. An official pre-trial brief prepared in London warned of the need to reconcile pressures for the release of information – 'particularly on the Australian side' – with the needs of security, and stressed: 'It will be important that the two countries march in step at all stages'.

Penney did not attend the Mosaic trials, although he kept in close touch with events from Britain. The man in charge of the whole operation was commodore Hugh Martell, the Royal Navy's task force commander at Monte Bello, and a crusty naval chief of the old school. The scientific director was Charles Adams, a senior member of Penney's staff on 'High Explosives Research' who had also attended Monte Bello for the Hurricane trial.

Martell ordered standby for the first Mosaic blast, called G1, on 14 May 1956, and the weapon, attached to a specially constructed steel tower, was fired just before midday two days later, giving a yield of 15 kilotons. Titterton, Martin, Butement and two other members of the Australian safety committee were on board the HMS Narvik, the headquarters ship stationed in the Monte Bellos, for the firing. During the afternoon, Martin, the safety committee's chairman, transmitted a message to Menzies that there had been no hazard whatsoever to life on the mainland, ships at sea or to aircraft: 'The whole operation proceeded with precision and was a complete success'.

The Australian public were subsequently assured that the cloud had drifted harmlessly out to sea. In fact, part of the cloud at altitudes between 4000 and 6000 metres did swing back over the mainland and deposited low level radioactive fallout across northern Australia. Fine fallout debris in this upper level wafted slowly across the continent and finally cleared the east coast about 60 hours later, leaving very small fallout readings at Daly Waters and Cloncurry in the Northern Territory and at Cairns, Townsville, Charleville and Brisbane in Queensland.

The highest measurements of contamination from G1 anywhere in Australia, however, were made at the West Australian coastal towns of Broome and Onslow, near the Monte Bello Islands. The measured doses were below the level set by the health physics people before the trials as being safe for the public; but the fact that there was any contamination on the mainland at all startled those in charge.

One of those who was surprised was James Hole, a radiological safety officer from Aldermaston, who had helped to develop the system of dosimetry used in the British tests to register radiation exposure among those involved. Hole also helped to initiate for the Mosaic trials a system of measuring contamination on the ground by taking readings from aircraft flying overhead. But he revealed to the Australian royal commission 30 years later that this system had a fundamental flaw: it actually underestimated by ten times the ground contamination. Hole said he discovered later that the measurements recorded in the aircraft had to be multiplied by ten in order to measure the proper contamination on the ground.

The RAF had assembled a group of Canberra and Varsity aircraft to conduct the same exercises for Mosaic as those at Totem – the Canberras to fly through the bomb cloud and take samples of it, and the Varsities to track the cloud later on. They operated from the Australian air force's base at Pearce, near Perth, from where they flew 1200 kilometres north at the time of each bomb test to be stationed at the small airfield at Onslow on the mainland coast about 120 kilometres south of the Monte Bello Islands.

It was one of these tracking aircraft about three days after G1 that alerted Hole and his fellow scientists to the fact that contamination had reached the mainland. This is how it happened. Stationed on board the Narvik, Hole received a signal from the

Pearce air force base down south that one of the aircraft which had just returned there from Onslow was registering contamination. Hole packed a laundry basket full of radiation detection equipment and two scruffy boilersuits for himself and took a helicopter across the water from the Monte Bellos to Onslow.

The choice of clothing and the laundry basket was quite deliberate. As Hole put it:

I had already had experience at Woolwich, and particularly at Aldermaston, of having to go to private houses and other places where, of course, emotions can play a very big role in radioactivity. The one thing you do not do is go somewhere dressed in a respirator, white clothing and hooded, and the other thing you do not do is take an instrument making noises. This only attracts attention. When I went to Onslow, I did not know what I was going to find. I suspected there was contamination.

Hole was right. An Australian security officer with an open-backed van met him at Onslow airport.

We found two or three bed matresses which we laid out on the back of this Holden van. I laid down on the back of this van on my tummy with equipment beside me, with the B12 geiger in its case held by a pair of pincers we used for holding radioactive material and with a pair of earphones to my ear. We divided the runway into four quarters and went up and down each quarter slowly. The response on contamination is instantaneous through earphones. It is not instantaneous when you use a geiger. The results of these traverses indicated there was some contamination on the airfield, but certainly very patchy.

This chap drove me in this van, in fact he found his way around the outskirts of Onslow better than a taxi driver in London, if you know what I mean. I never found any piece of contamination greater than the size of a tennis court. And it appeared from the evidence that this contamination I was measuring had come from the explosion.

That evening, Hole headed for the bar of Onslow's one and only pub, where he discovered the readings were no greater than ordinary background radiation. The pub was where everything happened in Onslow, especially at night. But although the bombs had given sleepy Onslow an unusual talking point, Hole's conspicuous appearance in the pub, with his boiler suit and instruments slung over his shoulder, did not. The customers in this frontier town simply carried on drinking.

But Hole himself ended up receiving a bigger dose of radiation than anyone in Onslow. He went into the bomb crater soon after the Mosaic G2 blast as health escort to a colleague whose job was to collect samples of the crater. 'It was virtually like a skating rink', Hole said. 'The sand obviously had been glazed and there were lots of colours in it. One of the problems in standing in this crater was you could get fascinated and forget you were receiving a dose. It was very pretty!' [11]

It was this second Mosaic bomb, G2, which caused a bigger row at the time than any other nuclear bomb exploded in Australia. Another month went by after G1 before G2 was fired – a month filled with tension, frustration, uncertainty and intrigue. There had been demonstrations against the tests in Perth at which protesters had carried placards stating that Australians were being used as guinea pigs. Joining the campaign, the Australian seamen's union threatened to go on strike unless Australian ships stopped taking supplies for the task force to Monte Bello. Later, they blacklisted the port at Onslow, and the supplies had to be flown in. The Royal Navy had two ships at the islands besides the Narvik, and five more stationed out to sea for weather duties, while the Australian navy had provided three ships for survey and logistic work.

In the weeks leading up to the trials, the boredom among the men on this large task force was partly broken by a secret visit from Earl Mountbatten of Burma. But as the delays grew between G1 and G2, the stress and disgruntlement built up. Bernard Perkins, one of the operators in the Narvik's wireless room, remembered the atmosphere as the day for G2 finally approached:

There were three or four abortive countdowns before the second explosion. Everybody was getting very fed up and one or two sailors were taken off the ship to hospital since they had had breakdowns. There was very great tension in the air. I remember talking to one scientist who was working on a timing device. He said that the long wait was because the weather had to be right, but that they had to hurry up because of time and money. [12]

In fact, after studying the behaviour of the G1 cloud and the weather reports, Martell had nominated Sunday 10 June as the first possible date when conditions would be right for the firing of G2. He ordered everyone to prepare. But, from his seclusion in the Monte Bellos, Martell had not bargained for the peculiarities of politics in Canberra. The strictures of Mammon from London may have dictated that the test be concluded swiftly, but God in Australia was about to intervene. At that time, the churches had a far greater hold over life in Australia than they do today. Ever the politician, Beale objected strongly on religious grounds when he heard that G2 was to be fired on a Sunday, and asked that it be postponed.

Martell was furious, but London grudgingly bent to Beale's request. Reginald Maudling, the new minister of supply, wrote to the Earl of Home, the secretary of state for Commonwealth relations: 'The objection was on religious grounds and Mr Beale felt he would have no adequate answer to the strong protests which would arise'. Maudling argued that the number of days when meteorological conditions would be suitable again would be limited, and that Martell should not be inhibited from firing when conditions were right – otherwise the task force could be there for weeks. 'We must, in view of the urgencies of the situation, hold ourselves free now to use the first suitable day and to face criticisms if it falls on a Sunday'.

Martell's concern at losing this opportune day was well grounded: one meteorological report had shown that since the Narvik arrived in March there had been no day which could have been categorically defined as suitable for firing the larger G2 bomb. The weather turned bad after Sunday 10 June and standby could not be ordered again for another week. Finally, at 10.14 am on 19 June, Mosaic G2, strapped to a 100-metre steel tower, was ignited. Seconds later, a spectacular mushroom cloud tore 16 000 metres into the air. The blast was terrifying. Buildings jolted at Onslow, more than 100 kilometres away across the sea. Windows and roofs rattled at Marble Bar, an inland town 400 kilometres to the east, where radioactive rain was later reported. The yield of G2 was 60 kilotons – the biggest and 'dirtiest' British atomic bomb of them all.

The true strength of G2 was kept a secret for years. Right up to 1984 the public in Britain and Australia were told in official reports that all the atomic bombs exploded in Australia had been in the 'low' or 'kiloton' range. Some of the bombs genuinely were low – between 1 and 10 kilotons. But 60 kilotons was not low. The true figure was not revealed until 1984, and then only casually in a letter from Geoffrey Pattie, the minister of defence procurement, to Lord Brockway, a Labour peer.

The main cloud from G2 moved, as predicted, northeast across the sea, but, after an unexpected wind shift, fine particles of fallout from the cloud at various levels swung back and drifted across the mainland. Reports of this started appearing in the press almost immediately, accompanied by heated speculation that the G2 bomb had gone seriously wrong.[13] The main reason for this was that Beale had made a statement in between the two Mosaic blasts which included the assertion that the second bomb would be smaller than the first. It was a remarkable comment in view of the information in Attlee's original message to Menzies a year earlier that the opposite would be the case, and it starkly demonstrated the shortfall in communications on the Australian side. The British tried to correct Beale's remark, but they were too late to stop it becoming public.

From the sheer force of the blast it was now obvious that the second bomb was many times bigger than the first, and the press travelling with Beale at Woomera the day after G2 demanded that he make a statement revealing the true state of affairs. Beale later described in his memoirs how one of his officials had promptly closed the Woomera telephone exchange to cut the journalists off from communication with the outside world: 'I was annoyed with him at the time for exceeding instructions but I was later to be grateful to him for his presence of mind'.[14] Beale's department in Melbourne pressed the Bureau of Meteorology for information, and the bureau in turn urged that it would be best to wait for an authoritative statement from the Australian safety committee before making any information available to the press. Beale, however, was not prepared to wait. On the basis of preliminary reports from the bureau, he told the press at Woomera that at

1600-3300 metres all significant particles had gone into the sea, but at 6000-6600 metres some cloud drifted inland although it was now tending to drift back towards the coast.

The next day, the Australian safety committee sent a message to Beale from the Narvik that the cloud was 160 kilometres out to sea, that all safety precautions had been met and that there was never any danger to the mainland. Beale made another press statement in a bid to reconcile his first announcement with this information from the safety committee, this time implying that the cloud had been over the mainland but had moved safely out to sea. Four days later, Sir Arthur Fadden, the acting prime minister, himself made a statement assuring the public he was satisfied that the whole Monte Bello operation was conducted without risk to life or property on the mainland or elsewhere. Fadden invoked the authority of the safety committee for this assurance – 'the only persons in a position to judge the matter'.

Leslie Martin, the safety committee's chairman, sent a report to the prime minister shortly after he and the committee's other members left the Monte Bello Islands. It was written in somewhat glowing terms which tended to play down the problems, a characteristic that was to feature in all the safety committee's reports of trials from then onwards. But the information it contained was discordant. It stated that the G_2 cloud had moved away from the northwest coast of Australia where it showed evidence of rapid dispersion. The cloud at no point approached the coast, and all 'immediate high activity' fell entirely into the sea. The report added, however, that there was 'some fallout of low level activity in a restricted coastal region, and to a lesser degree in a band reaching towards the centre of Australia'. This was near 'the low limit of detection', and the vast majority of Australians, including those in the big cities of Adelaide, Brisbane, Melbourne, Perth and Sydney received no radiation.

In the face of all these conflicting statements, the public could hardly be blamed for feeling confused or that they were being hoodwinked. Indeed, the G_2 affair marked a turning point in the acceptance of the British nuclear tests by the Australian press and public, and from that time onwards the British realised that falling confidence among Australians would be a serious factor threatening the future of the test program. Both the Australian safety committee and the British were alarmed and angered by Beale's incorrect pronouncement on the comparative strengths of G1 and G2, and by his statements at Woomera. Commodore Martell and Charles Adams, the two British figures in charge at Mosaic, visited Beale in Sydney on their way home, and during their meeting, Beale sought ways of extricating some measure of fact from his statement about G2 being the smaller bomb. But the British were unwilling to help him – they took the view that Australia had been told the correct information months earlier, and it was not their job to rescue Beale from his embarrassments.

Adams and Martell had visited Australia in mid-1955 for talks about Mosaic with members of the Maralinga Committee referred to earlier. Also known as the Australian Weapons Test Committee, this body had been set up under Beale's department to be responsible for organising the Australian side of the forthcoming tests. The Australian safety committee of scientists had also just been appointed, and Adams had a separate meeting with Alan Butement, one of its members. Adams indicated to Butement the probable yields of the two planned Mosaic bombs, confirming the original message from Attlee to Menzies that the second would be bigger than the first. After the event, Adams claimed that during this preliminary visit to Australia in 1955 he had spoken of probable yields of about 20 kilotons for G1 and about 80 kilotons for G2, and that Butement knew these figures.

On his return to Britain after the Mosaic tests, in August 1956, Adams wrote to a senior official in the British Ministry of Supply giving his account of the whole business, as well as some flavour of his and Martell's final meeting with Beale in Sydney.

Beale specifically asked me what I could suggest as a reconciliation of his statement [about G2's size] with the facts. What he wanted was to be able to quote, for example, 'the radioactivity was smaller' or that the effects in any sphere could be argued to be less than those resulting from G1. It was necessary for me of course to make it absolutely clear that no such statement could be made.

As regards the source of Beale's own statement, his account was that he had arranged a meeting which included members of his own department and 'somebody round the table' said that 'anyway the second explosion was to be smaller than the first'. Thus his attitude at my meeting with him was that he had been misinformed by somebody on Australian department of supply staff, but that he had authorised the statement.

Adams went on to discuss what 'the two Beale incidents', as he called them, could mean for communication between the British and the Australians before future trials. Was it sufficient for Britain to keep the Australian government in touch with matters of this kind through the Australian safety committee? He pointed out that, in this case, Britain had been entitled to assume that Beale would have been properly informed: Butement, whom Adams himself had briefed earlier, was a member of Beale's own department, as was the secretary of the safety committee, and it was a reasonable assumption that they would tell their own minister what they knew. 'I have no doubt we must stand firm in refusing to attempt any justification for Beale's statement', Adams wrote. 'I have personally told Beale we cannot do this and the only possible line is that we cannot be responsible for extricating him from his own spontaneous statements.'

Finally, he insisted that the true yields of the Mosaic bombs remain secret.

As regards any statement on the Mosaic yields I presume we should avoid making any comment as far as possible. If a statement had to be made it could only be on the lines, 'the second was bigger than the first, just as we expected and as the Australians had been officially informed'. I can see no security objection to such a statement but it would obviously discredit Beale. In my view no statement should be made unless specifically requested by Australia.

Australia did not request such a statement, and one was never made. Adams may have been strictly right in his advice that nothing happened at Monte Bello which conflicted in any way with the intentions of the trials as Britain had earlier stated them to Australia. But beyond these general intentions, the Australians, once again, had received very little pre-trial information. The Mosaic trials were the first since the Australian safety committee's formation, and the committee's members were considerably nervous about fulfilling their brief not to allow any bombs to be fired until they were satisfied that conditions were completely safe. This brought them into conflict with Martell, the man who gave the decision to fire the Mosaic bombs, because he was unaware of any arrangement that gave the Australian scientists the authority to question that decision. As far as he was concerned, it was a British responsibility and the final decision rested with him.

This revealed yet another gap in communications between the Australians and the British. Clearly, no-one in London had told Martell what the precise role of this newly formed Australian safety committee was to be, or, if they had, neither he nor Adams expected the Australian scientists to present a problem. But the Australians were concerned on two fronts. The first was the nature of the Mosaic weapons themselves. When the safety committee members – Martin, Titterton, Butement, Cecil Eddy and L.J. Dwyer – arrived at Monte Bello for the G1 firing, it was clear they had been told virtually nothing about the content of the bomb beyond the original message from Eden to Menzies that there would be 'the inclusion of light elements as a boost'. In order for them to make any realistic assessment about whether the upper and lower estimates of the weapon's yield were reasonable, they needed to know more than this.

Martell and Adams, faced with a possible further delay from this deadlock, decided to give the Australians more information, but on the strict condition that they confine it to their own use for security purposes. Martell told them that the major part of the yield from the tests would be from nuclear fission, and that the increase in yield from any thermonuclear processes would be small. The British scientists specifically wanted to know about the interaction of the light elements in an environment where nuclear fission happened – that is, the effect of the high temperatures produced in a thermonuclear weapon by the fission trigger.[15]

Even then, Martell and Adams gave away no significant information because Penney, back in Britain, had instructed them not to do so. Penney had cabled Adams:

Strongly advise not showing safety committee any significant weapon details, but would not object to their seeing outside of cabled ball in centre section. They could be told that fissile material is at centre of large ball of high explosive and that elaborate electronics necessary to get symmetrical squash. No details of explosives configuration or inner components must be revealed. Appreciate that the position is awkward for you and that you must make minor concessions.

The Australian scientists were, indeed, shown the G2 weapon, which no doubt gave them a sense that they were being kept informed even if they had not been told the details about its configuration. Titterton described that experience in fairly dramatic terms to the Australian royal commission in 1985:

Mr Butement, Sir Leslie Martin and I went and physically inspected that weapon just before it was armed. We stood, if you like, and admired it. I do not want that to be misunderstood. But, in truth, that weapon was a very beautiful piece of highly sophisticated engineering. I think the only word to describe it is beautiful.

Members of the Australian safety committee were justified in fearing that they were being kept in the dark on vital weapons matters at Mosaic. Six months before the trials, Penney had anticipated that the Australians were likely to ask for some of the filters from the aircraft which were planned to fly on missions to collect cloud samples from Mosaic and the later Buffalo trials at Maralinga. Clearly, Penney did not want to give too much information away that would enable the host country to calculate the actual yield from the weapons. So he wrote to Sir Frederick Brundrett, of the Ministry of Defence, to suggest a scheme that would involve delaying the Australians until the immediate post-firing contamination levels had partly died away, or, in scientific jargon, decayed: 'On balance I am recommending that if they ask us we give them a little piece of the filters, but that we wait a few days so that some of the short lived key isotopes have decayed a good deal'. Brundrett concurred: 'I do not quite see how on earth we could refuse such a request if they make it . . . I do not think there is any necessity to consult anybody else on this matter'.

Confronted with this correspondence at the Australian royal

commission in 1985, Penney justified his decision to be less than fully frank with the Australians because, on this point, the information could give away details on weapon design. 'This was weapon diagnostics, which was not the same thing as how big was the weapon', he said. 'On matters of weapon design, that was out.'

The second count on which the Australian safety committee was worried at Mosaic was the weather conditions at Monte Bello. When the safety committee held its first meeting after its formation in July 1955, one of the subjects it discussed was the vital question of meteorology. The committee members, three of whom, Titterton, Martin and Butement, had attended the Hurricane and Totem trials as observers, concluded that meteorological information had not been all it could have been at those trials, and they resolved to make it as complete as possible for future tests. To this end, they brought in as a member of the safety committee Dwyer, who was the director of the Australian Bureau of Meteorology. (Eddy died about a month after the Mosaic trials and Donald Stevens, the director of the Australian Radiation Laboratory, filled his place.)

The fact was that the Monte Bello Islands were unsuitable for firing atomic weapons because of their notoriously unpredictable weather conditions. The islands were prone to cyclones, unreliable winds and appalling rain storms.

Dwyer had produced some fairly alarming reports which showed just how limited the conditions were for testing bombs there. As early as 1951, when the British were conducting their reconnaissance of the Monte Bellos for their very first bomb trial, Attlee advised Menzies that British experts had concluded that 'for climatic reasons' an atomic weapons trial could be held there only in the month of October. The Hurricane trial was held in October 1952, but even then the unpredictable winds drove the cloud over the mainland.

Now, for Mosaic, the trials were held not in October but in May and June – months when the upper winds were predominantly from the west, that is, blowing towards the mainland, and when 'willy willies', or wild dust storms, were quite frequent. The Mosaic trial planners knew this, as did the Australian safety committee, because the previous year Dwyer had prepared a study of weather conditions at the islands for the years 1951 to 1955. He concluded that in a two-month period between April and July for any of those years only two to four satisfactory days would arise when firing conditions would be satisfactory. This proved to be an optimistic conclusion. Richard Fotheringham, a British meteorologist, conducted a study at the Australian Meteorological Bureau in Melbourne in January 1956, of the likely frequency of suitable wind conditions for the months April, May and June. He discovered a frequency of about 1 per cent – one day in three months. Dwyer produced his studies at a meeting of the Australian safety committee in January, 1956, four months before Mosaic began. The committee's conclusion was the most grim of all: it assessed from the evidence that the number of suitable firing days in the Monte Bello Islands amounted, on average, to only two a year.

It seems remarkable that, in view of this knowledge that the weather conditions were likely to break down, and with the experience of the Hurricane trial at Monte Bello four years earlier, the Mosaic tests were planned with no consideration by either the British or Australian authorities for Aborigines living on the northwest coast of Australia. Since the last Monte Bello trial in 1952, no-one had tried to find out about the Aboriginal population of the mainland adjacent to the islands, and the British were content to proceed with the comfortable assumption that there were no Aborigines there at all. When Martell was questioned before the Australian royal commission about whether he considered the possible effect of the Mosaic bombs on local Aborigines he replied tersely: 'Aborigines are nothing to do with Mosaic . . . The question does not arise. There were no Aborigines on the Monte Bello islands'. Martell also declined to admit that there had been radioactive fallout on the mainland from Mosaic, but, when pressed, said it was a measurable amount of fallout scientifically but not for practical purposes.

The Australian safety committee also ignored the Aboriginal issue at Mosaic. The whole question about whether more strict radiation exposure levels should be set for tribal Aborigines because of their open-air lifestyle and lack of clothing actually came before the safety committee at its meeting in April 1956, a few weeks before the Mosaic trials. But the committee did not set any special levels for Aborigines for Mosaic. It was only at the Buffalo trials at Maralinga later in the year that it adopted a new level for Aborigines which was five times lower than the general exposure level accepted for Mosaic. Colin Thackrah, an anthropologist working in Perth for the federal Department of Aboriginal Affairs, presented a report to the Australian royal commission which indicated that in 1956, almost 1700 Aborigines were recorded as being in the Pilbara region, the mainland area closest to the Monte Bellos.

And yet the trials went ahead because, as Penney explained to the Australian royal commission in March 1985, the information was needed urgently for Britain's hydrogen bomb program. Why, he was asked, were the Mosaic tests held when the weather conditions were so unacceptable? Penney replied:

All right, but let me tell you the other end of the story. The top priority job was thermonuclear. We wanted to see if we could make a few fast neutrons, and we wanted to do it in yields of 40, 50, 60 kilotons. [William] Cook [the deputy director at Aldermaston and chairman of its weapons development committee] said, 'Where can this be fired?' I heard all this later from him because he was doing the running job. Maralinga was not going to be possible; it was too early. And if we had said to the Australians, 50 kilotons at Maralinga, I think they would have said no. So we could not go there. The other possibility was to ask the Americans. Well, we had been through that hoop. And therefore it was either Monte Bello or wait – not to do it.

Not to do it at all was never really considered because, as a result of the Mosaic trials, Britain's thermonuclear tests, Operation Grapple, were able to begin on schedule at Malden Island in the Pacific in May 1957. In fact, the 'booster' theory appears to have worked so well in the first of the Mosaic bombs that questions were asked darkly in Whitehall afterwards as to why the second and much larger Mosaic bomb needed to be fired at all; it was even suggested that the G2 operation was a waste of between 3 and 4 million pounds – a huge sum in 1956. As Penney put it: 'I suppose it sounds a bit odd, but I was not worrying about money. Somebody else was.' [16]

After all the drama at Mosaic over misleading and conflicting statements, one lesson appears to have sunk in. Back in London, Adams and Martell reported on the trials to a meeting of civil service and military chiefs and suggested that much of the press outcry could have been avoided by providing wider publicity before the bombs about their likely behaviour. For instance, it was known that the explosions would produce 'a small increase' in radioactivity, and this should have been announced beforehand.

Martell was more characteristically blunt and defiant. He referred to 'the hysteria of the Australian Press'. He felt, according to the record of the meeting:

This was not unexpected and could be avoided if the population were taught the elementary facts about atomic explosions ... He felt that for future trials it would be necessary to provide educative information for the people of Australia ... He had made suggestions on this matter to Mr Beale who apparently took the view that only he, Mr Beale, should make statements on the tests and that the allegations of misleading reports were not true.

Penney returned to Australia in August 1956, to direct the first bomb trials to be held at the new Maralinga testing ground, under the codename, Buffalo. He was full of excitement and apprehension. On a technical level so far, Britain's nuclear tests had worked well, remarkably well. Britain had gone a long way towards closing the gap on weapons knowledge with the United States, and was within nine months of testing her first full-scale thermonuclear weapon. But the pressures to get the job done had been enormous, and they were now increasing – from many sources.

Here, at least, Britain had a 'permanent proving ground', but how long would Maralinga remain permanent? What would happen if there was another public relations disaster like Mosaic? The Australians had been compliant and co-operative enough up to now, but how much longer would they remain so? The public in Australia, as elsewhere, were becoming increasingly sceptical about these wondrous new weapons and alarmed at the build-up in the world's atmosphere of radioactivity from the tests in Australia, Nevada, the Pacific and Siberia. What if Menzies should take the unlikely course of bowing to public opinion on this question and ask the British politely to do their tests elsewhere? And what if Menzies should lose office to the Labor party, whose leader and deputy leader, Herbert Evatt and Arthur Calwell, were making public noises about halting the tests and calling for Australia, instead of making itself an atomic testing ground, to take initiatives towards negotiations by the three nuclear powers on a suspension of all tests?

These questions whirled through Penney's mind as he stepped off a Hastings aircraft at the freshly built Maralinga airfield on the afternoon of 24 August, dressed in a dark suit and the ubiquitous sweater, his usual modest, boyish grin belying the tension he really felt inside. One of Penney's first tasks was protocol – greeting the governor of South Australia, the Queen's representative, who had come to Maralinga especially for the famous scientist's arrival. Then he left for a quick inspection of Maralinga itself.

The place was hardly a picture of completeness. Even now, less than a month before the scheduled D-day for the first bomb test, Maralinga was still being built. The rush to get it finished on time had been so great that basic things like electricity and water supplies were being frantically installed up to a few days before the first bomb was fired. The plant to desalinate the water from bores sunk on the range was not finished, and thousands of litres of fresh water had to be imported by the transcontinenal railway to the Watson siding, south of Maralinga. Everyone, including Richard Durance, the Australian army colonel who had taken over as commander of the Maralinga range, took turns to drive relays, day and night, to haul the water up from Watson. Years later, Durance remembered the scene vividly: 'It was a bit of a mess'.

One curious side of the arrangement between Britain and Australia for the building of the range had contributed to the delays. As Durance explained:

The Australian side of that mess was a direction from the government of the day that the land could be made available, borrowed from the South Australian government, on the understanding that not one brick or power point or top of a gas stove or piece of metal for a tower came from the Australian market. It was all to be brought out. There were delays in the docks, trains in trouble. [17]

It was little wonder, then, that Beale's arrival at Maralinga with the press and the air hostess, Nan Witcomb, two months earlier, when things were even more basic, had caused headaches. Durance remembered that occasion very well:

It was a terribly awkward time to have a woman there. Most of the lads were frightfully busy working in filthy conditions and they didn't wear very much. She was kept out of the way because it was a completely male area. No-one even knew there was going to be a hostess on board the plane. If they'd warned us six weeks before we could have done something about it. But as things stood, there wasn't even a place for the poor girl to powder her nose, if you know what I mean.

What the scientists and servicemen who were on their way for the Buffalo trials thought they were going to find at Maralinga, and what they actually found when they got there, were two different things. Canada, which had sent representatives to the Hurricane trial back in 1952, obtained approval first from Britain and then from Australia to send a contingent of about 45 service officers, scientists and radiological experts to the Buffalo trials. The Canadians prepared a remarkable dossier for their people before they left, titled 'Life in the Village of Maralinga', which must have given some of them the feeling that they were heading for a relaxing tourist resort in the middle of the desert. It began:

The village has been planned with considerable care so as to make it not merely functionally efficient, but also a pleasant place to live. It is situated on a tree-covered hill about 900 feet above sea level, facing North with a fine view across rolling parkland.

The reality was different. No better account of the conditions many of the men lived through could be found than in a report of the experiences of the British 'indoctrinees'. This was the name given to a group of senior military officers sent out to witness a nuclear explosion, whose role is discussed further below. The indoctrinees had arrived amid the chaos of the last-minute rush to complete Maralinga, and had had to pitch in like everyone else to haul water, drive tractors, dig holes, and generally get the place in working order. It was the indoctrinees who finished building the Maralinga cinema, a job which might otherwise have lapsed.

The indoctrinees had their own living area, known as the Indoctrinee Force Camp, but it was hardly the stuff of tourist brochures. According to a report of life in the camp:

The wind was always strong and cold. If the sky was clear at night, there was usually a frost at dawn. As the camp was pitched on limestone rock, covered by only a few inches of orange-red sand, all tent pegs had had to be inserted with the aid of pneumatic picks. As a result insufficient pegs were inserted, and indoctrinees started by collecting rocks and fastening them to the brailing loops with wire and ropes to prevent their tents being blown away. The walls of the tents in most cases did not reach the ground, so that red dust was continuously blowing up inside and covering the beds, spare clothes, tables and chairs.

At Maralinga, four bombs were fired in Operation Buffalo and another three in Operation Antler the following year, the last of the major bomb trials in Australia. Their yields ranged from one kiloton to 25 kilotons. But the criteria for safe firing which Penney and his colleagues laid down were not met in all cases. Penney declared standby for the first blast, One Tree, on 11 September, but the weather suddenly deteriorated and stayed bad for another fortnight. The continuing postponements and frustrating delays for this, the first bomb to be fired at the much-trumpeted Maralinga ground, produced speculation in the press and questions in parliament suggesting that Maralinga, after all, may not have been a suitable choice. Were the delays and the extreme care that had to be taken, some people asked, not an indication of the terrible dangers from the radioactive content of these weapons?

The questions in parliament in Canberra continued through September up to the day of firing, and they came from government MPs as well as the opposition Labor party. Evatt joined the chorus of criticism and asked Beale in the House of Representatives whether the numerous postponments had made it clear that danger may be encountered and damage done if the wind changed direction during or after the test. Beale denied that last minute wind changes would cause danger, and blamed sections of the press for encouraging such stories. He had, he said, never heard greater streams of misleading statements on this point than those emanating from certain pressmen who had been cooped up at Salisbury, South Australia, over the last few weeks, waiting, and apparently not liking it. Evatt's deputy, Calwell, interjected: 'Hear, hear!' Beale once again invoked the authority of the Australian safety committee of scientists – 'The highest scientific authority in Australia assures us that when the decision has been taken the firing will be completely safe'. Another prominent Labor MP, Eddie Ward, of East Sydney, called for the tests to be discontinued.

The One Tree bomb was eventually fired from a tower at 5 pm on 27 September, more than a month after Penney's arrival at Maralinga. A correspondent from the *Times*, of London, who witnessed the first Maralinga bomb from 11 kilometres away, cabled a description back to his newspaper:

Already starting from the top of the fireball we saw a storming, threshing cloud that seemed to seek in the heavens its peace from man's intrusion. The noise made the endless expanse of Australia's central desert feel for a moment like the enclosed and claustrophobic inside of a six inch gun turret. The blast wave was disappointing, no stronger than the wind from London's Underground that strikes one in the street. The black flies returned to our shoulders. Within seven minutes vapour trails at more than 20,000 ft indicated the arrival of two Canberra bombers, one of which entered the cloud, which, within 10 minutes, was becoming not unlike an ordinary cirrus cloud. There was no trace of the tower, but where it had stood there was an ash-grey circle 500 yards in diameter, and not unlike the site of a camp fire after the coals have been swept away. There was little evidence of any crater. To the north – whither the wind had blown – trees as far as two miles from the point of the explosion were alight and smoking.

The fallout drifted eastwards directly across Coober Pedy, an opal mining town with a population then of 160. This had been predicted, and had allowed for the fallout to be at the level considered safe for whites – a level five times higher than the level recently decided upon as safe for tribal Aborigines. More than two thirds of Coober Pedy's population were Aborigines. Questioned about the fallout at Coober Pedy, Penney told the Australian royal commission: 'Not many people, though, were there'. Ronald Siddons, the senior Aldermaston mathematician who played a key role in fallout forecasting for the Antler trials at Maralinga, flatly disagreed at the royal commission with the decision to explode the One Tree bomb under the conditions it was fired. 'I would have said wait – until the prediction is more favourable.'

The second Buffalo bomb, Marcoo, was exploded on the ground a week later. Apart from being the first British atomic device tested at ground level, it was also the lowest yield so far, 1.5 kilotons. Nevertheless, the fallout was substantial, although it did not appear to spread much beyond the test range. It was the crater from the Marcoo blast next to which the Aboriginal family, the Milpuddies, camped when they wandered on to the test site a few months later.

The third bomb, Kite, was also a first – in this case, the first British atomic device to be released from an aircraft, the first operational drop by the Royal Air Force of a deliverable bomb. An RAF crew dropped the weapon from a Valiant bomber at 10 000 metres and it exploded precisely as scheduled at 165 metres above the ground with a yield of 3 kilotons. Because Kite was an air burst, the conditions for firing were not as restrictive as those set for the other bombs; the theory behind this was that the further above the ground a weapon is exploded, the less ground material it is likely to pulverise, suck up into its cloud and deposit back to earth as radioactive debris. But the path the Kite cloud took was not as scheduled: instead of travelling to the northeast it went southeast, because of a wind change, depositing fallout over the Maralinga village and low-level contamination on the outskirts of Adelaide.

The final Buffalo bomb, Breakaway, was exploded from a tower 11 days after Kite, on 22 October. Yet more bad weather had delayed the blast by four days. Breakaway, too, was a first: it was exploded at five minutes after midnight, to grab the best conditions while they lasted, and yielded 10 kilotons. Fallout again drifted over Coober Pedy.

In fact, none of the clouds from the four Buffalo bombs behaved entirely as expected because of the immense difficulty of predicting weather patterns with any certainty. As Siddons told the royal commission:

No meteorologist is going to put very much confidence in a forecast which goes more than 24 hours ahead in time . . . Therefore there was really little purpose in sort of straining to predict fallout at very long ranges.

A party of MPs and journalists had flown into Maralinga to witness the One Tree explosion when it looked like it may happen the day before it actually did happen. But when weather forced another postponement, the parliamentarians were put back on their aircraft, given a quick flight over the target area and flown back to Adelaide because there was nowhere at Maralinga to put them up for the night. The pressmen stayed on for the blast which finally happened the next day. However a group of 25 Australian MPs from all parties did eventually visit Maralinga during the Buffalo trials, Beale and Arthur Calwell among them. There was a little ceremony at the end of the visit at which Beale presented Penney with an inscribed cigarette case on behalf of the Australian government.

Durance, as range commander, hosted the visit, and he recalled at the Australian royal commission the speech Calwell made after the presentation to Sir William Penney:

He replied that he would like Sir William to know that his party and he were in full agreement with what was going on at the range. He also agreed with the fact that the British government were in no position to find other places to do this, that Maralinga was the only suitable spot and he thought this was quite correct that it should be so. He said: 'I would like you to know that my party and I support what you are doing, but it is not what I am going to say on Thursday night in the House when I move a motion of censure against it'.

The British were somewhat taken aback by the different public and private Labor party stands on Maralinga, something which they clearly had not expected. His spirits lifted, Penney wrote to the British high commissioner in Canberra after the visit to report that the party of MPs 'were all purring on eight cylinders' and that even the doubtful ones seemed convinced. A member of the high commissioner's staff reported the British perception of the Labor party's attitudes in a secret letter to the Commonwealth Relations Office in London soon afterwards:

Calwell, the deputy leader of the Labour party in the House of Representatives, and [John] Armstrong, a Labour senator, both said to him [Penney] that they were sure the tests must continue. This is of course directly contrary to the expressed views of their Leader, Dr Evatt.

The High Commissioner happened to see Calwell shortly after he had received Penney's letter and drew him on the subject of his visit to Maralinga, saying (innocently) that there was clearly no alternative to going on with these tests and it was quite obvious that Maralinga, like Woomera, was paying us all big dividends in relation to the possibility of war. Calwell wholeheartedly agreed. This is all rather surprising. It becomes, in fact, clear that the Labour party is split from top to bottom on the issue of atomic trials. Professor Titterton, who is deputy chairman of the safety committee, commented to the same effect to the High Commissioner on a subsequent occasion.

But the questions continued. The redoubtable leftwing Labor MP, Eddie Ward, alleged in the House of Representatives that 'something had gong wrong' with the One Tree explosion at Maralinga, and managed to add: 'The government has bungled and has not told the people of the dangers from the explosion' – before the Speaker ruled him out of order. Ward tried to raise the matter again later the same day, citing records of wind currents on the day of the explosion, but the government gagged him. Ward angrily told fellow MPs in an outburst reported in the press: 'They stopped me from telling how they bungled the bomb test'.

The most intimate view of that particular bomb test, One Tree, was experienced by the group of military officers mentioned earlier known as the indoctrinee force. Indoctrination was a favourite word of the fifties, but it was usually used to conjure up images of evil communist agents working on some victim from the West under heavy lights. The Australian safety committee, at a meeting in July 1956, discussed the need for, as they put it, 'the indoctrination of the public' over the nuclear tests, and Penney's forthcoming radio talk to Australians on the ABC, which Beale had arranged, was to be part of this public indoctrination.

The British had decided that a large group of military officers should be 'indoctrinated' on the effects of an atomic weapon actually exploding in the field, and its impact on the various target response items at Maralinga such as the tanks, vehicles, aircraft and specially constructed bridges and buildings set up near ground zero. The use of both the indoctrinee force and the target response experiments was a measure of how imminent and real the weapons testers considered the prospect of nuclear war in the mid-fifties.

The authorities in various British ministries considered the target response experiments to be vital in their planning of civil and military defence programs. The experiments were all designed to simulate the effects of an atomic bomb on a battlefield, above a city and through the food cycle. Flying glass from a bursting window was to be blown into a room and deliberately embedded in a telephone directory which could be studied afterwards to determine what may happen if the object struck was a human being instead. Sheep were to be fed grass contaminated with fallout from a bomb to discover the effects of such ingestion; caged goats, rabbits and mice were to be placed in pits at various distances from ground zero to study the effect of blast waves from nuclear explosions on living creatures. The Americans had already experimented at all these levels in their own trials – the use of indoctrinee forces, target response tests, experimenting with animals and exploding bombs at different heights on land and sea, and they had done so on a far more elaborate basis. The British had very little information from the American experiments and were now forced to duplicate them at vast expense.

One grim target response report came towards the end of 1956, after the Buffalo trials were over. Harry Turner, the Australian health physics representative, reported that a considerable number of rabbits near the Marcoo bomb site had died from ingestion of radioactive fallout. The rabbits had lost their fur and skin around the mouth, sometimes as far as their eyes. Their teeth were prominently exposed and many had gone blind. The rabbits were starving. One was caught and sent to Britain for further examination. Several hawks and other birds known as great Nullarbor eagles had been feeding off the dead rabbits, and one of the eagles appeared to be sick. No dingoes or kangaroos sighted so far appeared to be suffering from radiation sickness.

As for the indoctrinee force, more than 280 officers eventually had been chosen, 178 of them British, 100 Australian and 5 New Zealanders. The Canadians had been allowed to send indoctrinees to the American tests in Nevada, so they did not feel any need to take part in this exercise. The indoctrinees were stationed 8 kilometres upwind from the One Tree bomb when it exploded, and were taken up to the target point over the next two days where they witnessed a scene of total desolation. All trees were reduced to stumps less than 1 metre high. Vehicles were overturned and some were still burning. The dummies which had been dressed in protective and non-protective clothing were blown about, the clothing ripped from their bodies and the respirators burnt off their faces. A Centurian tank, its engine still running, had been blown more than 1 metre sideways. The tank could still be driven, but a real crew would have been dead.

A report on the indoctrinees' reaction to the One Tree blast noted:

The vital moments were over so quickly that one hardly had time to absorb the effects. Most people felt that they would have liked to witness a second explosion shortly afterwards in order to see it all again.

Penney was impressed by the enthusiasm, and agreed to a smaller group, 110 of the indoctrinees, staying on for the Marcoo bomb. After all, the indoctrinees had helped muck in to get Maralinga ready on time, and they had then been forced to wait around for weeks in miserable living conditions until the weather was right.

This time, though, none of them was allowed into the target area after the blast. A ground burst like the Marcoo bomb is, by its nature, a 'dirty' bomb because it dumps its radioactive contamination down quickly in a more concentrated form than air bursts. The military chiefs had asked for a ground burst to be included in the Buffalo trials because, as Penney explained to the Australian royal commission:

The military, as I keep stressing, were thinking about nuclear war, and in nuclear war the nuclear weapons would be to attack the enemy and do as much harm to him as possible. A ground burst was a very likely way. They dump the stuff all around, and if, in combat, there are men to be attacked, a ground burst will dump stuff on them and it will be in military terms a successful explosion.

The indoctrinees at Marcoo were split up. Four were put inside a Centurion tank stationed a mile from the blast, 24 watched from a series of covered trenches in the ground nearby, and the rest stood in the open 3 kilometres from ground zero. The indoctrinee officers were impressed by what they had seen because, in sheer military terms, they reported that they were more ready to accept a nuclear missile as a tactical weapon after their experience than before. They were dispatched back to their various units in Britain, Australia and New Zealand to report to their fellow officers on what to expect when Armageddon came. And they had been well looked after: the radiation film badges they had used were more sensitive than the types issued to the workers and servicemen who stayed on at Maralinga far longer.

A great deal of planning and attention had gone into the indoctrinee programs and the target response experiments, as well as the actual monitoring of radioactive fallout from the Buffalo trials. Apart from the usual cloud tracking flights by aircraft, some 86 ground stations had been set up around Australia to monitor fallout using sticky paper equipment and air filters to catch samples of airborne contamination. These preparations were in stark contrast to the rapidly improvised measures for Aboriginal safety.

The Aborigines, as we have seen, had been given a low priority at all the previous trials, Hurricane, Totem and Mosaic. Now that the tests had moved back to the mainland for Buffalo, and looked like staying there for a long time, the question finally began to occur to the Australian safety committee about the effects of radioactive fallout from atomic bombs on Aborigines living in their tribal state, virtually naked and with bare feet. As mentioned earlier, this question was never really considered before 1956.

The radiation experts at Aldermaston had produced a report at the end of 1955 on safety levels for radioactive contamination for the forthcoming Buffalo trials, but it had failed to take into account Aboriginal lifestyle and habits. The Australian safety committee asked that these factors be addressed, and in April 1956, the Aldermaston report was republished with an appendix which analysed conditions for fixing contamination levels for Aborigines who lacked clothing, would be likely to sleep on contaminated ground and eat contaminated food and unlikely to wash contamination from their bodies. This led the Aldermaston people to conclude that the permissible levels of contamination for tribal Aborigines would have to be reduced by a factor of five from the levels allowed for the rest of the population.

The Australian safety committee considered this at a meeting in April 1956, and noted what this meant: that for a nominal burst (20 kilotons), the acceptable level would occur at a distance of about 240 miles (400 kilometres) from ground zero. The committee viewed this as 'a very serious matter' and decided it would need further consideration before any final pronouncement could be made.

One reason why they were troubled was that Penney had set down a condition for the British tests, based on American practice at the Nevada tests, that there should be a 100 mile (160 kilometres) radius around ground zero which was free of any population. Now, here was a new report saying that tribal Aborigines, the people who actually inhabited the test zone, should not be any closer than 240 miles if their health was to be safeguarded. A whole host of settlements and mission stations where Aborigines lived lay well within this radius – Commonwealth Hill, Coober Pedy, Ernabella, Everard Park, Granite Downs and Mabel Creek, to name a few. The implications of this for the test program were obvious. Alan Butement, the Australian government's chief scientist and a member of the safety committee itself, told the committee at a meeting the following month that the tests might have to be restricted to relatively small atomic devices in the air or on high towers with low effective wind speeds. Butement also suggested that further restrictions may have to be imposed so that winds blew the cloud to the northwest; the chances of obtaining such suitable winds, he acknowledged, were slight.

While the safety committee was considering these disturbing

new factors, the Mosaic tests at Monte Bello were allowed to go ahead without the latest information on Aborigines being taken into account. It was not until May 1956, four months before the scheduled start of the Buffalo trials at Maralinga, that the safety committee received a report which indicated there were about 1600 Aborigines living in the region of South Australia where the tests were to be held. The committee eventually sent to the Australian cabinet in August, a month before the trials started, a report on what it described as 'the Aboriginal problem'. It was a confusing document whose language seemed designed more to reassure ministers that Aborigines were being considered, something from which the government could derive important public relations value, than to come to grips with the real situation at this late stage.

The report told ministers that Aborigines would be exposed:

To a bigger radiation dose than normal human beings whose clothes and homes provide shielding. In order to ensure protection for these people (who also pose the added difficulty that they are migratory) the safety commitee has determined a radiation level – 'A' – which can be accepted in any region where aboriginals are likely to be. This level is lower than that which would be acceptable for the white population. This will impose a further restriction on the choice of suitable firing conditions, beyond those already agreed with the UK. We also wish it to be clearly understood that such a dose can be delivered only once in the Buffalo test series to any one area. That is the dose contour from test three at distances beyond 100 miles must not overlap that from test one.

What did this mean – that if level A was reached at one place from one test, then a lower level from another test at the same place was acceptable? Or that the total dose from all four tests at one place must not exceed level A? Or something else? The answers were never provided and the cabinet apparently never asked for them. On 4 September, just one week before Penney ordered his first abortive standby for the Buffalo trials, the cabinet in Canberra approved the lower radiation levels for Aborigines, in a decision whose wording simply compounded the confusion. The cabinet approved that 'the level of radiation to be permitted for both

Aboriginal and white population be Level A with no overlap of dose contours'. This decision showed how perplexed ministers had been by the whole issue or how cursorily they had treated it, or both. The whole point about level A was that it was meant to be five times lower than the level for whites. But it was never indicated precisely what the level was, nor was any radius set for level A fall-out. In other words, despite the apparent flurry of belated concern on this question, there was never any real prospect of making sure that the new restrictions worked.

One reason for this was that those in charge of the tests, including the Australian safety committee, remained remarkably ignorant of the location and lifestyles of Aborigines in and around the range. The scientists' minds were on other things: would the bombs ignite as planned, would the target response experiments work, and would the fallout stay away from the big white population centres to the east? We saw in Chapter Four how hopeless the arrangements were for ground patrols of the vast Maralinga range.

The air patrols to locate Aborigines, despite the efforts of those who flew them, were largely ineffective. The man in charge of the air operations at the Buffalo trials, and at the Mosaic tests earlier that year, was RAF Air Vice Marshal Stewart Menaul. Menaul himself was in the aircraft that flew through the clouds of the first Mosaic bomb and the first Buffalo bomb, and was in the Valiant which dropped the third Buffalo bomb, Kite. Twenty-four years later, in 1980, Menaul wrote a book called *Countdown: Britain's Strategic Nuclear Forces*, which purported to tell 'the whole story for the first time' of Britain's efforts in designing and producing atomic and thermonuclear weapons, plus the V bomber force as the delivery system, entirely from national resources without outside help. His book was certainly optimistic, and critical of the opponents of nuclear weapons, but it was not the complete story. For example, this is all Menaul revealed about the true purpose of the Mosaic bombs: 'The primary object of the trials was to test two nuclear weapons designed by the Atomic Weapons Research Establishment at Aldermaston'. Again, he dealt with the controversial and troublesome G2 explosion at Mosaic in one sentence: 'The second test was completed satisfactorily on 19th June, 1956, and at the beginning of July the entire task group moved from Pearce Field in Western Australia to Edinburgh Field in South Australia . . . '

In 1972, Menaul wrote a letter to the *Times* in London containing a scarcely concealed attack on Australia and New Zealand for their opposition to French nuclear tests in the Pacific. He found opposition to the French tests somewhat hypocritical:

Australia, New Zealand and other Commonwealth countries took part in British nuclear tests, both on the Australian continent and in the Pacific, and gained valuable experience and knowledge in the process. It is partly surprising, therefore, that senior politicians in Commonwealth countries should join in the general chorus of protestation against the French government's actions, and even invite the British government to lend its support.

Menaul's book contained nothing about the air patrols for Aborigines at Maralinga, an indication of the low priority this job was given. He was questioned closely about the patrols when he appeared before the Australian royal commission in London in March 1985, and he insisted that the patrols were done conscientiously. A report which Menaul wrote at the time recorded a single air search before the first and last Buffalo bombs, but did not record any searches before the second and third bombs. Menaul refused to concede that this meant no searches were done on those occasions: 'Aborigines do not travel 100 miles a day, I am afraid. They sleep most afternoons. If you searched the area on Wednesday you would not really expect to search it on Thursday.'

Menaul maintained he was familiar with the way Aborigines lived, and to stress this he told the royal commission how he had taken some visiting Americans, two generals and two scientists, by helicopter to visit a tribe of about 20 Aborigines who lived in the bush about 160 kilometres from Maralinga. The Americans had told him they wanted to see some Aborigines. 'We took them gifts', said Menaul. 'We took them beads and we took them food'.

The man to whom Menaul was obliged to give a final assurance that the air patrols for Aborigines had been effective was Richard Durance, the Australian army colonel, later brigadier, who was commander of the Maralinga range for Buffalo. Durance, in turn, had the ultimate responsibility for reporting to Penney before Penney gave the orders to fire. Durance certainly matched Menaul in his colourful assessment of Aboriginal living habits and customs.

Durance told the Australian royal commission he believed the reason for sending out air patrols at night was to look for 'shy' Aboriginal tribes who hid from the ground patrol officers, MacDougall and Macaulay, during the day. Here is Durance explaining how he understood these tribes lived:

They were sufficiently shy and could not be contacted, but one of their traits was that they wakened in the mornings, as I was informed, early and were concerned with evil spirits that would enter them during the night. This could be offset by – a silly word to use when you are speaking of human beings – but offset by lighting the spinifex all round them and jumping in the smoke. Now, they did light the spinifex, for what reasons, really, I would not know, and that is what the planes were looking for at night.

Penney's major preoccupation during the Buffalo trials in September and October 1956 was political – how to keep the Australians happy so that Maralinga would remain in British scientific and military hands. 'I think that it is very important that we take whatever steps we can to strengthen our friendly relations with Australian politicians and officials in order to have the best chance of keeping the use of the Maralinga range', he wrote to Sir Frederick (Freddie) Brundrett of the Ministry of Defence in London.

Penney proposed several steps to keep the Australians on the British side, one of which was to give the Australian safety committee an idea about the construction of the Blue Danube and Red Beard weapons and to tell them how much fissile material was in any weapon that was to be tested on the range. This would amount to allowing them to see the test weapons and to them being given a short statement about their construction. This was, indeed, a radical departure from previous practice and it caused a good deal of agonising in Whitehall. The information Penney proposed giving may not have been sufficient to enable the Australians to make completely accurate calculations of the weapons' yields, but it was certainly more than they had been given before and it was, some British officials felt, flatly contrary to Britain's postwar understanding with the United States.

On the other hand, the row over the Mosaic tests, the rising public opposition to nuclear tests in general and the increasingly hostile public statements by Evatt and other Australian Labor politicians had begun to strike a raw nerve in London. As one Whitehall official wrote: 'The Australian situation is getting distinctly messy. I am sure Penney is right in thinking we should be wise to take out an insurance policy.' There was the added complication of the Australian safety committee which had come into being for the 1956 trials, and which itself was acutely aware that the whole testing program could be jeopardised if something went wrong at Maralinga. The safety committee shared Penney's political worries about the future of the trials, but it also had to be seen to be doing its job for public consumption at home. It was a strange dichotomy: the safety committee was set up to monitor and, if necessary, veto the tests in the interests of safety in Australia; yet it knew that any delays it initiated could throw Britain's entire nuclear weapons timetable into chaos. Penney himself summed up the safety committee's odd self-conflicts when he cabled London from Australia three days before his arrival at Maralinga: 'Australian safety committee solidly with us but are conservative and apprehensive'.

Penney's secret messages to London during the frustrating weeks leading up to the first Buffalo shot reveal the pressures he was under. In late August he cabled:

Everything is going well. Greatest problem is to relieve public apprehension about radioactive fallout. Definite progress has been made but there are small hostile groups trying to make mischief . . . I am confident that we can handle these matters.

A month later, as the weather continued to delay the firing, he cabled Cook at Aldermaston:

We have had a tough night . . . Could not prejudice future of range and therefore cancelled without last minute fight with safety committee . . . At any rate I have done my best to win confidence of Australians and keep long term use of Maralinga . . . Everyone of people here behaved magnificently and took the disappointment like men.

By October, another pressure had arisen: the Olympic Games were due to open in Melbourne in late November and it would not do for the British to be letting off atomic bombs in Australia as the sporting world flocked into the country. The trials must be over by then – bad weather or good. Penney cabled Cook:

Grateful advise if my number one priority not to prejudice future of Maralinga is correct. Difficult for me here because I cannot fully assess political strength of troublemakers raising scares by rainwater counts. We can never guarantee that activity will not be found in rain 500 or more miles away.

There is no evidence that, in the end, the British went as far as Penney's suggestion in giving the Australian safety committee what Freddie Brundrett described as 'sufficient information to enable them to carry out their job'. The Australians were told the likely maximum yield of each weapon in advance of firing, but they were never given the actual yields. Their report to the Australian prime minister after the Buffalo trials was based on what they had been told beforehand about the expected yields, and it gave the misleading impression that these were the yields actually achieved. Even though Britain was now well established as a nuclear power in its own right, the lingering perceptions of its obligations to the United States and of future Anglo-American atomic collaboration had once again dictated its policy of secrecy towards Australia.

Penney did well to be worried about the sureness of Australia's ongoing co-operation with the nuclear tests, nevertheless. Britain had sought Australia's help in the form of logistic contributions to the Mosaic and Buffalo trials in 1956 and to the Grapple hydrogen bomb tests which began in the Pacific in May 1957, not to mention the provision and preparation of the Maralinga ground itself. The Menzies government had agreed to all these requests, at a cost of several million pounds to the Australian taxpayer (the precise figures have never been published). But Australian officials were becoming increasingly irritated by the open-endedness of the British requests and the unwillingness of the British to make available details of the tests for which Australia was being asked to provide support.

When, in September 1956, a request arrived in Canberra for Australia to agree to a further program of British nuclear trials for 1957, the Menzies government, for the first time, refused to give its assent straight away. The British request gave no information except that the trials were planned from October to November 1957, and that there might be up to five tower tests 'on a somewhat similar scale to the four rounds in the Buffalo series'. Australia asked for more details about the nature of the tests, such as the yields of the bombs and the likely fallout, before it gave agreement in principle, but none were forthcoming. A standoff ensued for the next seven months while Britain brought diplomatic pressure to secure Australia's agreement and Australia continued to ask for more detailed information before giving it.

When Britain finally responded to Australia's request for more information, in April 1957, it was in the form of a pesonal message to Menzies from the secretary of state for Commonwealth relations. In somewhat lofty tones, it referred to the original proposal sent to Australia the previous September, adding: 'I understand that it would be helpful to you in considering these proposals to have a general outline of the scope of the tests we would wish to carry out'. The cable revealed that Britain was preparing to explode six bombs at the new trials, not five as mentioned in the original proposal, and that the maximum likely yields would range from 3 kilotons to 80 kilotons, bigger even than Mosaic G2. But there was a qualification: 'Whether we shall wish to explode all six depends on how the work goes between now and October'. This ambiguous statement, it appears, was a reference to the British hydrogen bomb tests which were due to begin at Malden Island in the Pacific the following month and to continue until late in the year. The message to Menzies about the proposed new round of trials in Australia carefully avoided using the word atomic and referred only to 'major trials', 'tests', or 'rounds'.

Australia delayed still further before responding to this latest request. There were two issues at the heart of Australia's growing concern, both of them inextricably linked. Australian officials had begun to suspect after all this time that Britain may not, perhaps, have been fully frank with them about the nature of all the trials held so far and those now being proposed. Already it was clear to some Australian officials that the Mosaic tests, with their inclusion of light elements, had had a thermonuclear connection. They now suspected the same about the proposed new tests at Maralinga. In particular, the large yields which the British had forecast for these trials, plus the possibility that the number of bombs fired could be reduced from the maximum number of six, made the Australians wonder if there was some connection with the hydrogen bomb tests about to start in the Pacific. One clause of the memorandum of arrangements between Britain and Australia for setting up the Maralinga range stated that no thermonuclear (hydrogen) weapon would be tested on the site. The question was now asked in official Australian circles whether Britain may be secretly flouting this clause.

The proposed new tests at Maralinga had been given the codename, Antler, after the Australians had objected to an earlier name, Volcano. With its implications of death and destruction at a time of growing worldwide protest against nuclear tests, Australian officials feared a possible outbreak of public alarm if the Volcano name was used and they told the British bluntly that it was completely unsuitable.

This concern was not surprising in view of the other issue which the Australians were confronting at this time. This involved a revision of the arrangements for managing the Maralinga range and for monitoring the safety of the bomb tests themselves. With the arrival of the original British request for approval of the Antler tests in September 1956, Menzies decided that in place of the ad hoc administrative arrangements set up for the Buffalo trials, some more permanent organisation was needed which gave Australia political as well as administrative control over the Maralinga range. The result was a new body, the Maralinga board of management, with an Australian chairman and British and Australian members, but under the control of the Australian Department of Supply.

At the same time Professor Leslie Martin, chairman of the

Australian safety committee, had proposed that the safety committee's functions in future should be divided between two bodies – one to be in charge of weapons safety at Maralinga itself, the other to examine the broader radiological hazards to the Australian people resulting from weapons tests. Martin had argued that radioactive contamination of the atmosphere and the ground from nuclear trials had become a major political issue. There was every chance that nuclear tests might be suspended as a result. He felt it was desirable to have a second group of people, independent of the safety committee, to advise the government on measurements of radioactive products around the country, leaving the safety committee the principal role of investigating the safety aspects of the weapons on site. In short, Martin wanted a stricter set of monitoring safeguards governing contamination hazards to the Australian public than he believed could be achieved through the safety committee alone.

The new body, created in May 1957, was the National Radiation Advisory Committee, with Martin as a founding member. Titterton took over from Martin as chairman of the Australian safety committee, whose membership was now reduced to three. Martin's concern about nuclear radiation as an issue was no doubt genuine; but the changes introduced as a result of his recommendations were also partly political, a move by the Menzies government to reassure a worried public. The Menzies government waited until all these changes over the Maralinga management and the safety bodies had been put in place before it sent Britain, on 16 May 1957, its approval in principle of the Antler trials.

As events turned out, the Australians had been right to be suspicious about the nature of the Antler trials and the contents of the weapons. Antler was always presented as part of the atomic weapons test program, but Penney revealed in early 1985 that, like the Mosaic trials, Antler was really linked with Britain's thermonuclear experiments. He told the Australian royal commission:

Scientific tests of the Antler series were needed to confirm understanding of the triggering mechanism for the high yield thermonuclear explosions conducted at Christmas Island in the Pacific.

As a result of weapon design information obtained from the Pacific tests, in May and June 1957, Britain decided in the end to limit the Antler trials to three bombs – two mounted on towers, and the third suspended from balloons. The first two Antler tests, called Tadje and Biak, were fired on 14 and 25 September, both of them delayed by bad weather. They yielded 1 and 6 kilotons respectively. The final shot, Taranaki, was fired a fortnight later from balloons suspended 300 metres above the ground, and yielded 25 kilotons, the same strength as the very first British atomic bomb, Hurricane.

The fallout pattern went awry from predictions in all three cases. The centreline of the Tadje cloud moved north when it had been expected to move east. The main fallout concentration from Biak was deposited to the northwest of ground zero instead of to the northeast. The Taranaki bomb was exploded from a greater height than any others in all the British tests: the tethered balloon system's advantage was that it could take the weapon to an altitude not reached by towers, with the expectation that the fallout would be reduced. In fact, there was less fallout near ground zero than expected, but more fallout at long distances: radioactive rain was reported once more in Adelaide. Ronald Siddons told the Australian royal commission that the fallout was higher than expected essentially because of a failure to model accurately the falling velocities of the radioactive particles and their distribution in the cloud.

The Australian safety committee, now under Titterton's chairmanship, sent a characteristically glowing and reassuring report of the Antler series to the Australian prime minister:

The safety committee has satisfaction in reporting to you that, after analysis of all these data, it can assert that the safety measures taken were completely successful. The fallout on the occasion of this trial was considerably less than in any previous trials and there was absolutely no risk to any individual, livestock or property at any time.

What the safety committee did not tell Menzies was that the highly radioactive component, cobalt 60, had been secretly included in the Tadje bomb. The secret was sprung almost a year after the explosion, in July 1958, when Doug Rickard, a member of the

Australian health physics team at Maralinga, and then aged 19, was conducting a routine survey of the bomb sites. At one area of Tadje, he came across radiation levels so high that his instruments could not measure them. Rickard dug the dirt about with his feet and discovered several metallic-looking particles which were undoubtedly the source of the activity. He put them in a tobacco tin and drove in his Land Rover 48 kilometres back to the health physics laboratories at Maralinga.

His arrival caused great consternation and intrigue because the pellets were more powerful than anything his team had ever detected. In fact, the staff were waiting for him outside because, as he approached, the instruments in the laboratory had gone haywire. They had to leave the pellets outside when measuring them, otherwise the the the gamma spectrometer scanning instrument would have become saturated. The pellets were quickly analysed to be cobalt 60. The Australian health physics team got in touch with the authorities at Aldermaston in England, and Rickard described what happened next:

Immediately a heavy security blanket went into effect. I was interviewed by a security officer and it was impressed upon me not to speak to anyone about this at all, particularly any Australians, no matter what their position at Maralinga. As the person who actually discovered the particles, and was involved in their recovery, I was under the distinct impression that the British authorities did not want the Australian government to know anything at all about what happened. [18]

Over the next four months, the health physics team found many more cobalt pellets lying on the range. Several were returned to the UK for study and the rest were put in lead cases which were buried in concrete pits near the Maralinga airfield, along with a great deal of other radioactive debris. Although most of the pellets were recovered from the range, there were many bits of cobalt fragments which had broken up into pieces too dangerous or difficult to handle and which had to be left there. Rickard said:

There were problems because the level of radiation was so high that it was obvious that the existing health physics group personnel could not do it because by this time we were already over our limits.

Rickard himself went to Britain the following year, 1959, to work for a time in health physics at Aldermaston. But at the time of the Maralinga cobalt 60 incident, he did more handling of the cobalt pellets than anyone else, packaging them into lead containers and measuring them for heat. Records show that he received higher radiation doses during the time he spent at Maralinga from October 1957 to June 1959, than other members of the health physics staff. He told the Australian royal commission that, while monitoring the fallout path from the Antler trials on one occasion, he ended up with so much fallout in his hair that his head had to be completely shaved. Rickard has since suffered permanent bone marrow damage and other physical disabilities, and doctors in Brisbane and Townsville, in Queensland, have told him his symptoms are consistent with high exposure to ionising radiation. Because of his deteriorating health he has been unable to work full time since 1981. Rickard launched a claim for compensation against the Australian government, on grounds that his health breakdown was due to radiation exposure during his employment. The federal compensation commission recognised his claim and held the Australian government liable, although the amount of compensation had not been settled at the time of writing.

Rickard's boss at Maralinga as head of the Australian health physics team was Harry Turner, whom we first met at the time of the Pom Pom incident involving the Aboriginal family, the Milpuddies, earlier in 1957. When Turner realised what Rickard had found, he complained to the Australian safety committee. Turner later explained:

Our measurement showed that these pellets were a substantial number of millicuries [a unit used to record radiation strength] in each case. It was conceivable that such a pellet could be accidentally transferred to one's clothing and for a period of time relatively high doses could be incurred. For about nine months we had walked in that area where the cobalt 60 pellets were, not knowing that they were there, meaning that it was possible that by some mischance somebody may have collected one of those pellets and not realised what it was. [19]

According to Turner, Titterton, as head of the safety committee, conferred with the British after Turner had complained, and then saw Turner again:

He [Titterton] said that he had been told prior to the test that cobalt 60 would be involved but they didn't tell me because they knew that I would find out anyway. I couldn't quite understand the logic of that argument, but now that it was known to be there we wanted it removed.

When he was asked at the Australian royal commission if he believed what Titterton told him, Turner replied:

Look, pardon me, but I have got to introduce a scientific probability into it. I cannot say I believed or did not believe, but I was suspicious that it was not necessarily true.

Turner was a physicist who trained at the university of Western Australia, and later spent two periods working with the UK atomic energy research establishment at Harwell, before returning to Australia in 1956 when he was posted to Maralinga as the Australian health physics representative. He worked at Maralinga for eight years and, like many scientists whose life's work was spent with nuclear radiation, he was not prone to overplaying the dangers from it. But for Turner, the cobalt 60 incident was 'probably the most embarrassing episode on the range'. He said: 'It left us a little bit unhappy as to why the British did this without informing us'.

Titterton's appearance before the Australian royal commission came six months after Turner's. When Titterton was asked why he did not warn Turner about the presence of cobalt 60 on the range, this is what Titterton replied:

When a group like this is involved on a deadly monotonous problem like surveying a range for large intervals over a large number of years, they get a bit bored. They get completely accustomed to what they are going to see. They begin over time to get lax. Now, it was possible – and this, I think is what Harry [Turner] resented, quite reasonably – it was possible by this curious circumstance to give Harry and his workers a bit of a test, quite a small test because the radioactivity of the cobalt was quite trivial compared to the radioactivity in the weapon. That meant for a period of time the radioactivity emanating from the weapon completely blotted out the residual cobalt, and, as time went by and the radioactivity decayed down and down, the cobalt emissions began to stand out. Now, they were very easy to find because there happens to be a unique signature for cobalt 60 in gamma ray terms.

Greg James, the Sydney QC appearing for several Australian nuclear veterans groups, asked Titterton if this was some test exercise of concealment.

No. It was absolutely a guaranteed situation that Turner and his group would find it. It was interesting to us, who were responsible for this operation, to see how quickly they found it. They came out of it with flying colours, actually. They did the job really very well.

Titterton's explanation did not sit easily with the contents of correspondence he conducted with Aldermaston at the time of the cobalt incident. In August 1958, Charles Adams, the Aldermaston scientist who had played senior roles at the Hurricane, Mosaic, Grapple and Antler trials, wrote to Titterton in the wake of the cobalt discovery:

You will probably remember that I told you at Antler that one of the assemblies had some Co 60 in it for tracer purposes. I have now heard that Turner in the course of routine surveys has found some small pellets in which he has identified Co 60. In order that this may not cause any disquiet to him he will be informed by signal that Co 60 was used as a tracer and that you, as chairman of the safety committee, knew and approved the action.

Personally I regard this as a matter of information that need go no further than the safety committee and Turner. However, I should be guided by your judgment here as to whether it should be passed on to anybody in the Department of Supply. There is of course nothing to worry about in the mere presence of Cobalt in the quantities used, but the name has a political flavour to it and I would consider it inexpedient to extend the chance of its being raised as a political issue. I hope your personal plans are becoming clearer and that you did not find your stay at Geneva too tedious.

This was the year that America, Russia and Britain held a conference in Geneva on the suspension of nuclear tests, something that resulted in an agreement by the three powers to a test moratorium. Titterton wrote back to Adams that he had taken up with the safety committee the matter in Adams's letter.

It will be minuted as a formality without the material being named. To keep everything straight, I brought Turner up from Maralinga and talked with him in the presence of the committee and I do not think he has done anything indiscreet; he did, however, inform Durance of the nature of the material and he tells me that Frank O'Connor [of the Australian Department of Supply] was also informed. I will have a word with O'Connor when I am next in Melbourne, and I do not see any reason why the information should go further than that.

At the Australian royal commission in Sydney in May 1985, Greg James put to Titterton that, on a reading of this correspondence, Titterton's explanation to the royal commission about a little test on the range to find the cobalt 60 was nonsense. 'Are you calling me a liar?' Titterton demanded. 'Yes, Sir Ernest, I am calling you a liar', James replied. Titterton said: 'I find that whenever people lose arguments that they cannot win logically they resort to shouting outrageous things at the person that they were unable to beat. That is all I wish to say.'

What were the British scientists doing with cobalt in the Tadje bomb? In the early days of nuclear weapons technology, some scientists envisaged the idea of a cobalt bomb, or 'doomsday' weapon. This had to do with the fact that cobalt 60 has a half life of 5.3 years – that is, the time taken for half its radioactive products to decay – and is an emitter of gamma rays, the most penetrating form of ionising radiation. As Turner explained the principle of such a bomb, nonradioactive cobalt 59 would be used as a tamper and in the explosion it would absorb neutrons and become cobalt 60. This meant that with cobalt 60 pulverised and injected into the atmosphere the fallout would last for a long time, and the people in the fallout zone could continue to be contaminated for several years after the blast.

If this was the nature of the British experiment it must have failed because the cobalt, instead of volatilising in the weapon as it would be expected to do, was left lying in pellet form on the ground. Titterton did concede under questioning at the Australian royal commission that the cobalt 60 was originally inserted into the bomb in order to assist in the diagnosis of the yield; he admitted he did not tell other members of the Australian safety committee about the cobalt before the explosion. Dr John Symonds, who, in 1985, wrote a history of the British atomic tests for the Department of Resources and Energy in Canberra, gave this explanation of the cobalt in his document:

The cobalt 60 sample was placed in the Tadje device for the purpose of assisting in the determination of the energy released at the time of the explosion. In many instances, it had been previously possible to obtain such data through the radiochemical examination of particulate matter collected on filters by aircraft flying through the cloud, though the results were often found to be heavily dependent on a number of rather obscure factors.

Symonds continued:

With some of the experimental tests at Maralinga and elsewhere, it was determined that analysis was likely to be more reasonable if a known amount of radioactive material could be added to the device as a tracer which would not depend on a variety of difficult assumptions. Other tracer methods had been tried though not very successfully. The cobalt 60 tracer used at Tadje was thrust away from the main fireball without very much mixing being achieved and was, in consequence, almost a complete failure.

The full story of the use of cobalt in the Maralinga trials still requires an answer. Titterton refused to give it at the royal commission, and added to the air of mystery, when he said: 'I cannot tell you that. That is weapons information.' Significantly, Menzies had been questioned in parliament on at least two occasions as early as 1953 about the possibility of Britain testing a cobalt bomb in Australia. He was asked to give an assurance that this would not happen. Menzies replied: 'I have stated repeatedly that the important tests that will take place from time to time at the Woomera range will not be associated with any danger to Australian lives'.

Britain continued to test hydrogen weapons in the Pacific during 1958, but the Antler trials at Maralinga turned out to be the last nuclear bomb tests she ever conducted in Australia. The moratorium on nuclear tests between Britain, America and the Soviet Union came into being at the end of 1958 after a spate of atmospheric weapons tests by each of the three powers during that year – 5 by Britain, 25 by the Soviet Union and a staggering 48 by the United States. The US conducted a further 18 nuclear tests either underground, underwater or at high altitude in the same year.[20]

By the time the moratorium ended in 1961, so had Britain's nuclear estrangement from the United States. The goal Winston Churchill had set on his return to office in 1951, of restoring full Anglo-American atomic collaboration, was finally achieved in July 1958, under another Conservative prime minister, Harold Macmillan, when the United States amended its Atomic Energy Act to permit the exchange of information about the design and production of nuclear warheads and the transfer of fissile materials between the two countries. Britain had succeeded in her long drive to revive, as Churchill had put it, 'her former influence and initiative among the allied powers' – or so it seemed. The British independent nuclear deterrent, so agonisingly and successfully developed, henceforth would become an adjunct of the massive United States strategic nuclear weapons machine, and, after 1961, Britain would conduct her nuclear tests jointly with the United States underground at the place Penney had wanted from the very beginning: the Nevada test site.

The British had never lost sight of this objective during all the tribulations and uncertainties of the testing program in Australia.

The Hurricane test at Monte Bello in 1952 had been deliberately conducted as an all-British affair, with no American observers invited, just so the British could make the point that they were capable of making and testing a bomb without anybody else's assistance. Churchill played up this essentially political point of the Monte Bello test when he said afterwards: 'We have conducted the operation ourselves, and I do not doubt that it will lead to a much closer American interchange of information than has hitherto taken place'. [21]

When that full interchange was restored six years later, it was the result of several key factors. First, the growing military and scientific strength of the Soviet Union had convinced the Americans of the need for greater co-operation within the Western alliance to match the Soviet advances. The Soviets' launch in October 1957 of Sputnik, the world's first space satellite, was a shattering revelation to the Americans and the British, just as the first Soviet explosions of an atomic bomb in 1949 and of a thermonuclear device in 1953 had been. Sputnik, launched by a rocket, signalled the onset of a new race between the two superpowers for a new means of delivering their nuclear warheads, on medium range and intercontinental missiles. Henceforth, Britain and America decided that the concept of national self-sufficiency in military matters was now out of date, to be replaced by a concept of interdependence which meant combining resources and sharing tasks in many fields.

Second, the leaders in office by the late fifties, Harold Macmillan of Britain and President Eisenhower of the United States, were particularly attuned to giving currency to this new mood and to restoring full atomic collaboration between their two countries. For his part, Eisenhower had always believed that the McMahon Act, passed before his presidency began, had treated America's old wartime ally too unfairly. Macmillan, like Churchill before him, believed in giving the Anglo-American alliance top priority and in trying to recapture some of the old spirit of the 'grand strategy'.

The most important reason for the restoration of full atomic relations, however, was the sheer success of Britain's independent nuclear weapons program. Britain's atomic tests in Australia and her explosion of her first hydrogen bomb in May 1957, deeply impressed the Americans. The British achievements dramatically demonstrated the point that America had no more secrets to keep from the British. Moreover, from the point where Britain had decided to manufacture H-bombs to the time when she independently tested one had taken her no longer than it had taken the Americans for the same task. American officials came to the conclusion that there was really no point in continuing to refuse to share their nuclear knowledge.

On his way home from the Buffalo trials at the end of 1956, Penney made a stop in New York. Ever conscious of the need to drive this point home in Washington, he gave an interview in which he tactfully boasted about what the British had achieved from Maralinga:

We have made substantial advances in weapon design. We have learnt a lot about the effect of explosions on military equipment, indoctrinated a lot of service officers into atomic warfare, and learnt a lot of things important in civil defence. We have learnt how much protection shelters give, how blast damages various types of structure under accurate control conditions – all knowledge which we did not have very accurately before. [22]

Maralinga was remembered somewhat differently by those people who actually worked in the army or civilian construction teams on the bomb sites, oblivious to the highly charged political nature of the whole exercise. One of them was Robert Southwell, a Briton who went to Australia in 1955, when he was 21, to travel the world and earn money. Southwell and a friend answered a newspaper advertisement and ended up with jobs at Maralinga, which took them into the ground zeros after explosions to retrieve the battle dresses and boots from the experimental dummies propped up there for the bombs. Unlike the dummies, Southwell and his mates were never issued with protective clothing. What was his conclusion of the whole business? 'I regard the whole Maralinga episode as a very well-paid adventure, and had no idea at all of the risks involved in dealing with radiation.' [23]

Chapter Six
'MINOR TRIALS'

'What is going on at Maralinga?' – Question to Howard Beale, the
Australian minister for supply, in the House of Representatives, Canberra,
September 1956.

Maralinga today looks much as it must have done in the mid-fifties,
at the height of its fame. The airport with its huge runway is still
there, complete with the decaying arrival hall, which no-one now
uses, giving it the strange air of a scene from a Nevil Shute novel.
The remarkable network of sealed roads radiating out from the
village to the bomb sites is still there, almost as good as the day it
was built, but it carries no traffic. Maralinga village itself has lost
none of its beautiful setting, on a red hilltop surrounded by plains
of dense mulga overlooking a distant range of blue hills. But the
abandoned village has an eerie feel. Most of the buildings have been
dismantled and taken away, leaving only a home for the resident
policemen who patrol the range in Land Rovers every day. They
live in what was once the hospital, which still contains the original
wooden stretchers with canvas coverings. In the mornings and
evenings, the trees around the building are alive with hordes of
dazzling pink and white Major Mitchell cockatoos, and at night a
dingo creeps up to feed on scraps left especially by the policemen,
then slinks back into the scrub. The tennis courts, their markings
just visible, have been almost overtaken by weeds. The open-air
swimming pool has been filled in with dirt, but a dilapidated
fountainhead remains at one end with a faded sign advising
swimmers to shower before entering the pool.

If you left the village and drove 30 kilometres north to the
forward area, where the trials actually happened, and walked across

the range carrying a geiger counter at a site called Taranaki, the only sound that would disturb the silence and tranquility would be the wild clicking of the machine registering radioactivity from fragments of plutonium mixed crudely in the dirt. The plutonium is a legacy not of the atomic bomb that was exploded at Taranaki in October 1957, the very last of the British atomic weapons to be tested at Maralinga. Rather, it came from a series of secret experiments that were carried on long after the bomb trials were over, and which went under the inoffensive title of 'minor trials'.

The minor trials actually began at Emu Field in 1953, and transferred to Maralinga in 1955 where they continued until 1963. In the early days, Britain had considered holding some of these minor trials at Wick, on the northeast coast of Scotland, but the idea was abandoned because the damp weather would have upset the delicate monitoring equipment. Penney explained to the Australian royal commission another reason why Wick was spared the minor trials:

I think any minor trial in the UK would have taken a lot of careful thought. If it had a dangerous material in it, a radioactive material, in the UK you cannot get away from water running into rivers and that sort of thing, whereas out in Maralinga there was nothing like that.

Their name was later changed to assessment trials and, finally, to the Maralinga Experimental Programme, largely so that it would not appear as if Britain was cheating during the weapons test ban from 1958 to 1961. (The full bomb tests, by contrast, came to be known as the 'major trials'. For convenience, the name minor trials has been retained in the text to cover all the other experiments, whatever they were called at the time – assessment tests, experiments or minor trials.)

Most of the minor trials involving plutonium took place at Maralinga during the period of the test moratorium from November 1958 to September 1961. Because of their nature they would appear to have violated at least the spirit of that ban, to which Britain claimed to have adhered, hence the great secrecy surrounding them. As we shall see, this problem was rationalised because any explosions involved were kept below a level that could be detected by the Russians and Americans, so that Britain was able to continue its weapons development program in Australia while the moratorium was on.

The minor trials went under the code names Kittens, Tims, Rats and Vixen – names which, as Penney later admitted, were designed not to inform people about their true nature. The Kittens, Tims and Rats trials basically were tests on component parts of nuclear weapons. With Kittens, the tests were designed to refine the initiator, the source of the neutrons that actually trigger off an atomic explosion, and to measure the output of neutrons from the initiator. Tims and Rats were tests of a key aspect of the implosion technique of achieving nuclear fission: both series of tests used different methods to measure how the central fissile core of an implosion weapon behaves when compressed, or squashed, by the impact of chemical explosives.

The Vixen trials began in 1959 and were conducted in two stages, Vixen A and Vixen B. They were designed to see how a fully assembled nuclear weapon, and the fissile material it contained, would behave in an accident, such as an aircraft crash or a fire in a weapons store: would a nuclear explosion be triggered off in such circumstances? For this reason, the Vixen trials were known as safety assessment tests, a curious name in view of the highly radioactive plutonium they left behind.

The precise number of minor trials has never been fully documented, but it seems from information the British government supplied to the Australian royal commission in 1985 that there were up to 700, from the start of Kittens in 1953 to the finish of Vixen 10 years later. The earlier minor trials, Kittens, in which plutonium was not involved, were announced to the press, but they were usually described uninformatively in terms similar to those used by Penney in Sydney in September 1953, as 'merely tests to obtain scientific information'.

The Tims and Vixen trials differed from the others in that they used plutonium: in the case of Vixen, plutonium was actually burned in petrol fires to see how it would behave in an accident. But many of the other minor trials involved the dispersion on the Maralinga range of radioactive uranium and polonium and toxic beryllium.

The plutonium is the greatest hazard remaining at Maralinga today. It is present in the topsoil at four sites where plutonium trials took place after 1959: Taranaki, Wewak, TM100 and TM101. In fact, the Australian royal commission confirmed from evidence that Maralinga is probably the only place in the Western world where plutonium is dispersed without precise knowledge of how much is above and below the ground (there is no information about the condition of former Soviet nuclear test sites). By far the most significant plutonium contamination is at Taranaki where it was dispersed in plumes along the ground and carried in fine powder form by winds around the site. The precise amount of plutonium used in these trials had always remained a mystery because the available records were incomplete and the British authorities had refused to give details.

But in 1984, the UK Ministry of Defence provided information on the plutonium used in the Tims and Vixen trials from 1959 to 1963, giving a total amount of plutonium used as 24.4 kilograms. About 900 grams of this was later returned to the UK – about 400 grams from a Vixen A trial, returned in 1959, and 500 grams from a Tims trial, returned in 1979. The remainder, 23.5 kilograms, is still at Maralinga, either scattered on the range or in burial pits mixed in with other radioactive debris. These figures, of course, do not include the plutonium used in the earlier major bomb trials. [1]

Plutonium is one of the most dangerous substances known. It has a long half life, more than 24 000 years – that is, the period taken for one half of its radioactivity to decay. It is particularly hazardous if inhaled in particle form because of its propensity for causing cancer if it lodges in the lung. To give an idea of its toxicity, experiments have deduced that 16 milligrams of insoluble plutonium in the lungs would cause death within one month; put another way, 0.3 milligrams, about the same size as a speck of dirt, lodged in the lung would give a 50 per cent probability of cancer induction. [2]

In 1967, after Britain had decided it had no further use for Maralinga as a testing site, it sent a team of royal engineers to Australia to clean up the range. Operation Brumby, as this exercise was called, was cursory because any plutonium that could not be recovered and buried in pits was simply mixed into the soil by ploughing and grading; in some places, several centimetres of fresh topsoil were then thrown over it. Some of the contaminated areas were fenced off, although others were left completely open, and Maralinga was quietly forgotten until it shot into the headlines again in the late seventies.

Operation Brumby took little account of the winds and duststorms that prevail at Maralinga. Penney was asked at the Australian royal commission whether those who conducted the plutonium experiments in the minor trials would not have assumed that, over a period of time, the plutonium would be likely to spread outside the range itself. He replied: 'If plutonium were the same density as dust, I would say yes. Plutonium is not heavy stuff. I do not know. I have to concede it might spread.'

When scientists from the Australian Radiation Laboratory (ARL) conducted a survey during 1984 and 1985 of radioactive contamination at the Maralinga sites, using detection equipment more sophisticated than that available in 1967, they found plutonium dispersed across a wider area than previously realised; they also discovered that a considerable number of fragments were scattered outside the fence erected years earlier at Taranaki which encloses 19 shallow burial pits containing plutonium mixed in with radioactive debris. There were no fences around the contamination at the other sites, Wewak, TM100 and TM101, until the ARL scientists ordered temporary fences to be put up during their survey in July, 1984. The ARL presented a report of its survey in April, 1985, during the royal commission's visit to Maralinga. Its findings are worth summarising because of the light they throw on the plutonium hazards and the enormous task facing the British and Australian governments if the range is to be properly cleaned up – especially as the contamination extends over land to which the traditional Aboriginal owners now wish to return.

At Taranaki, the ARL scientists found many areas of very high plutonium activity, or 'hot spots'. Most of them came from metal fragments contaminated with plutonium – in fact, the scientists concluded there were up to 100 000 of these tiny fragments lying on the ground or buried just below the surface. They consisted mainly of fractured pieces of steel or light alloys ranging in size from 0.5 mm to a few centimetres. The scientists also detected a large plutonium plume at Taranaki which, apparently, had not been isolated before and which they called the northwest plume because of its direction. Their probes detected contamination in this plume 18 kilometres from the firing pad, and even soil samples taken 32 kilometres away revealed some light contamination. The ARL scientists concluded that their ground surveys could not account for more than 10 to 20 per cent of the plutonium used in the minor trials at Taranaki; they assumed the rest was in the Taranaki burial pits. The scientists also found plutonium on the surface at Wewak, TM100 and TM101, but in much smaller concentrations than at Taranaki.

They discovered at other minor trials sites remnants of natural uranium, uranium 235 and uranium 238, as well as small amounts of beryllium. Although it is not a radioactive substance like uranium and plutonium, beryllium is a toxic chemical which can cause serious illnesses when inhaled into the lungs in particle form.

It can lead to beryllicosis, a lung disease, as well as pneumonitis and bronchitis. Beryllium is used as a reflector to increase the efficiency of the chain reaction in a fission bomb. According to evidence presented to the Australian royal commission, at least 101 kilograms of beryllium was used in the minor trials, only a fraction of which has been accounted for since. Indeed, the ARL admitted its survey was never intended to be an exhaustive discovery of the beryllium still at Maralinga – 'only a feel for the magnitude and extent of any beryllium contamination'.

The ARL scientists concluded in their 1985 report that plutonium was present in high concentrations over large areas at Maralinga, and now represented the major hazard on the range because of the dangers of humans inhaling fine particles of it. The main risk to a casual visitor to Maralinga, they believed, was probably from souvenir hunting: 'A fragment of metal picked up and handled could be contaminated with plutonium, and such actions could result in the ingestion or inhalation of substantial quantities of radioactive material'. The scientists also concluded that the way in which plutonium had been disposed at Maralinga, even in shallow burial pits sealed with cement, was not acceptable by current practice.

How, then, did the plutonium get there – and how did the

governments and scientists at the time of the minor trials allow it to be disposed of in such a careless way?

The minor trials were always shrouded in even more secrecy and mystery than the major bomb trials themselves. Britain gave Australia even less information about the minor trials than it gave about the major trials, excluded any Australian representatives, including the Australian safety committee, from attending the minor trials and pointedly asked the Australian government to give the minor trials no publicity at all because of the embarrassment Britain could suffer over the nuclear test moratorium after 1958. Australia went along with all these arrangements, but not as willingly as it had with the earlier, major bomb trials.

Up to 1959, the Australian safety committee recommended that all the minor trials be allowed to go ahead, and the Menzies government accepted its advice even though the information available to Australia had been particularly scanty. From 1959 onwards, the minor trials involved far deeper political tension between Britain and Australia than any trials that had gone before – major or minor – because Australian government officials realised that some of these trials could involve a nuclear explosion in Australia at a time of a moratorium on nuclear weapons tests and when discussions were under way in Geneva on a possible complete cessation of tests.

From that point onwards, the Australian government began to intervene far more than it had done in the past, insisting that Britain make information available directly to Australian ministers and senior bureaucrats, as well as to the Australian safety committee of scientists. So, for the first time, the Australian government declined to rely exclusively on the safety committee to keep it informed. Titterton's role was particularly important at this time because, as chairman of the safety committee, he was usually the first point of contact with the British and, as such, he usually received information in advance of other safety committee members and the Australian government.

The problems really began in 1959, when the British decided to include plutonium in the minor trials for the first time, with Vixen A. Even before the full nature of these trials was known, Titterton appears to have told the British that there would be no problems in principle about conducting them. Early in 1959, a British official in Australia cabled to London that Britain could expect to receive formal consent from Australia for the forthcoming trials soon. The message added:

A difficulty arose because the safety committee whose advice was sought had been given no information on the proposed trials. Fortunately Titterton took it upon himself to agree in principle even though he had no details. I think it important that [Aldermaston] should follow the previous practice and should release to Titterton as much information as they can about the forthcoming series. Can you press them to do so?

The British were worried about the possible political sensitivity of the Australian government to the inclusion of plutonium in the Vixen trials. As mentioned in Chapter Three, they discussed the best way of approaching Australia on this question. They agreed that Penney should write personally to Titterton seeking his advice on how to get Australian government approval, which Penney did on 15 June 1959. Penney explained in his letter that, as part of the Vixen safety tests, the British wanted to conduct two trials to determine the dispersion of plutonium under 'representative field conditions', in other words the sort of fire that may result from an accident. Originally, the plutonium trials were planned for 1960, but it had been decided to bring them ahead one year. The proposal was to carry out two trials in each of which about 200 grams of plutonium metal would be burned in a controlled petrol fire. Penney outlined the safety conditions under which the trials would be held, including the estimated amount of plutonium that would become airborne, and concluded: 'We hope the results will be of general interest, and we should, of course, make them available to Australia'.

It is clear from British documents at this time that the British saw Titterton as their best channel for riding through any political problems with Australia. Captain F. B. Lloyd, a senior official in charge of atomic weapons trials in the British Ministry of Aviation (formerly the Ministry of Supply), had a meeting lasting one hour with Titterton in Canberra and reported back in London in May

I am convinced that our best way of getting through any possibly awkward proposals is to brief Titterton in the first place and then, if required, go through official channels. Indeed, Titterton may well get this through without any additional action.

Titterton cabled Penney that he believed there would be 'no serious problems in obaining agreement'; he then wrote a letter recommending such agreement to Alan Hulme, the successor as minister for supply to Beale who, by now, had taken up residence as Australia's ambassador in Washington. Titterton recommended that approval of the Vixen trials be given subject to certain conditions, including that the results be made available to Australia and that no material used in the trials should escape beyond the restricted area at Maralinga – although, based on past experience, it seems difficult to understand how either condition could be guaranteed in advance. He told the minister that while the safety committee had no reservations about the trials from a safety viewpoint,

I should perhaps mention that they do differ from normal 'minor' trials in that, for the first time, fissile material would be used in them and this has some slight political overtones in view of the discussions in Geneva relating to nuclear weapon tests.

Hulme sent Titterton's comments to Athol Townley, the minister for defence, saying that he, Hulme, felt inclined to agree to Penney's approach. Townley was concerned about the political implications of the Vixen A trials, and advised that he and Hulme should discuss the question urgently with Menzies. When he learned of the British proposals, the prime minister consulted his senior departmental advisers who warned him that Australia had very little information about the trials and should seek more in view of the discussions going on at Geneva.

The political significance of the British trials had now become a prime Australian government concern, even greater than the question of radiological safeguards, and it remained so until the minor trials ended in 1963. But it was almost as if this political concern had intruded too late. Arrangements once made between friendly governments, such as the memorandum of 1956 giving Britain use of Maralinga for ten years, are difficult to undo, especially when the conditions that attach to them are less than stringent.

In spite of the nagging worries, the Menzies government approved the Vixen trials of 1959, just as it approved all the following requests for minor trials. Townley wrote back to Hulme in July 1959:

I am quite happy as to the technical and scientific aspects as outlined by Professor Titterton, and, having complete confidence in him and his Committee, I am not troubled very much by the trials in themselves. This assumes that the recommendations of the safety committee are accepted by the United Kingdom.

The Australian defence minister's letter continued:

The political aspects, however, can be potentially dangerous. The Geneva meeting which you mention has a bearing on it. There is also the fact that for the first time it is proposed to use explosives on the Woomera range which will bring the usual howl from the 'Ban the H Bomb' section of the community – Communist and otherwise.

It is my view, therefore, that there should be some political discussion on it. This might be done by yourself and the Prime Minister, or perhaps the Prime Minister and one or two others. I would hesitate to put it into full Cabinet, purely on the 'need to know' basis.

As the years went on, ministers and their advisers raised objections, caused delays and exchanged terse correspondence with British officials and the Australian safety committee itself; but they never followed their concerns to their logical conclusion and stopped the trials. The Australian minister for supply approved a further round of Tims, Rats and Vixen A trials for 1960, although the proposal from Britain had not named specific materials to be used in them, saying only that 'radioactive and toxic materials similar to those employed during 1959 will be used'.

It was in early 1960 that the British first raised with Australia, through Titterton, their wish to extend the Vixen program that year with a more elaborate series of tests known as Vixen B. British officials on a visit to Australia sought Titterton's view on the problem of creating long-term contamination on the Maralinga range from the trials. Titterton told them that, in his view, such contamination was acceptable as long as the British were able to give assurances that contamination would not go outside the range boundaries. [3]

But the Vixen B proposals were to signal a significant change by Australia in its manner of dealing with the British. Australian officials, particularly those in the Department of Defence, had become increasingly worried over the way that all scientific information about the trials was concentrated on a small number of people, the Australian safety committee, and particularly its chairman, Titterton. Because of his regular visits to Britain where he discussed the minor trials at first hand with scientists at Aldermaston, Titterton held more information than anyone else in Australia on which the safety and political judgments of the trials had to be made.

Australian officials had begun to realise that the existing arrangements for communicating with the British had been set up years earlier when the political sensitivity of the British tests had not weighed in Canberra so heavily if, indeed, at all. For its part, Britain at this time took the view that it was simply fulfilling the letter of the original arrangments, set up when the safety committee was formed back in 1955, to pass on to Titterton, as safety committee chairman, such details as it chose to reveal. It had never given safety information directly to the Australian government when seeking approval for the major bomb trials in the past, and it saw even less reason to do so now for the minor trials. As one senior Whitehall civil servant wrote confidentially to a colleague at this time:

We do not specify, nor does the Australian government enquire into, the details of our experiments when seeking formal approval. Such approval is always subject to Titterton's safety committee accepting a detailed safety statement... I agree, therefore, with Titterton that we should avoid formal communications on these contentious experiments and propose that we proceed without going through the normal channels.

By the middle of 1960, Australian officials in the Defence, Supply and Prime Minister's Departments, as well as the ministers for defence and supply, were deeply involved in discussions on two key issues: the adequacy of the information available from Britain to Australia over the proposed trials, and possible new arrangements for approving the trials. Until now, the formal channel of communication had always been the safety committee signalling its approval of any trials to the prime minister, through the minister for supply, who, in turn, gave final approval to Britain. But the political and bureaucratic concern about this arrangement that had now built up was reflected in a note filed in the Prime Minister's Department, at the time of these discussions, that 'we had some doubts as to whether enough information had been passed to the safety committee in relation to the Vixen B series to enable the safety committee to form a considered judgment'. Titterton and the other safety committee members strongly objected to what they took as this implied criticism of their professional integrity.

But although there were these secret ministerial and bureaucratic concerns in Canberra about Australia being kept in the dark, Athol Townley, the minister for defence, was displaying a more sanguine view in public. In August 1958, he referred in parliament to the projects at Maralinga and Woomera as being carried out 'jointly by the Australian government and the United Kingdom government', and told MPs: 'We have access, of course, to everything in the nature of tests carried out at the two places'.

The result of all this was a new arrangement which gave the minister for defence final responsibility for advising the British, through the Prime Minister's Department, of final approval of the new trials. In addition, Sir Leslie Martin and another senior defence department official in future would have access to the same information as that which the British passed to the safety committee before each trial. The safety committee would continue to advise the government on safety questions, the possible damage or injury to persons and property and so on; but Martin and his colleague were to examine the proposals and advise on the wider political ramifications of the trials.

Martin was still the scientific adviser to the Department of Defence, putting him in a key role. He had been, of course, the inaugural chairman of the safety committee but had left it in 1957 to become a member of the new National Radiation Advisory Committee, a body whose formation he himself had suggested. Martin's concern at that time appears to have been to have a body separate from the safety committee which could concentrate on the biological questions arising from fallout from the atomic tests, following the rows over the Mosaic and some of the Buffalo explosions. He and others at the Defence Department were now concerned about the proposals for the Vixen B trials, which, from the little information they had, could possibly appear to involve a complete weapon as assembled for storage or transit undergoing a 'safety' test. Martin explained to two British atomic weapons officials who visited Australia towards the end of 1960 why the Australian government now felt it must have political advice on the minor trials, apart from the advice it received from the safety committee: there was, he said, no question of distrusting the safety committee, but they were not in a position to assess the political as opposed to the technical risks.

As a result of the new arrangements, Townley was eventually told that the aim of Vixen B was to find out what would happen to certain types of nuclear weapons if they were damaged by fire or bombing while in storage or transit. The test device would be an operational weapon complete with firing mechanism, but assembled in such a way that the core could not become critical. Nevertheless, considerable quantities of plutonium would be involved, and the radioactive danger area for the Vixen B tests had been set down as a radius of 38 kilometres.

Townley approved these, the first Vixen B trials, and they took place at Taranaki over a month from early September 1960. Although the weapon was designed not to achieve full criticality, the question of what did and did not constitute a minor nuclear explosion in these and other Vixen trials – which were taking place at the time of the nuclear test ban agreement – is a delicate one. Penney took the view that as long as any explosion in these trials was achieved predominantly by chemical means, and the fissile reaction was kept to a small level which could still be detected by instruments, then the exercise could be termed an experiment and not a proper nuclear test.

Penney was questioned about this on the final day of the Australian royal commission's hearings in London in March 1985, when he was asked whether the Vixen B experiments involved very small nuclear explosions. He replied: 'Yes. No, wait a minute. The difficulty was no-one could define what a nuclear explosion was. We discussed this with the Russians and we tried definition after definition and in the end everyone gave up.' Penney was also asked about the position which he and his colleagues took about holding these trials during the test ban. He agreed that the British eventually decided that any fission explosion kept to a power of less than 10 tonnes of TNT equivalent would not be a breach of any treaty, and that part of the reason for adopting that definition was because anything below 10 tonnes could not be detected by outsiders. 'We are now talking about tiny little things which may be defined as an explosion or not', he said.

The proposal which Britain sent to Australia for further Vixen trials in 1961 was as vague as all the earlier statements, containing no specific information on the purpose of the trials, their nature and the materials and equipment to be used. At one point, as defence officials in Canberra sought more details, the British high commission suggested that the simplest way for them to fill in the gaps would be 'to have a chat with Titterton'. The Prime Minister's Department in Canberra later tersely rejected this advise, and pointed out to the high commission that the information on which the minister for defence made his decision to approve the trials should be official UK information.

In fact, Townley refused to approve the 1961 trials until Britain had sent two senior atomic weapons officials to Canberra to brief him. He eventually gave his approval after requesting that any device be eliminated from the trials which, from its external configuration, might be taken rightly or wrongly as an operational weapon. The 1961 Vixen B trials went ahead at Taranaki during April and May. There were no minor trials at all the following year because, by then, Britain had resumed full-scale nuclear testing at Nevada after the breakdown of the three-power test moratorium, and could not stretch its resources to a Maralinga program concurrently.

The final trials of any sort took place at Maralinga in April-May, 1963, when four Vixen B tests were performed at the Taranaki site. Britain had advised Australia earlier that plutonium and beryllium would be involved and that a fissile reaction was possible which could produce a quanitity of fission products which would give rise to radiological effects only of a comparable magnitude to those from the parent material, plutonium. [4]

Again, the Australian government approved the 1963 program; but it was against a background of mounting Australian concern, not to say alarm in some quarters, that two senior British officials visited Australia in October and November 1962, to discuss the final round of trials and the future of the Maralinga range itself. These two British officials were Roy Pilgrim, the head of safety co-ordination at Aldermaston, and L.T. Williams, the director general of atomic weapons in the Ministry of Aviation. We are fortunate in having a detailed confidential report which Pilgrim and Williams made of their visit, plus an impressionistic account of the visit which Pilgrim prepared separately, both of which go a long way towards explaining the deep political undercurrents in Australia and the tensions between Canberra and London at that time.

The British reports reveal a remarkable degree of political cynicism and power play on both sides regarding events at Maralinga – the Menzies government being concerned, more than anything else, with its own survival and the British with keeping their options open about using Maralinga for further trials without giving Australia any guarantees or commitments.

The British visitors arrived in Australia at a time when the Menzies government was acutely conscious of its knife-edge political survival. At the 1961 general elections a year earlier, called in the middle of an economic credit squeeze, Menzies' conservative Liberal-Country Party coalition had scraped back to power with a working majority of only one – and even that seat had been decided on the distribution of preferential votes from a Communist candidate. The MP who won it was James Killen, a Queensland lawyer, who, since his election to parliament six years earlier, had emerged as one of the most conservative figures in Menzies' party on questions of defence and foreign policy and who, himself, was to be hurled into the spotlight of the Maralinga story some 17 years later.

Pilgrim and Williams began their visit in Melbourne with a meeting with the British high commissioner, Sir William Oliver. The high commissioner pointed out that the agreement with Australia for the operation of the Maralinga range was due to terminate in about three years, and that the British needed to work out their future policy if they wanted to negotiate a new one. Pilgrim and Williams reported:

He was convinced that these negotiations would be difficult and indeed might fail altogether unless the UK was able to give the Australians much more information about the object and nature of the experiments and also a somewhat greater share in the control of the Range.

After lunch they went to see Sir Leslie Martin in his Melbourne office.

Sir Leslie made some very blunt observations during this talk; his main point being that Australia gained no benefit whatever from the Maralinga Experimental Programme and that while he had agreed to the Programme for 1963 he would never again agree to a Maralinga Experimental Programme unless it were preceded by a much fuller exchange of information. [5]

We took the conventional line, trying to convince Sir Leslie that the UK had in fact provided all the relevant information which could reasonably be expected, short of detailed diagrams of the devices to be functioned, but the most that could be secured from Sir Leslie was the statement that while they did not expect to see detailed weights, dimensions and layouts, they did expect to learn a good deal more about the general plan behind the experiments and a general picture of the procedures.

It must be said at once that these comments of Sir Leslie, which bore out precisely the anticipations of the UK High Commissioner, were repeated to us in virtually every interview we had during the whole visit. The rationale behind them appears to lie in the fear of the Australian Government, which has the slenderest possible Parliamentary majority, of some untoward incident occurring at the Range in circumstances in which they could be depicted to the Australian public as having wholly inadequate control of events taking place on Australian territory.

In this respect, one incident which Australian officials kept raising with the two British visitors was an unfortunate escape of balloons from Maralinga which had happened during the Vixen B trials in September 1960. Balloons were used in some minor trials to support equipment and measuring devices as a means of picking up a broad range of information about the spread of material from the experiments. On this occasion, eight balloons had been prepared to gather data and had been tethered by cables at different distances from the firing site, but on the night before a planned trial seven of them broke away from their moorings during a wind squall. Five balloons were recovered a few kilometres from the trials area, but the other two managed to drift as far as Cobar, an outback town of New South Wales, and Hungerford, on the border between New South Wales and Queensland – some 1400 kilometres from Maralinga. The incident was deeply embarrassing, and led to a committee of inquiry into how it could have happened. The committee found there had been no safety plan for the balloons, that the self destruct mechanism on the balloons was not reliable and that there were no markings on the balloons warning that they were filled with hydrogen and that an explosion was possible.

The balloons affair inevitably cropped up when Pilgrim and Williams went to Canberra the next day. At a meeting with officials from the Prime Minister's and Defence Departments, they reported:

The opportunity was taken once more to remind us of the concern felt by the Minister of Defence over safety, particularly since the memory of the balloon incident was still very much alive with him. In fact, it is reasonably certain from what was said that the Minister of Defence is less concerned with safety, which he is satisfied to entrust to the Safety Committee, than with political embarrassment. At all these interviews the narrowness of the Government majority was stressed and the consequent sensitivity to even the slightest possibility of any kind of Maralinga incident which could come to the ears of the public.

Some of the senior Australian public servants took the two Britons into their confidence about their views on Australia's stand on Maralinga and nuclear weapons generally in the post-Menzies era, which they rightly predicted was now on the horizon. At their meeting with two top men from the Prime Minister's Department, J.F. Nimmo and A.T. Griffith, the British reported that,

stress was laid on the possibility that the Government may change in which case, in Mr Nimmo's view, we should not assume that the incoming Government would necessarily demand the closure of Maralinga as an Experimental Range . . . This advice assumed that such an incoming Government would be formed by the Labour Party. Similarly, Mr Kingsland of the Defence Department gave his personal view that in the event of a Liberal-Country Party Coalition Government without Mr Menzies as Prime Minister succeeding the present government, then Australia might favour the possession of her own nuclear capability.

Pilgrim and Williams went on to the Australian National University for talks with Titterton, whom, they reported, showed no particular anxiety about the amount of information he was getting from Britain on the minor trials.

Professor Titterton gave us his usual reassurances that the political worries of the Department of Defence are not to be regarded too seriously and there is no doubt that he continues to press his view on the Minister that the Department's doubts are unjustified. Elsewhere, however, views were expressed to us that Professor Titterton had probably overplayed his hand in this respect and he is now having little influence other than on questions of safety.

One of the British officials, Roy Pilgrim, wrote his own separate and secret account of his impressions about the British relationship with Australia over Maralinga when he returned to London. He concluded that Australia's policy of seeking tighter control over events at Maralinga was at least partly prompted by the feeling that Maralinga was not giving either side value for money.

Australia considers that she is getting nothing from her contribution and, as a result of the cancellation of the 1962 programme and the very few firings proposed for 1963, she is beginning to express doubts as to whether UK is making enough use to justify the continued existence of the Range.

Pilgrim concluded that Sir Leslie Martin's blunt threat not to approve any more tests there without receiving more information 'showed that he was suspicious of our behaviour and that in the future he intended to force us to "come clean" '.

Pilgrim then weighed up the advantages and disadvantages of any possible future government in Australia and its implications for the British at Maralinga. He concluded that Menzies conceivably could be defeated at any time, although the opposition Labor party was still suffering from a recent history of turbulence and could need time to become sufficiently united before winning an election.

Quite apart from this aspect it should also be realised that Mr Menzies must be approaching the time when he will decide to retire. This is significant since, from our point of view, a Liberal-Country Party Coalition Government would be likely to have a different policy according to whether or not it is headed by Mr Menzies.

As far as the British were concerned, Pilgrim noted, a government led by Menzies gave a reasonable measure of co-operation and assistance 'without excessive insistence on information'. But a future Liberal-Country Party government not led by Menzies would adopt a different attitude and might favour Australia possessing a nuclear capability of her own, and joining the nuclear club.

Under such circumstances there could be strong pressure on UK to give Australia warhead information and an attempt to turn Maralinga and its activities into a combined project on the lines of Woomera and W.R.E. Salisbury.

(It is interesting that at this stage, late 1962, three years before Menzies' eventual retirement, these British reports contained no names on which of Menzies' colleagues might succeed him as leader or their likely stands on policy.)

Pilgrim concluded by considering what the Labor party and its leader, by now Arthur Calwell, might do if they became the government.

There is some feeling in the Prime Minister's Department that . . . it would not be out of the question for Mr Calwell to accept advice leading to a maintenance of something like the present situation as far as we are concerned. On the other hand, it has to be recognised that the Australian Opposition has for some time hoped for support for Brazil's proposal that South America and Africa should become a nuclear free zone and, in the event of such support being forthcoming, to want to extend the zone to include all the Southern Hemisphere.

This prediction, at least, was borne out. In 1985, the Labor government in Australia led by Bob Hawke did support a declaration by South Pacific nations to make the Pacific Ocean a nuclear-free zone, although Australia retained the right to accept visits from American and British nuclear armed warships. But in almost every other respect, the Hawke Labor government's stand on nuclear issues – including the mining and selling of uranium and the operation of United States secret defence bases in Australia – had become almost indistinguishable from that of the conservative Liberal party.

In spite of Penney's original assurance in 1959 to make results of the Vixen trials available to Australia, data on the results from all but one of the trials were not made available to Australian authorities in report form either straight after the trials or later. Titterton probably received some information verbally when he met with British officials from time to time in Australia or the UK. The British could argue that the results of the trials related to weapon design, which was a subject off limits as far as Australia was concerned. The British had also resumed their long sought atomic collaboration with the Americans during the Vixen series, and if the information was to be shared with anyone it was with the Americans. [6]

When the Soviet Union began resuming atmospheric nuclear weapons testing in September 1961, thereby ending the three year moratorium, Menzies denounced the decision in parliament. He certainly did not allude to the fact that Britain's secret Vixen tests in Australia over the previous two years had probably gone against the spirit, if not the letter, of the same moratorium agreement.

Britain had continued to keep its options open with Maralinga, and not just as a place to conduct the minor trials. Even before the advent of the test moratorium in 1958, the prospect of a longer term international ban on nuclear testing in the atmosphere had prompted a search for a place near Maralinga where weapons tests eventually could be conducted underground. But a preliminary survey turned up no suitable site within 160-300 kilometres of Maralinga. The only place that looked at all worthwhile appeared to be Mount Lindsay, 400 kilometres from Maralinga, but this created a problem because it was on an Aboriginal reserve. 'Some notice in gazette will be legally necessary before any actual excavation took place and there would be problem of devising suitable cover story', the British high commission in Canberra told London. The Menzies government asked at that stage that any further survey for an underground test site be put off until after the Australian general election due at the end of 1958 because they were nervous about any controversy over the nuclear tests entering the campaign. The British agreed.

But the idea of an underground test site in Australia continued to be floated in talks between British and Australian officials up to 1963, when Britain, the US and the Soviet Union agreed to a partial test-ban treaty, ending nuclear tests in the atmosphere. Perhaps the British had in mind an underground site near Maralinga to conduct more minor trials. In any case, the proposition petered out because Britain already had begun testing its nuclear weapons underground in Nevada.

With the decision to close Maralinga, Britain sent a team of royal engineers from Aldermaston to conduct a final clean up of the range in 1967, known as Operation Brumby. A senior Aldermaston scientist, Noah Pearce, prepared a top secret report of this operation soon afterwards, describing the state in which the range was left and acknowledging that the cleanup had been designed to reduce the possibility of inhalation of plutonium from its 'resuspension' in dust. The Pearce report, as it came to be known, was kept under wraps in Britain and Australia for 11 years until 1979 when Prime Minister Malcolm Fraser's Liberal government in Australia released a sanitised version, deleting references to some radioactive and toxic materials buried there, including cobalt 60, natural uranium and beryllium; the full version was released by the Hawke government in Canberra in 1984 – both releases having been prompted by sensational press leaks over what the report revealed.

The Pearce report described how the ground at Taranaki, the most heavily contaminated site after the minor trials, was treated during the Operation Brumby cleanup. A tractor was used to tow a scraper over the most badly contaminated parts making a cut in the soil to a depth of 10 centimetres, which was then mixed by a grader. Even then, some sections were still heavily contaminated, so they were covered with 7.5 centimetres of clean topsoil. You can still detect some of the original 1967 furrows at Taranaki today, looking a bit like a lightly ploughed field or the neat rows of sand left behind after the cleanup of a Sydney beach.

About 180 hectares were treated this way by scraper. There were 19 burial pits at Taranaki, containing about 20 kg of plutonium mixed in with steel plates and girders, lead and concrete bricks, cables and other debris from the trials. The pits were sealed with a cap of concrete 30 centimetres thick and reinforced with a series of mild steel bars. They were buried just 30 centimetres below ground level.

Scrapers were also used to mix the soil at two other sites with plutonium contamination, TM100 and TM101. At a fourth site, Wewak, contaminated soil was dug up and used to fill in the crater at Marcoo, the site of the ground burst during the Buffalo bomb trial series. Two more burial pits containing highly radioactive debris were stationed at TM101.

Operation Brumby appears to have been designed to render Maralinga as featureless as possible and to remove evidence of the place as a vast testing ground. All fences were taken down around the contaminated areas, with the exception of the burial pits at Taranaki and TM101, leaving the place open to anyone who may wander into the area unaware that plutonium was still mixed in the topsoil. Remarkably, fences were not put up again around these contaminated areas until the Australian Radiation Laboratory conducted its 1984-85 survey. Pearce reported: 'With the passage of time and the eventual removal of the fences at Taranaki and TM100-101, the debris pits . . . will have lost their identity'.

Pearce also concluded from measurements done at the time that by scraping and grading the soil, the possibility of plutonium contamination from 'resuspension', or churning up in dust, had been reduced to a level which did not constitute a risk. As he put it:

The plutonium which was originally deposited on the surface has been thoroughly dispersed through the top few inches of surface soil. Hence the concept of a surface layer of plutonium available for resuspension is not appropriate.

Pearce's optimistic conclusion took no account of dust storms and soil erosion, both of which prevail in this region of South Australia, and which would leave the plutonium free to be scattered across heavily populated areas of the state. Indeed in 1979, the Australian Ionising Radiation Advisory Council (AIRAC) produced a report on radiological safety and future land use at Maralinga which, although it strongly sought to play down the dangers, identified this very problem. [7] AIRAC noted a 'heavy loss of top soil' at Taranaki and a 'massive loss of surface soil' from most other trial sites dating from 1972; it reported: 'There is little doubt that grading and ploughing the soil in the ground zero environs in Brumby in 1967 rendered the activated soil available for dispersal by wind'.

The Australian safety committee certainly knew about the plutonium contamination at the time of Operation Brumby, but the question is, how much did they know? The committee reported to Menzies in July 1967, after inspecting the work at both Emu Field and Maralinga during Brumby, that they were satisfied both ranges were now radiologically safe. They told the Australian prime minister: 'Permanent and unrestricted access could be made to all but a few small areas and even they could be occupied on a short term basis without risk'.

In addition, Titterton wrote to the head of the Australian Department of Supply in July 1967, that 'the cleanup has been more effective than we had requested and the UK team have more than met our requirements for decontamination as these were laid down in our agreement with them'. Titterton added in a second letter that, as for the few small areas where there was still radiation, 'the levels of radiation are such that anyone, aboriginal included, would suffer no hazard through short term occupancy of the area. However, we would not permit anyone to build a home on one of these sites.'

The Australian safety committee received a copy of the secret Pearce report after it was completed in 1968. So even then, neither the safety committee nor the British appeared concerned that the land had been left in such a way that it was not fit for permanent, long-term occupation. In fact, both sides seem to have accepted the view that it was then good enough to leave some parts of the land contaminated to such an extent that access by humans would not be considered advisable for more than a few days each year.

John Moroney, who was secretary of the safety committee for ten years from 1957, was questioned closely about this when he appeared before the Australian royal commission in Sydney in June 1985. Moroney, a physicist who had once worked with Sir Leslie Martin at Melbourne University, explained that the safety committee had not insisted that the British leave Maralinga safe for permanent human occupation because the committee never believed that could be achieved by the ploughing and grading cleanup method the British had proposed.

There was another reason, as Moroney explained: the safety committee never expected that anyone, including the traditional Aboriginal owners of the Maralinga lands, would want to live there permanently. In fact, the safety committee fully anticipated, according to Moroney, that public interest in Maralinga would have petered out within 15 to 20 years of Operation Brumby – or, as Moroney put it more bluntly himself in a letter to Titterton in July 1964: 'The range is a long way from anyone, no-one will go there so why worry'. The British and Australian governments appear to have shared this view.

Although the Australian safety committee approved the results of Operation Brumby, it seems clear that all the committee's members did not know at the time of Brumby the full extent of the plutonium contamination, through the dispersion of metallic fragments on the ground. That contamination was really only revealed in 1985, after the Australian Radiation Laboratory's survey conducted by scientists using more sophisticated equipment and in a political climate where there were pressures to be more vigilant about the plutonium contamination than in 1967.

Why did the Australian safety committee not take more steps at the time, however, to discover the real extent of contamination left at Maralinga? Moroney told the Australian royal commission that the Australian safety committee of scientists did not have the proper resources to make its own checks, that it had to rely on information provided by the British scientists. Would that have made a difference, Peter McClellan, the counsel assisting the royal commission, asked him? 'No, because I had faith and trust in my British colleagues'. If Moroney had known then about the contaminated plutonium fragments on the range, McClellan asked, what would he have done? 'I would have put it before the safety committee that the measures taken to treat the range may not then have been the best methods'.

The British government suggested at the royal commission through its counsel, Robin Auld, QC, that the Australian safety committee should have been in a position to deduce at the time of Brumby the possibility that there were more plutonium 'hot spots' around the place than the ones identified in the cleanup. It cited as evidence a message which Noah Pearce himself sent to Moroney in June 1967, towards the end of the cleanup, in which Pearce talked of the British scientists' concern about an area of Taranaki containing 'three smaller areas where the activity is higher and is associated with large particles unevenly distributed over the surface'.

Was Pearce not indicating here an element of uncertainty about possible extra hot spots, asked Auld? Moroney replied:

Not at all. I am sure my exchanges with Noah were such that . . . if he had come across a problem wherein he saw a very large number of these fragments posing an unattended pathway to risk, he would have told me. That was my belief. He would not have done it obliquely like this. There is nothing in that signal which says, 'Look, John, there is a major problem here which we have to re-examine'.

So Maralinga was closed up and abandoned. The assumption by the British and Australian scientists at the time of the Brumby cleanup in 1967 that the place would naturally rehabilitate itself with vegetation never came to pass. The bomb sites are as desolate today, the trees as broken and dead, as the days after the bombs went off. As everyone in Whitehall and Canberra had hoped, Maralinga quickly faded from the public mind.

Then ten years later, in December 1976, Tom Uren, a Labor opposition frontbench MP in Australia, and later a minister in Hawke's government, made what appears to be the first call for a royal commission into events at Maralinga. Uren asked in parliament if it was true that Australia had co-operated with Britain in conducting secret atomic 'trigger' tests at Maralinga during the moratorium on nuclear weapons tests, and if waste and debris from them was buried there. By now, rumours and allegations had begun to surface among ex-servicemen and others about nuclear waste, and even an unexploded nuclear weapon, being buried at Maralinga. Uren demanded that if what he had asked was true, then a royal commission be set up to establish the facts.

Uren issued another statement outside parliament in which he said:

During [the test] moratorium period the Australian government co-operated with the British government to secretly carry out certain atomic tests in the Maralinga area . . . The explosions caused by these tests were so small that they could escape public scrutiny and international detection.

James Killen, the MP whose election in 1961 had saved Menzies' government, was now the defence minister in Malcolm Fraser's administration. Killen replied to Uren that, as far as he knew, the last explosions at Maralinga had been conducted in 1955-56. He said: 'Urgent inquiries have been set in train to establish precisely what has been buried at Maralinga'. The press did not take up the story.

Killen's cautious reply was in stark contrast to that of a colleague, Vic Garland, four years earlier. Garland, as a former Liberal government minister for supply, had said in September 1972, in response to allegations about radioactive waste at Maralinga: 'We know what is there'. It had become clear by the mid-seventies, however, that the Australian authorities were definitely far from clear about what was there or how it had got there.

Soon after Uren made his call for an inquiry, Killen wrote to him, in February 1977, saying that the Maralinga matter had 'become confused and distorted by several unfounded allegations', one of which was 'that about 800 tonnes of nuclear waste material, including plutonium, is buried at Maralinga'. Killen went on to say there was no evidence to support or substantiate these allegations in any way. Later, the minister was forced to retract these remarks when his department advised him of the true situation, no doubt after consulting the Pearce report which Canberra had been given in secret almost 10 years earlier.

In 1977, the Australian Ionising Radiation Advisory Council embarked on a field study of radioactive waste at Maralinga, which culminated in the 1979 report referred to earlier over the loss of topsoil at the sites contaminated with plutonium. The AIRAC study was remarkable for the way it either glossed over or failed to detect the extent of the contamination which was turned up in 1985. One of the most interesting things about this AIRAC exercise was the announcement that it was about to take place by another Fraser government minister, Kevin Newman, in August, 1977. Newman's imprecise statement said: 'Its [the AIRAC probe's] purpose is to study the possible dispersal by natural agencies of radioactive substances remaining after the low yield atomic tests at Maralinga from 1955 to 1963'. Here, for the first time, was any minister in Britain or Australia admitting, intentionally or not, that the minor trials probably involved fission explosions. Again, the press did not follow the story.

The Maralinga affair did not really hit the headlines until October 1978, when the *Australian Financial Review* published an article based on a leaked submission which Killen had made to cabinet warning that some of the plutonium buried at Maralinga could be stolen by terrorists. [8] The report disclosed that Killen's submission had said that as well as the 20 kilograms of plutonium buried at Taranaki, recovery of which was impractical because of its dispersal among radioactive debris, there was another half a kilogram of plutonium buried near Maralinga airport in a 'discrete mass' which could be recovered; that because of its extremely toxic properties this plutonium could be used as a weapon in the hands of terrrorists who could threaten to disperse it in a city; and that the way the plutonium had been left at Maralinga was probably a breach of Australia's obligations under the International Atomic Energy Agency because it was not properly safeguarded under IAEA rules.

The Fraser government at the time was preparing to enter the nuclear industry through the opening up of uranium mining in vast new reserves in the Northern Territory. It had become secretly worried about the plutonium because it represented a potential source of embarrassment in view of the government's public claims that it would apply the strictest safeguards to the selling of Australian nuclear fuels. So the Killen submission presented the Australian cabinet with three options: dig the plutonium up and rebury it at Woomera, where there was more security than at Maralinga; take it officially into Australia's inventory of plutonium under IAEA rules; or – the favoured option – ask Britain to take it back.

The revelation of the cabinet submission created a furore. Killen made a blistering attack on the *Financial Review* for publishing details of the submission, the leaking of which he described as a criminal act: 'It is a day for regret when a journalist and a newspaper, aided by a criminal act, have published a story which is against the interests of the nation and its people'. Killen confirmed the existence of the half kilogram of plutonium, then accused the journalist, Brian Toohey, of alerting potential terrorists to its presence. He failed to mention that his own cabinet submission itself had warned the government that the plutonium was a potential target for a terrorist raid.

The half kilogram of plutonium in the so called 'discrete mass' was actually buried along with other radioactive products with shorter half lives, such as cobalt 60, among debris in an underground dump known as the cemetery near the Maralinga airfield. Its presence was recorded in the Pearce report. This plutonium had been used in a Tims trial at the TM101 site in 1961 as part of a series of experiments to test the behaviour of plutonium metal when it was shattered by an explosion. On this occasion (the only one, it seems), the scientists had constructed six containers each with a narrow throat into which the products of the explosion could be fired, thus making most of the plutonium recoverable. The airfield cemetery also contained, in 360 steel drums, radioactive waste from RAF aircraft which had taken part in the British hydrogen bomb tests at Christmas Island and which had been decontaminated afterwards at an air base in South Australia, Edinburgh Field.

Australia was now in a particularly delicate diplomatic position if it wanted Britain to take the recoverable plutonium, or anything else, home again. Back in September 1968, after Operation Brumby, Australia had signed an agreement with Britain terminating the original memorandum of arrangements of 1956 which had given Britain the use of Maralinga as a test site. The 1968 agreement had released Britain from 'all liabilities and responsibilities' at Maralinga, except for certain strictly defined claims which had nothing to do with any cleanup of the range (see Appendix Two).

The *Financial Review's* disclosure about the half kilogram of plutonium sparked a spate of letter writing and interviews by politicians and scientists. Don Dunstan, the premier of South Australia, Maralinga's state, wrote to Fraser in Canberra the same day expressing 'my concern at the disturbing nature and implications of this report', and asking for full details of what the federal government knew about wastage from the British tests at Maralinga. (A secret submission to Fraser from the Prime Minister's Department in Canberra a few days later said that Canberra had passed a copy of the Pearce report to the South Australian government in 1973, when Gough Whitlam's Labor government was in power in Canberra, and Dunstan's Labor government was in office in South Australia).

More significantly, perhaps, both Penney in England and Titterton in Australia were interviewed separately about the plutonium on the same radio program by the Australian Broadcasting Commission. Their answers, like their locations, were a world apart. Penney said: 'There must be some plutonium contamination in the immediate area of where the explosions occurred, yes, there must be some'. Asked about the source of the plutonium, Penney replied: 'This testing ground was used not only to test weapons but to test some components. The components had very small quantities of radioactivity in them.'

Titterton, by contrast, cast doubt on whether there was a recoverable lump of plutonium at Maralinga even though, like Penney, he knew the contents of the Pearce report: 'I think if there was a lump of plutonium it would have been taken away', said Titterton. 'I mean, material which is worth three times its weight in gold would not be allowed to lie there. Somebody would have taken it away for useful purposes.' The interviewer told him Killen had confirmed there was a discrete mass of half a kilogram. Titterton: 'Well, I know nothing about that . . . Even if that is correct it still is incredible that anybody could find that small piece of plutonium in the immense desert of Maralinga'.

Three days after this interview, Titterton, by now returned full-time to his work as a professor of nuclear physics at the Australian National University, wrote to both Fraser and Killen in a tone of urgency and agitation. He told Killen he had tried unsuccessfully to contact him as soon as the Financial Review's leak appeared. 'Apart from the seriousness of the leak, which your Thursday night statement dealt with effectively, I was concerned with the content of the Cabinet submission itself, if this was as reported in the Financial Review'. To both Fraser and Killen, Titterton sent a copy of an article he had written for publication in the Sydney Morning Herald about the Maralinga controversy; the article, he pointed out to Fraser, 'may be of interest to you as the Opposition is likely to continue to pursue the matter over the next week'.

Titterton's article debunked the suggestion that Maralinga was an attractive target for terrorists. But, unlike in his radio interview, he appeared to acknowledge the existence of the half kilogram of plutonium which, he wrote, 'would be a piece about the size of a hen's egg' and 'therefore is hardly a cause for hysteria or fears'. Clearly, Titterton's role as a scientist-politician had not diminished since the days of the Maralinga tests.

On 6 October 1978, the day after the Financial Review's article appeared, Ian Sinclair, Australia's acting minister for foreign affairs, sent a secret message to David Owen, the British foreign secretary in James Callaghan's Labour government. He said Australia had been planning to approach Britain eventually about the exhuming and removing of recoverable plutonium, but pointed out 'that the question has now assumed greater urgency because the matter has unfortunately become the subject of public concern in Australia'. Sinclair's message somewhat delicately described how international awareness and sensitivity over such weapons grade material had heightened since the burial of the plutonium 'more than two decades ago' (it was, in fact, even less than that – in 1961).

A closer reading of his message, however, revealed the real source of his worry: the Fraser government was acutely conscious of the potential political problems the fifties weapons plutonium now posed to its bid in the seventies to sell uranium for peaceful purposes in compliance with the Nuclear Non Proliferation Treaty, and it was seeking a way out of the 1968 agreement that absolved Britain from any further responsibilities at the Maralinga range. [9] Sinclair explained that in 1976 Australia had advised the IAEA that debris contaminated with plutonium was buried at Maralinga, and had undertaken to report if any of the material was in a recoverable form. He then came straight to the point – that Australia considered repatriation of the recoverable plutonium to the UK 'would represent the appropriate solution'.

Britain responded by sending a team of Aldermaston experts to Australia, including Noah Pearce, to examine the burial pits, but it refused to agree immediately to Australia's request to take the half kilogram of plutonium away. When Britain eventually did agree to the request the following month, November, it did so under a set of strict conditions which it insisted Australia accept first. They included an agreement that Britain would decide the timing and mode of transport of the six drums containing the half kilogram of plutonium from Australia to Britain; that Australia give a firm undertaking that the operation would be conducted with maximum secrecy; and that Australia pay all costs of the operation within Australia and be responsible for the provision of anti-terrorist protection while the plutonium remained on Australian soil (the operation ended up costing Australia almost $162 000).

Most important, Britain told Australia that no basis remained for any further request for repatriation of nuclear waste and there was, therefore, no question of Britain having any further responsibility to repatriate waste from Maralinga. It asked for a clear statement that the Australian government accept this. Australia agreed to all these conditions, and they became the basis for a further agreement executed between the two countries in January 1979 (see Appendix Two.)

The actual removal operation took place in strict secrecy in February 1979, and was not announced until 22 March, when the half kilogram of plutonium was back in Britain, at Aldermaston. A team of 22 British and Australian scientists and engineers from the Australian atomic energy commission, Aldermaston and the Australian army flew to Maralinga and spent two days setting up camp and opening the pit at the airport cemetery which contained the dreaded plutonium. Three Hercules aircraft were needed to bring in their equipment, which included a bulldozer, a cement mixer, an air compressor and various radiation monitoring devices.

It could not have been a worse time of the year: the temperature hovered from 45 to 50° C and the winds on most days blew at up to 120 kilometres an hour, which meant the pots containing the plutonium could not be opened in the free air. But the political pressures were such that the job had to be done as soon as possible. Because of the intense heat, the scientists, clad as they were in stifling protective suits, were able to work only early in the mornings or at night. Even then, some of them lost up to 4 kilograms in weight from sweating inside their suits as they delicately prepared the plutonium pots for transportation.

The job took 12 days to complete. The plutonium was in six pots, each of which, in turn, was inside a steel drum. When they started to remove these drums from the burial pit, the scientists discovered that the drums had rusted considerably, so they had to prepare a new base for each of the pots as it was taken from its drum. Then the pots had to be filled with cement grout and placed in large containers where they were embedded in a special concrete mix. Much of this concreting was performed at night under floodlights, to escape the heat, and in a tent, to escape the wind. When it was all over, the tent, contaminated plastic used in the sealing of the pots and other equipment were thrown in the pit and the whole thing sealed over with concrete again. The large containers in which the plutonium had been sealed weighed a total of almost 12 000 kilograms. They were flown out of Maralinga on a Hercules aircraft early on the morning of 16 March and transferred to an RAF VC10 at Edinburgh Field which left for Britain the same day.

A month before this secret operation, Malcolm Fraser had written to the South Australian premier saying he agreed 'that as much information on Maralinga as possible should be made public'. Four months later, in June 1979, Fraser's government released the Pearce report, albeit a censored version with references to the burial sites and some of their contents deleted. In May 1984, the classified, original, version of the Pearce report was leaked to the *National Times* of Australia, which published a long article about the surface plutonium contamination at Maralinga based on its contents. [10] Soon afterwards, the Hawke government released the full Pearce report.

Still more alarming evidence about the state of the range at Maralinga filtered out around the time that the sanitised Pearce report was released. In the same month, June 1979, the state government of South Australia issued a report based on a biological and botanical survey by its department for the environment of the most contaminated test sites at Maralinga.

The South Australian scientists had collected 19 rabbits and a dingo which were running wild around Taranaki and some of the other sites. They discovered that plutonium, caesium and strontium had been taken up on the fur, in the gut and in the respiratory system of all of them. One of the rabbits had actually been picked up outside a warren right next to the Taranaki burial pits containing the 20 kilograms of plutonium, making it almost certain that the rabbits had burrowed their way into the pits. In fact, the South Australian report said:

It is possible for rabbits, that are rather notorious for their ability to excavate burrows in almost any material, to gain access to the pits by simply burrowing under the six inch concrete slabs. Calcrete capping of a tabular type occurring naturally in the Nullarbor Plain is often used by rabbits as the roof of their warrens. As we are discussing products which have a half life of 24,000 years, it would seem almost a statistical certainty that in some time in the future the rabbits may have access to a pit.

How much plutonium really remains at Maralinga? The Pearce report, still considered a basic reference point on the state of the range, gives the figure of 20 kilograms lying in the pits at Taranaki. The Ministry of Defence in London gave information to Australia at the beginning of the royal commission's hearings, in September 1984, on the amount of plutonium used in the minor trials 'based on data available in UK files'. These figures gave a total of 24.4 kilograms of plutonium used in the minor trials, of which about 900 grams had been returned to the UK. This left not 20 kilograms, but 23.5 kilograms still at Maralinga.

The Australian Radiation Laboratory's report of 1985 was even more ambiguous on this question. It said its discoveries of plutonium on the ground at Taranaki accounted for no more than 10 to 20 per cent of the total plutonium used, and that it was assumed that the remainder was in the burial pits. This implied yet a different total of 25 kilograms of plutonium still at Maralinga; the ARL, indeed, admitted there was 'considerable uncertainty' about its figures.

The Australian royal commission did not shed a great deal of light on this question. It seems probable that the authorities today do not know precisely how much plutonium has been left at Maralinga, the full extent of its dispersal on the ground or the manner of its disposal in the Taranaki burial pits. A large range of debris lies in the pits at Maralinga – not just cables, drums and metal but contaminated Land Rovers, lorries, caravans, observation towers and even bits of aircraft. Somewhere among all this, the buried plutonium is dispersed.

At the sites of each of the major bomb trials at Maralinga, Emu Field and the Monte Bello Islands, a pyramid-shaped, squat, concrete plinth was erected on each of the ground zeros in 1979, recording, in the fashion of a memorial, the explosion that happened there in the fifties and warning that the site was still a radiation hazard.

For many years, both Maralinga and the Monte Bello Islands had been the prey of salvagers. At Maralinga, Aborigines from Yalata had gone in with the tacit agreement of the federal and South Australian governments to dismantle buildings from the village and take them away. But they also dug up contaminated debris which had been buried, including copper wire, trailers, hydraulic jacks and lathes, apparently without having been warned of the dangers beforehand. In 1979, when the authorities finally woke up to what was happening, Malcolm Fraser, the prime minister, wrote to the premier of South Australia saying it was 'undesirable' and asking for it to be stopped.

At the Monte Bello Islands, the salvaging was of a more swashbuckling kind. Although the ground zeros of the two Mosaic bombs of 1956 had been clearly marked, many of the warning signs erected back in the fifties, and updated in the sixties, had long since rotted and decayed. The islands remained a prohibited area under the Defence (Special Undertakings) Act of 1952, passed at the time of the Hurricane bomb; but with no-one there to police it the law was useless as a means of deterring sailors from landing on the islands over the years and plundering the remnants from the nuclear tests which had been left strewn about the sandhills.

One man who has made several salvaging expeditions to the Monte Bellos was Ian Blair, a large, jocular businessman from Onslow, the coastal town about 130 kilometres from the islands. Blair first went to the Monte Bellos searching for green turtles in a boat called the *Will Succeed* in 1959, the year he became sergeant of police at Onslow. He resigned from the police force in 1966 to concentrate on various business enterprises.

Blair approached a company in Perth, Western Australia, which, he learned, had the franchise from the Royal navy for salvaging scrap, and began sending them whatever he could find. He made three salvage expeditions, collecting by hand scrap which included heavy armour-plated copper wire running from the ground zero sites to various points around the islands. Later, he returned to the islands many times accompanying parties from survey companies, the national mapping authority, the West Australian museum and groups who were simply looking for shells. Blair told the Australian royal commission in July 1985:

There was not a great deal of scrap metal left to salvage after I finished. On many of these trips I camped on the islands. On one occasion, I think it was with the museum party, we actually camped almost in the bomb site for about a week. We camped there because it was close to the beach and it was sheltered. As far as salvage is concerned I was issued no warnings about dangers in being on the islands or handling the scrap metal. I was given no safety procedures.

Nor did Emu Field escape the clutches of the souvenir hunters. Frank Smith was a member of the Australian army's radiation detection unit who was stationed at Emu for the radiation monitoring from some of the early Maralinga bomb tests. He told the royal commission in June 1985:

Souveniring was a big thing right from the start. One incident was that a Land Rover was taken from Totem One or Totem Two at Emu by an air force gentleman and taken back to Laverton air base in Victoria. During the commanding officer's inspection it was found. The gentleman was, I believe, subsequently court-martialled. It was handed over to the Department of Supply in Melbourne. From what I have been advised, but I cannot justify this, it was eventually sold at auction in South Australia.

Smith also reported that target response items from the Maralinga bombs were also snapped up – the clothing, clocks, guns, brasswork, and a whole host of goods laid out near the ground zeros to record the impact of an atomic bomb. 'Quite a lot of those disappeared. I should imagine there are a few houses around the country that have got them as ornaments in their doorway.'

The contamination levels at several of the major bomb trial sites in Australia, at Maralinga, Emu Field and the Monte Bello Islands, remain today above the levels which the International Commission on Radiological Protection consider safe for members of the public. But the Australian Radiation Laboratory, in its report of 1985, forecast that the radioactive nuclides will have decayed at all of them after between 40 and 50 years, making permanent occupation at each of the bomb-trial sites possible by about 2025.

The more lasting problem is the ground surface plutonium at Taranaki and three other Maralinga sites. By the mid-eighties, it seemed that no Australian government would be able to ignore the question of dealing with this waste. Since the fifties and sixties, public opinion had become more demanding on environmental and nuclear questions, and Australia's attitude towards the treatment of its Aborigines had changed radically. Even sections of the otherwise pro-nuclear scientific world had come to the conclusion that the state in which Maralinga had been left was wrong. One of these people was Keith Lokan, a member of the Australian Ionising Radiation Advisory Council, the director of the Australian Radiation Laboratory, and a principal author of the ARL's 1985 report on the state of Maralinga.

Lokan was asked by the Australian royal commission about the wisdom of the minor trials which dispersed the plutonium. 'My view is that they should not have been conducted', he said. 'Because plutonium has a very long half life and the problem is with us then for a very long time'. How long, then, would a health risk remain for people intruding on the range, Lokan was asked – 24 000 years, the period of the half life of plutonium?

It would be a longer period of time because 24 000 years is what is needed to reduce the quantity of radioactivity to one half, and another 24 000 years to one quarter and so on. A rough-and-ready guide might be to say: by the time it has decayed through ten half lives, which means it will have reduced to one thousandth of its present level – and that would take 240 000 years. [11]

John Moroney, another scientist from the Australian nuclear establishment and a former scientific secretary of the Australian safety committee, was prepared to admit to the royal commission that the cleanup which the safety committee approved with the knowledge it had in 1967 was inadequate. 'With these plutonium fragments, dilution is not a solution', Moroney said. 'You have to take them away'. [12]

Sir Ernest Titterton has been the only scientist to disagree with the renewed assessments in the mid-eighties about the extent of the plutonium contamination at Maralinga, when he said, in one of the most remarkable statements made at the Australian royal commission: 'There is no hazard from plutonium on the range'. [13]

Taking away the plutonium, as Moroney termed it, and any other debris inside the burial pits, would be an enormous enterprise costing millions of dollars. Some scientists have argued that, even accounting for the needs to satisfy environmental and Aboriginal aspirations, the costs of such an exercise would outway the benefits of putting the money into something else, given the remoteness of the site and the uncertainty about how the land may be used in future years as a place to live or work, or, indeed, whether it will be used for any other purpose at all.

The British government adopted the substance of this argument in September 1985, when it put its final case before the Australian royal commission over the crucial question of the future of the Maralinga range. Through its counsel, Robin Auld, QC, Margaret Thatcher's government acknowledged that there was some hazard from the Taranaki plutonium contaminated fragments, but went on to argue that the royal commission did not have sufficient evidence on which it could base any reasoned recommendations about what, if anything, should be done about it. The British government reminded the royal commission that Australia itself had known there would be a contamination problem when it permitted Britain to do the tests:

In April 1956, when the Australian and UK governments entered into the memorandum of arrangements for the establishment of the permanent proving ground at Maralinga, the area was then, as now, little used by Aborigines. The Australian government knew that the nuclear tests to be carried out there would cause residual contamination and that, for that reason, public access to it would need to be restricted for the foreseeable future . . . Scientific knowledge is not now, and certainly was not then, sufficiently advanced to enable a complete decontamination of an area in which nuclear explosive tests have taken place. In 1955 the Australian government did not seek such an onerous, if not impossible, undertaking from the UK government, nor would the UK government have committed itself to the use of the Maralinga range if it had contemplated any such requirement.

There was an element of disingenuousness in this argument because, when Maralinga was set up in 1955-56, Britain did not warn Australia that it planned to conduct tests there five years later which would leave plutonium dispersed over 2.5 square kilometres of land. Some might say that, in view of the Menzies government's open-door policy on the nuclear tests, it would have made no difference if Britain had alerted Australia to this likelihood.

The British government also put forward at the Australian royal commission the proposition that there was no real evidence about the living patterns and movement of Aborigines in the Maralinga area, either before 1955 or since restrictions on entry were partly lifted in the eighties. Therefore, it suggested, no cleanup could be justified simply on the basis of Aboriginal need. It argued that the test sites were unsuitable as camping places for Aborigines: there was no water, little firewood and no ready food supplies. The British argument cited another disadvantage of the test sites for Aborigines: '[They have] been polluted in a physical, and for them, a spiritual sense'.

This was an astonishing remark since it went to the very heart of the whole matter; it seemed to imply that, having had their lands polluted with radiation, the Aborigines should be content to forget about them. In claiming there was no information about the Aborigines' lifestyles in the area, the British government's argument also ignored the evidence which many Pitjantjatjara Aborigines themselves gave to the royal commission about the manner in which they lived in various parts of the central desert of South Australia at the time of the bomb trials, as well as the remarkable discoveries of the patrol officers, Walter MacDougall and Robert Macaulay, that Aborigines had lived within the prohibited range throughout the years of the testing.

Britain's final word was to leave things as they are: that the burial pits at Maralinga were safe, that fences should be left around Taranaki to stop visitors straying into the plutonium fragments and that the radioactivity at the ground zero bomb sites at Monte Bello, Emu Field and Maralinga was decaying at such a rate that permanent occupation of them would be possible in 50 to 60 years – 'in the unlikely event of it ever being sought'.

The Australian government, by contrast, took a more low-key stand before the royal commission. It declined to recommend any specific conclusions that the royal commission should draw. But the Australian government, represented through its counsel, James McIntyre, did acknowledge in its final argument: 'As a minimum . . . action will need to be taken to improve the radiological safety of the sites'. Having said that, however, the Australian government then cited money as a major factor in determining what should be done about the contaminated sites. Any benefit to be derived from returning these sites to their Aboriginal owners, Australia argued, had to be balanced against the cost to Australia of cleaning up the area.

Indeed, money looked like being the major sticking point on this vital question. In December 1984, the South Australian government went some way towards redressing the disruption and damage of earlier years when it had proclaimed the Maralinga Tjarutja Land Rights Act, returning to the Aboriginal traditional owners more than 76 000 square kilometres of land surrounding the Maralinga and Emu Field test grounds. The legislation deliberately excluded substantial sections on the actual testing sites at both locations because the South Australian government did not want to hand over land which was still contaminated until the cleanup question had been resolved.

The Aborigines, however, want to have this land back ultimately as well, and it is for this reason that they argued at the Australian royal commission through their legal counsel, Geoff Eames and Andrew Collett, that a further cleanup of the ranges should be launched, removing the contaminated material above and below the ground. The Aborigines' submission did not say exactly where it should be removed, but the trend of their arguments throughout the royal commission's hearings implied that the rest of the recoverable plutonium, at least, should be repatriated to Britain. Moreover, the Aborigines advanced what appeared to be the only logical argument, politically and historically, that Australia and Britain should share the cost of cleaning up the range, and of any research that would be needed on how to handle the operation. British and Australian authorities were equally to blame for the inadequacy of the Operation Brumby cleanup, they argued; and British and Australian authorities ignored to an equal degree at the time any possible aspirations the Aborigines may have had for the land in the future. Their final argument to the royal commission was:

Accordingly, in political terms, there is no reason why a range cleanup to a certain risk standard (i.e. less than complete removal) should be acceptable to Aborigines. Expressed in another way, Aborigines can quite legitimately ask why should the government be telling them that it thinks it is acceptable to return to them land that has on it contaminated substances which will cause the death of (say) one in one hundred thousand people. It is clear ... that any cleanup option chosen will be very costly. This is inescapable. However the decision whether to spend the money and clean up the lands properly is fundamentally a moral question.

By 1986, the only cost estimates on cleaning up Maralinga had come in a report which the Australian government asked the Australian Atomic Energy Commission to prepare over seven weeks from May to July 1985, and which was presented to the Australian royal commission the following September. The Australian Atomic Energy Commission's report has been criticised for the time limits on its preparation, but it offered several options and estimated costs, including:

An 'emu parade' of special retrieval teams to collect plutonium and other debris from the ground (less than $100 000); fences to be erected around areas of 'significant plutonium contamination' with warning signs ($800 000); collecting plutonium contaminated surface soil from three Maralinga sites, estimated at 480 000 tonnes of dirt ($10 million); burying this soil 2 metres under the ground ($4 million); burying it 10 metres under ($33 million); chemical treatment of the soil to extract plutonium from it – even then the recovery efficiency would be only 50-70 per cent ($60-$150 million); stabilising the plutonium already in burial pits at Maralinga by concrete grouting of the pits to cut off gaps which have opened up and to stop water entering ($2 million); exhuming the present pits and cutting and crushing the waste they contain ($8 million); treating this material on the spot with a plant to recover the radioactive particles ($20 million).

After all its deliberations on this, one of the most pressing problems it was asked to investigate, the Australian royal commission was unable to decide what should be done. 'The royal commission has neither the resources nor the time to enable it to consider properly all of the options and possibilities for cleaning up the Maralinga range', it concluded in its report in December 1985.

• NO CONCEIVABLE INJURY

Instead, the royal commission proposed that another body be set up to take the problem on, called the Maralinga Commission, to consist of the traditional Aboriginal owners and the Ausralian, British and South Australian governments.

But on one question, the royal commission was categorical: who should actually pay for what, if anything, was eventually done. It ignored the Aborigines' argument that the cost should be borne equally by Britain and Australia, which had both permitted the contamination to take place. The royal commission recommended that Britain should pay for the lot.

There is an overwhelming moral obligation on the UK. It has become clear to everyone that Operation Brumby was neither prudent nor effective . . . It would, in the opinion of the Royal Commission, be grossly irresponsible of the UK Government if it did not now accept that it has a continuing obligation to clean up the contaminated areas so that they are acceptable for unrestricted access. [See Appendix Two.]

The royal commission did not relinquish Australia from responsibility over the future use of the Maralinga lands although, curiously enough, it did not chastise Australia in this respect to the same extent as it did Britain. It said Australia should compensate the Aborigines for the loss of their lands during the British nuclear tests. The compensation should not take the form of putting a monetary value on the lands, but should consist of aid to help the Aborigines to return there to live as and where they wished with a reduced level of hardship. Thus, the Australian government should provide water supplies, medical aid posts, schools, stores, shelter and communications for Aborigines who want to set up outstations on the Maralinga lands and water bores for those who want to return to a semi-nomadic lifestyle. The royal commission concluded:

The traditional owners of the Maralinga lands are eager to re-establish their traditional relationships with their lands and are responding keenly to attempts to make this possible.

This, too, involved a moral responsibility, no less than the cleanup of the range. Both issues were the legacy of a very political exercise between the British and Australian governments years earlier; but by the mid-eighties their resolution seemed destined to remain a source of diplomatic and financial tension between the two countries for the rest of the decade and beyond.

Chapter Seven
NO CONCEIVABLE INJURY?

'The number of children and grandchildren with cancer in their bones, with leukaemia in their blood or with poison in their lungs might seem statistically small to some, in comparison with natural health hazards. But this is not a natural health hazard and it is not a statistical issue. The loss of even one human life, or the malformation of even one baby – who may be born long after we have gone – should be of concern to us all. Our children and grandchildren are not merely statistics towards which we can be indifferent' – President John F. Kennedy, July 1963.

Even up to the mid-1950s, well after the British began testing nuclear weapons in Australia, the phenomenon of radioactive fallout was still something of a mystery to nuclear scientists. They had a good idea what went up into the atmosphere when a nuclear bomb was exploded, but they were not so certain about what came down again – or where, or in what concentrations or over what period of time. More significantly, doctors and scientists were still uncertain about how much exposure to radioactivity was dangerous to human health. They certainly knew from the appalling experience of the victims at Hiroshima and Nagasaki just how dangerous massive doses were; but they were still feeling their way on the vital question of how much harm could be caused by exposure to low levels of radiation. That question is still hotly debated today.

When Aborigines and British and Australian veterans from the fifties tests began alleging in the late seventies that their health had suffered as a result of exposure to radiation from the bombs, the governments in Britain and Australia instinctively denied any culpability. Their arguments rested on the assertion that the precautions taken to safeguard those exposed to the tests were adequate and that they were in line with international safety standards at the time. But the somewhat turbulent history of those safety standards is enough to show how questionable the governments' comfortable claims are liable to be. Even the Australian royal commission, after taking evidence from many scientific and medical experts in an inquiry lasting more than a year, was unable to come to any firm conclusions on this question, as we shall see later.

Yet by the mid-eighties, the law elsewhere was beginning to take a critical stand on the safeguards employed at nuclear tests in the fifties. In May 1984, a federal judge in Salt Lake City, Utah, found that radioactive fallout from atmospheric, or above ground, American nuclear tests in the fifties had been responsible for the cancer deaths of nine people and that the US government had been negligent in its conduct of the tests. The ruling ended a long court action brought by plaintiffs on behalf of hundreds of cancer victims in Nevada, Utah and Arizona who claimed their illnesses were caused by fallout from the Nevada Test Site, where the US conducted 93 atmospheric nuclear tests between 1951 and 1962. It was the first time the government of any Western nuclear power had been held liable for damages resulting from nuclear tests and the first time that a court had directly linked cancer to radiation from the tests. The American ruling, to which we shall return later, came after years of furious controversy among scientists about the dangers of radiation.

Until 1963, all the nuclear powers, the US, the Soviet Union, Britain and France, conducted their weapons testing in the open atmosphere. In that year, the Americans, the Russians and the British signed the limited test ban treaty agreeing to confine future nuclear tests underground, thus putting an end to the careless and wilful dispersal of radioactive fallout over land. France ignored the ban and continued testing weapons in the atmosphere, mainly in the Pacific Ocean, until the mid-seventies. China, the fifth nuclear power after 1964, also carried on with atmospheric testing until the early eighties. There is almost no information about the behaviour of Soviet underground tests, but there have been several reports of Anglo-American underground weapon explosions in Nevada since

1963 leaching radioactive clouds into the open environment. So although putting the tests underground has not entirely eliminated radioactive pollution, it has at least drastically reduced it. And there have been many more nuclear weapons tested since the atmospheric test ban treaty than before it.

Several authorities have attempted the highly difficult task of estimating the effect on human health worldwide of fallout from the atmospheric nuclear tests of the fifties and early sixties. Up to the start of the 1963 test ban treaty, there had been 362 nuclear weapons exploded in the atmosphere; the Americans had tested 193 of these, the Russians 142, the British 21 and the French 6. [1] One health damage estimate has come from Robert Alexander, of the US Nuclear Regulatory Commission, the Washington-based government agency in charge of regulating standards in America's nuclear power industry. Like many government bodies elsewhere involved with setting and policing nuclear safety standards, the NRC tends to be conservative in its outlook. Robert Alexander has estimated, on the basis of the average radiation doses to the world's population from these atmospheric tests, that the effects are as follows: up to 84 500 cancer deaths and up to 168 000 genetic effects, 7200 of which are classified as 'serious'.

Professor Joseph Rotblat, of London University, has made a similar estimate. Rotblat reports that past tests of nuclear weapons are likely to give rise to nearly 100 000 additional deaths from cancer in the world, plus half that number of premature deaths due to genetic damage. As Rotblat points out, since most of the tests took place in the northern hemisphere, most of the radioactive fallout remained in that hemisphere; the dose commitment for the population in the northern hemisphere is about three times greater than for that in the southern hemisphere. [2]

Any attempt to put meaning into estimates of this sort, and to apply it to the British tests in Australia, must take account of the controversy over low-level radiation dangers – the groundwork for which was laid fifty years before the first atomic bomb was exploded at Alamogordo, New Mexico, in July 1945.

In 1895, a German professor called Wilhelm Roentgen discovered a source of rays which, unlike light rays, were capable of penetrating sheets of card and metal and even human flesh, but not bones. For want of a specific term, Roentgen called them X-rays. The following year, the Frenchman, Henri Becquerel, discovered that uranium spontaneously emitted similar rays which, like X-rays, could penetrate cardboard and blacken a photographic plate. The phenomenon which Becquerel had discovered was known as ionising radiation: the energy of these penetrating rays was such that they knocked electrons off the atoms of the material through which they passed leaving them as charged 'ions'. These ions, in turn, were capable of causing great chemical changes and damages, particularly in the cells of the human body – hence the harmful effects of ionising radiation.

Marie Curie and her husband, Pierre, were fascinated by Becquerel's discovery. Madame Curie gave the name 'radioactivity' to this characteristic of spontaneously emitting ionising radiation. The Curies went on to discover and isolate the highly radioactive elements, polonium and radium, and before long the medical profession had seized upon both X-rays and radium as tools for diagnosing and treating patients.

Meanwhile, much pioneering work on the nature of the atom was being performed at Cambridge University under Ernest (later Lord) Rutherford, the New Zealand-born physicist. Rutherford conducted experiments with uranium and discovered that the radiation it emitted consisted of more than one kind, which he named alpha and beta particles. A third type, gamma rays, was isolated soon afterwards. These ionising radiations are discussed further below.

Almost from the very beginning radiation was known to be dangerous although it took some time before the real extent of the hazards was realised: it could not be detected by feeling, smelling or seeing and many of its effects did not become manifest until after a latency period of several years.

The fate of the French pioneers themselves illustrated the different effects radiation could have on the body. Becquerel carried a vial of radium around in his pocket for several days and discovered it gave him skin burns. Madame Curie tragically succumbed to the more insidious, long-term effects of radiation when she died of leukaemia some years later at the age of 67, contracted through her long exposure to radioactivity from radium and its products. Over the first three decades of the twentieth century, radium become quite a fashionable thing. Doctors prescribed it in medicines to treat various illnesses, and radium was in big demand for a variety of cosmetic, consumer products including luminous-dial wristwatches. Gradually, the number of cancers and other illnesses among radium and X-ray workers began to grow. In America, for instance, a large number of women were employed in factories to paint a mixture of zinc sulphide and radium on the digits of wristwatch faces to make them glow in the dark. It was usual for the women to lick their paint brushes in order to give them a finer point before applying them to the watch; inevitably, they swallowed some of the radium which, instead of passing through their bodies, lodged in the bone structure, and eventually an epidemic of bone cancer broke out among these women, crippling and killing many of them.

By the mid-1920s experts in Britain decided the time had come to collect evidence about radiation exposure and to try to set some sort of standard for doses to be 'tolerated', as new jargon put it, by X-ray and radium workers. An International X-ray and Radium Protection Commission was set up, and by 1928 the unit of radiation exposure dose was defined and agreed upon internationally as the roentgen, named after the discoverer of X-rays. By 1934, the experts had agreed on a recommended maximum external dose rate for workers exposed to radiation of 1 roentgen (r) a week. But it was still not a burning public health issue at this time, and any further moves to probe deeper into the mysteries of radiation and its effects on the human body were suddenly put aside after the outbreak of the Second World War.

After the war, the whole scene changed drastically. Up to the 1940s, the major source of exposure to ionising radiation had come from medical radiology. But with the discovery of nuclear fission on the eve of the war, the invention of the atomic bomb during the war and the planned development of nuclear reactor programs after the war, the range and types of radioactive materials to which the public would be exposed was about to increase dramatically. The old prewar standards of safety, such as they were, clearly were inadequate to cope with this new situation. So in 1950, a new body was set up in London called the International Commission on

Radiological Protection (ICRP), to succeed the old X-ray and Radium Protection Commission. The ICRP consisted largely of scientists from Britain, the United States, Canada, France, Sweden and Germany. It was theoretically independent of any government, its members having been chosen for their scientific expertise rather than their nationality. The ICRP's recommendations, however, were adopted by most Western governments, and its advice remains the standard measurement for radiological protection in most Western countries today.

The ICRP in its first year, 1950, adopted a more cautious standard than the prewar levels by lowering the maximum recommended dose to 0.3 roentgen a week. This was the standard applying at the time of the first British atomic bomb test in Australia in October 1952 – and, as Lord Penney told the Australian royal commission, the British regarded the ICRP's recommendations as the Bible.

All radioactive substances undergo a process of disintegration, or decay. It is during this process that they give off radiation, until they cease to decay and reach a stable state. The time for that to happen can range from a fraction of a second to millions of years, depending on the substance. Radiations, in turn, take four different forms. There are alpha particles, which have high energy but can be stopped quickly, even by a sheet of paper; beta particles, which tend to have greater energy and can penetrate human tissue up to a few millimetres; gamma rays, which have the greatest penetrating power of all, equal to X-rays, and are capable of 'irradiating' the entire human body; and neutrons. Ordinary human clothing is usually enough to prevent alpha and beta particles from entering the body, but gamma rays can be stopped only by a much greater shield, like a wall of concrete.

The roentgen measurements adopted in the ICRP's first recommendations after the war applied only to external exposure of gamma and X-radiation, because this was considered to be the most dangerous. Health physics, as the new discipline concerned with the impact of radiation came to be known, was still in its infancy and, as more information accumulated, a bewildering variety of extra units were adopted to measure more closely the impact of radiation on the body. The rad ('radiation absorbed dose') became the measurement for radiation actually absorbed by human tissue. Another unit, the rem, stood for 'roentgen equivalent man' and was designed to measure the biological impact of the radiation absorbed. The latest unit in use is the sievert, one sievert being equal to 100 rems. For the sake of simplicity, the unit r is retained here, referring to roentgens and rems which may be taken as roughly numerically equal.

The international recommendations at this time still applied only to occupational workers, or those people actually working in the radiation industry, who were aware of the dangers and could take precautions. No separate exposure levels had been set for people involved in or living near nuclear weapons tests, and it was not until 1953 that the ICRP addressed itself to laying down still separate recommendations for exposure levels for the general public – a level initially set at roughly ten times less than the maximum permissible level for those working with radiation. Over the years that the British were conducting atmospheric nuclear tests in Australia, the ICRP's recommendations were being gradually tightened as radiation experts learned more about the dangers. The ICRP's annual dose limits for whole body exposure in 1950, at the outset of the British tests, had been decreased by a factor of about three from those applying in 1934. They have been reduced by a further factor of three since 1950.

The implications of this for the exposure levels accepted by the British at the tests in Australia are obvious. The Australian royal commission calculated from records of the exposure levels adopted for each of the British tests that those applying at the Mosaic tests in May and June 1956, were three times higher than revised ICRP levels set in 1959. Sir Ernest Titterton grudgingly admitted to the royal commision that the exposure levels adopted for the earlier British tests were not acceptable internationally by the time the bomb tests were over in 1959: 'Now it does not say that anything that happened on the previous higher levels is dangerous or damaging. It just says that in the light of the present knowledge it would be prudent to accept the low levels.'

The new ICRP recommendations of 1959 set a maximum permissible dose for workers in the radiation industry of 5 r a year, corresponding to 0.1 r a week. This maximum exposure recommendation has been effectively retained since then, with variations for individual body organs such as the gonads, the thyroid and the blood-forming organs. By way of comparison, a dose of 400 r administered over a few hours is considered sufficient to kill those unfortunate enough to receive it.

For the first time, the ICRP in 1959 set down recommendations to allow for higher doses than the permitted maximum to be accumulated in a short period, say over a few weeks, with a corresponding reduction in the lifetime dose. The British had actually predated this idea with the radiation exposure levels they had adopted for the Hurricane bomb trial back in 1952. The exposure levels for the Hurricane and Totem trials had been set by Penney and David Barnes, a senior health physicist from Aldermaston, in consultation with the British Medical Research Council. Barnes told the Australian royal commission in London: 'In 1952, the ICRP limits were inflexible. The [weekly] dose was too restrictive to allow records to be recovered.' Barnes was referring to the problem, mentioned in Chapter Two, which the British saw: that if they stuck to the ICRP exposure guidelines, the test could turn out to be a scientific flop. For instance, they would not be able to send men into 'hot' areas soon after the bomb blast to recover vital records on fallout, blast, heat and so on.

So Barnes and Penney sought, and received, approval from the British Ministry of Supply for what was called an 'integrated dose' – in fact, a special dose much higher than the ICRP limits to be administered to a few men in special circumstances, where the success of the scientific enterprise justified it. There were two 'integrated dose' levels: a lower one of 3 r of gamma radiation and a higher one of 10 r. The men who received these were not to be exposed to radiation again for up to a year.

The way the whole outlook on radiation dangers was becoming more cautious during the 1950s is reflected in the terminology of the ICRP at the time. The decade had begun with the concept of a 'tolerance dose', implying that there was a threshold of radiation exposure below which no harm would result. In 1950, the ICRP introduced the notion of a 'maximum permissible exposure' and warned in a policy statement:

In view of the unsatisfactory nature of much of the evidence on which our judgments must be based, coupled with the knowledge that certain radiation effects are irreversible and cumulative, it is strongly recommended that every effort be made to reduce exposures to all types of ionising radiations to the lowest possible level.

The 'lowest possible level' still left room, it seemed, for a 'tolerance dose'. But by 1958, just after the close of the British bomb trials in Australia, the ICRP had begun to speak in policy statements of new dangers, such as genetic effects. It said: 'The objectives of radiation protection are to prevent or minimise somatic injuries and to minimise the deterioration of the genetic constitution of the population'. And, speaking of the higher, 'integrated' exposures, in cases of emergency work, which it had just approved, the ICRP added: 'Women of reproductive age shall not be subjected to such emergency exposure'.

Behind these latest strictures lay an emerging debate, which continues to this day, on the key question of the dangers posed by low levels of ionising radiation. This discussion specifically revolves around ionising radiation to which greater numbers of people began to be exposed with the expansion of nuclear power programs in the fifties. This is quite apart from the natural, background sources of radiation, to which everyone has always been subjected, such as cosmic radiation from outer space and radioactive substances in the earth's crust.

Radiation can have three main types of effect on people: acute, long term and genetic. The acute and long-term impacts together are known as somatic effects, because they relate to effects on the body of a living person. Acute effects result from heavy exposure to radiation, and produce the sort of symptoms so graphically illustrated by the victims of Hiroshima and Nagasaki and, in 1954, by inhabitants of the Marshall Islands in the Pacific Ocean who were subjected to large fallout from an American hydrogen bomb test. These symptoms are also sometimes known as radiation sickness. They result from immediate effects of ionising radiation on the gastro-intestinal and neuro-muscular systems, and include nausea, vomiting, diarrhoea, cramps, weight loss, fatigue, sweating, fever and headache. There can also be skin burns and loss of hair.

Aborigines at Wallatinna and Welbourn Hill described experiencing some of these symptoms after the passage of the Black Mist from the Totem One bomb in 1953. The number of acute symptoms experienced depends on how high the dose is; death from acute radiation effects can occur up to two months after exposure, although evidence from the Japanese victims suggests that it can even take several years. For acute radiation effects, there is a threshold of exposure: the dose has to be particularly high enough to produce these symptoms. If you receive a low enough dose, you will avoid them.

The same cannot be said for the long-term effects of radiation, which include cancer, leukaemia and eye cataracts. Nor does it hold true for the genetic effects, the damages to the body's gene structure caused by ionising radiation which are then passed on to future generations. As early as the 1920s, biologists had shown with experiments how ionising radiation could alter the genes of plants and insects such as the fruit fly. Experiments on animals involving radiation and genetics were stepped up after the Second World War, and the results extrapolated to human beings.

It is now almost universally accepted among scientists and geneticists that there is no level of radiation which can be considered safe, as far as long-term and genetic effects are concerned – no 'threshold'. But this was not the case in the 1950s, when doctors and biologists were discovering more about radiation and its effects as each year went by.

One of the unfolding debates, for example, revolved around not just the level of radiation to which people were exposed, but the precise nature of the dose. It was quickly realised that external guards against the highly penetrating forms of radiation, gamma and X-rays, were not enough. For instance, alpha and beta particles may not be able to enter the body easily through the skin, but they can cause great damage if inhaled through breathing or ingested by eating food. Plutonium 239 is one of the most toxic substances known: it emits alpha particles and has a very long half life – the time taken for half its radioactivity to decay – more than 24 000 years. If fine particles of plutonium are taken into the body on air or food, they lodge in the lungs and body tissues where they continue to emit alpha radiation and where, as we noted in the last chapter, only a minute quantity of plutonium is sufficient to cause cancer.

The advent of nuclear weapons brought hundreds of radioactive 'fission products', all of which had different half lives and which behaved in different ways in the human body. Some, like strontium 90, lodged in the bone and the bone marrow, a key blood-forming tissue. Another product, iodine 131, concentrated in the thyroid gland. If particles of these substances were deposited on grass, which was then eaten by cows, they could contaminate the milk, thus finding their way into the human body via this 'critical pathway'. Consequently, children, as big milk drinkers, were more vulnerable than adults to these particular radionuclides.

If lodged in certain parts of the body, these products continue to emit radioactivity causing damage to the cell structure, almost invariably resulting in cancer. The intestine and the reproductive organs, as well as the thyroid and the blood-forming tissues, are among those parts of the body more sensitive than others to radiation. There are still great uncertainties about the relationship of radiation to cancer, the principal one being due to the fact that it is impossible to distinguish cancer caused by radiation from cancer caused by any other agent. What is certain is that no level of radiation exposure should be considered safe in terms of avoiding long-term effects such as cancer.

The detonation of the Americans' first large thermonuclear device, Bravo, in the Marshall Islands in the Pacific in March 1954, produced heavy fallout from the 15 megaton weapon – 750 times more powerful than the Hiroshima bomb – on the inhabited atolls of Uterik, Rongerik and Rongelap, almost 200 kilometres downwind from ground zero. The islanders were evacuated two days after the test, but by then many had received sufficient whole body doses to give them skin burns on their necks, backs, arms and faces and to cause vomiting and diarrhoea.

The heaviest fallout was on Rongelap: 1000 r was measured on the northern tip of the island two days after the explosion, more than enough to kill anyone who lived there. Fortuitously, the island's population lived in the south which received about 175 r. This was still enough apparently to produce serious long-term effects years later. More than 65 per cent of those on Rongelap who were aged under ten when Bravo was exploded have since undergone surgery for the removal of thyroid cancers. Radioactive iodine ingested through water on Rongelap led to radiation doses in the thyroids of children which were between three and eight times larger than the entire external doses to their bodies; in the case of adults, the thyroid contamination was about the same as the external doses. In the four years after Bravo, women on Rongelap had a miscarriage and stillbirth rate more than twice that of unexposed women.

The bizarre and tragic experience of the Marshall Islanders illustrated how the age at the time of exposure and the sex of victims can be equally significant factors as the size and type of dose in determining the effects of radiation; children and young pregnant women can run greater risks than other people from exposure to some forms of radiation. Studies on these sorts of variable risk factors continue today, notably by the US National Institute of Health.

The Marshall Islanders, like the Australian Aborigines, were given no warning about the dangers of radiation or advice on how to protect themselves. Also like the Australian Aborigines, the Marshall Islanders today are afraid of the contamination which makes their homelands dangerous to live in. Both people use the same word to describe the radioactive debris at Rongelap and Maralinga: 'poison'. In June 1985, more than 200 people from Rongelap evacuated the island on the *Rainbow Warrior*, a ship owned by Greenpeace, the environmental group. They moved to Mejato, a previously uninhabited island in the Marshalls, declaring they would never return to Rongelap because it was too contaminated. The US government declined their request for help with evacuation, saying it was unnecessary.

Unlike the Australian Aborigines from Maralinga, the Marshallese from Rongelap have been the focus of a sustained medical probe since the fifties. Medical teams from the US Atomic Energy Commission (now the Department of Energy) began examining the islanders straight after the Bravo blast and have returned to do follow-up tests at least once a year since then. Indeed, many Marshallese later became convinced they were being used in some planned experiment on radiation. A secret document from the

Brookhaven National Laboratory in New York, produced three years after Bravo, noted: 'The group of irradiated Marshallese people offer a most valuable source of data on human beings who have sustained injury from all possible modes of exposure'.

As we saw earlier, the scientists in charge at the British nuclear tests in Australia did not begin to consider until the tests had been going for three years that the radiation exposure levels adopted at the earlier tests may not be adequate for desert Aborigines. The levels initially laid down at the British tests applied to white people protected by clothes and houses. They ignored the Aborigines whose lifestyles made them far more susceptible to all types of radiations. This was one of the most graphic illustrations of the way radiation protection standards in the fifties were being adapted on the run.

By the mid-fifties several international studies on radiation and human health began to get off the ground, partly in response to growing public concern about fallout from atmospheric nuclear tests. Both the British Medical Research Council and the US National Academy of Sciences embarked on research into the biological effects of radiation, looking particularly at genetics. The United Nations general assembly set up UNSCEAR, the United Nations Scientific Committee on the Effects of Atomic Radiation. UNSCEAR has since played a significant role in gathering worldwide information about human exposure to radiation and had issued eight major reports up to 1982.

Some of the most spectacular results, however, came from the less high-profile studies on the effects of low-level radiation. One of these began in 1955 under Alice Stewart, an epidemiologist then at Oxford University. Stewart's department had noted that the number of children dying of leukaemia had risen by almost half in the few years since the end of the Second World War. She set out to discover why. After two years' research, involving almost 1300 cases, Alice Stewart concluded that children whose mothers had had pelvic X-rays during their pregnancies were twice as likely to develop leukaemia, or some other form of cancer, before the age of ten as children whose mothers had not been X-rayed.

Initially, other scientists dismissed Stewart's work, arguing that it relied too much on probability and the memories of the mothers. But a few years later, in the early sixties, a study at Harvard University examined her claims by looking at almost three quarters of a million births from 37 hospitals in the United States. The Harvard study found that children whose mothers had been X-rayed during pregancy ran a 42 per cent higher risk of leukaemias and other types of cancer than those whose mothers had avoided pre-birth irradiation. Nonetheless, it took 20 years from the time of her study for Stewart to recieve a final blessing from the scientific community. It came in 1976 from Sir Edward Pochin, a consultant to Britain's National Radiological Protection Board and a former chairman of the ICRP. Pochin said: 'It now appears likely that absorbed doses of only a few rads in the foetus may induce malignancies of various types'.

Studies such as Stewart's created enough concern among radiologists for them to conclude that X-rays should no longer be used on pregnant women, and to be more cautious about the use of X-rays for diagnosis generally. Stewart's work had also begun to confirm what many experts had suspected for a long time: that there is a 'linear' relationship between radiation and cancer, that the risk of cancer or some other long-term effect is proportional to the dose received.

In 1976, Alice Stewart became involved in another highly controversial but revealing study of low-level radiation. Thomas Mancuso, a professor at the University of Pittsburgh, invited her to America to assist in an examination of the incidence and cause of death among workers at the Hanford nuclear plant in the state of Washington. Hanford had been set up during the Manhattan Project to produce plutonium for the US weapons program, and had remained one of America's prime nuclear installations, with nuclear reactors, reprocessing plants and vast waste disposal areas.

Stewart was accompanied by George Kneale, a mathematician colleague from Oxford. They and Mancuso applied a statistical analysis, which was heavily criticised later, to data which had been collected on about 25 000 workers between the years 1944 and 1971. Their results were initially published in 1977, with an updated version following a year later. The Hanford study eventually focused on about 5000 deaths among men and women workers, and compared cancer rates for those who had been exposed to radiation at Hanford with those who had not been exposed. Even for the exposed group, the levels of radiation exposure were very low: an average lifetime dose of just over 2 r. Alice Stewart and her colleagues concluded that there was a significantly higher rate among exposed Hanford workers for cancers of the lung and pancreas and for multiple myeloma, a rare type of bone marrow cancer. Their results suggested that the current ICRP recommendations on radiation exposure had underestimated the risk level by a factor of between 10 and 30.

Around the same time as the Hanford results were published, more disturbing figures emerged from another study in Portsmouth, New Hampshire, where researchers had looked at the death patterns among men working on the maintenance of nuclear submarines in the naval shipyard there. They examined more than 1700 cases and concluded that among those who had been exposed to radiation, the death rate from cancer was 38 per cent compared with 21 per cent for workers who had not been exposed. Again, this study was heavily criticised. Unlike Hanford, where the radiation exposure records for the workers were actually available, the Portsmouth researchers had been obliged to determine whether dead workers had been exposed to radiation by asking next-of-kin: the US Navy steadfastly refused to release the exposure records.

The low-level radiation row had blown up in Australia years earlier, in 1956, at the same time as Alice Stewart was embarking on her study in Britain of leukaemia rates among children. Hedley Marston, a senior biologist at one of Australia's leading research bodies, the Commonwealth Scientific and Industrial Research Organisation, was chosen to conduct a biological survey revolving around the movement of fission products in the fallout from the British nuclear tests. It was intended to be one of those rare cases of Anglo-Australian collaboration during the tests where results were actually shared: besides Australia's CSIRO, Britain's Medical Research Council and Agricultural Research Council were also involved.

Marston and his fellow workers collected thyroid glands from sheep and cattle in areas of north and northeastern Australia which were considered likely to be traversed by fallout plumes from the Mosaic and Buffalo tests between May and October 1956. They were particularly keen to examine the uptake of iodine 131 in the animals' thyroids in a bid to measure the movement of fission products into the food chain. Marston eventually published his findings in the Australian Journal of Biological Sciences in August 1958 – two years later. In the intervening period he had become embroiled in a furious row with the British scientists at the tests and with the Australian safety committee over his planned publication. The reason: Marston's conclusions flew in the face of the bland assurances the safety committee had given to the Australian government and, through it, to the public that there had been no danger to mainland Australia from the 1956 tests at Monte Bello and Maralinga.

Marston's survey indicated:

That extensive areas of Australia have been contaminated, and that some of the more heavy precipitations occurred on terrain situated over 1500 miles [2400 kilometres] from the site of the explosions, in areas more or less thickly populated.

After the second Mosaic explosion, G2, he found that iodine concentrations in the animal thyroids rose by up to 100 times above those recorded from the first Mosaic test a month earlier. The thyroid studies after the second Mosaic bomb indicated to him that some of the areas most heavily contaminated were up to 3000 kilometres away from the test site, on the northeastern seaboard and in central western Queensland. In fact, Marston concluded, the effects of the the second Mosaic bomb could be detected in a band about 1600 kilometres wide, stretching west to east across the continent. Marston's findings contradicted the report of the Mosaic tests which the Australian safety committee had sent to Menzies, assuring him: 'Incontrovertible evidence had been obtained which shows that all contamination of the mainland was near the low limit of detection . . .'

Marston also reported that the plume from the third bomb in the Buffalo tests at Maralinga in October 1956 contaminated Adelaide and the countryside surrounding the city. The safety committee advised Menzies of this bomb: 'The lower cloud ... dropped its active material almost entirely in the restricted area. The small, higher cloud ... produced virtually no fallout over the continent.'

Marston was quietly fuming at the discrepancies between his team's discoveries and the version being given to the public that fallout across Australia was, to quote two descriptions often used by the safety committee, innocuous and trivial. In July, after the Mosaic tests, Marston wrote to a senior colleague at the CSIRO:

These (our thyroid findings), taken in conjunction with various 'official' announcements in the Press, can only lead to one of two conclusions, viz. either the monitoring set up in use at present is incapable of doing what it aims to accomplish, or someone is lying.

But what caused more of a row than anything was Marston's conclusion that the presence of iodine 131 in the animal thyroids indicated that they had also taken up radioactive strontium 90 and other bone-seeking isotopes. He feared a transfer of strontium to the human food chain, via milk, and then a lodging in the human bone marrow where it could cause leukaemia. The rate of transfer to human beings would be at its peak, he reported, during the periods when the radioactive debris remained on the grazing pastures.

Marston did not record any specific measurements of strontium in his report. His concern, as a biologist, was simply to point to what he believed were the dangers from strontium based on his records of iodine uptake. It is now known that iodine and strontium behave differently after a nuclear explosion, iodine tending to travel further in the fallout than strontium. Marston's findings were published in full by the Australian Journal of Biological Sciences, except for two figures on gamma fallout which Penney insisted he delete on grounds that they could be used to reveal bomb-design information. Apart from that, Penney did not appear to object in any way to Marston publishing his report.

The Australian safety committee, however, were less pleased. The safety committee, by now under Titterton's chairmanship, prepared a reply in which they dismissed Marston's conclusions: 'He offers a number of opinions, unsupported by scientific evidence'. The safety committee particularly attacked Marston's interpretations of his measurements of iodine and his speculations about a parallel danger from strontium, and declared: 'Strontium 90 fallout in Australia is among the lowest in the world and..the contribution to it from the British tests in Australia is very small'. The safety committee were also angry at Marston's implied criticisms of their own earlier statements about safety on the tests.

The safety committee's attack on Marston, and a reply by Marston himself, were submitted for publication to the Australian Journal of Biological Sciences, but both papers were withdrawn at the last minute. Sir Macfarlane Burnet, the distinguished chairman of the new National Radiation Advisory Committee, and a member of the journal's editorial board, had tactfully suggested in a letter to Titterton:

I am frankly worried by the situation because of its latent potentialities to give rise to action which could be labelled by the Press as an attempt by Government to interfere with scientific integrity, or on the other side, as an attempt by left wing scientists to interfere with defence preparation. All concerned are fully aware that neither is the case.

The row, however, simmered on beneath the surface for some years.

At the time of the Marston controversy there was growing worldwide concern about the effects of strontium from the mounting number of hydrogen bomb tests. In April 1957, the Association of Atomic Scientists in Britain, under the chairmanship of Professor Joseph Rotblat, issued a report on the problem. Like Rotblat, the association's members were 'rebel' atomic scientists who had turned against the weapons applications of atomic energy. Their report encapsulated the division which reigned in the scientific world then on the 'threshold dose' question:

There is here a fundamental difficulty in that the relationship between the damage produced and the amount of radiation is not known. 'If this relationship is such that there exists a threshold dose below which cancer cannot be induced, then it can reasonably be inferred that the small amount of strontium 90 which will accumulate in bone from the current H bomb tests would not result in any harm.

If, however, the number of additional bone tumours resulting from radiation is directly proportional to the dose, then even a very small dose will give rise to a small but definite probability of bone cancer. This means that in a very large population a certain number of people would contract this disease as a result of their having a small amount of strontium 90 in their bones. The evidence is as yet inconclusive.

Doubts of this sort about the harm caused by even low levels of radiation were finally put to rest in 1972, when a committee appointed by the US National Academy of Sciences reported on a long study of the question. The Committee on the Biological Effects of Ionising Radiations, or BEIR, as it was known, rejected the 'threshold' concept and went further than any previous major study in arguing that no dose of radiation, however small, could be considered to carry no risk to human health. The BEIR report also laid down as a general philosophy that no exposure to ionising radiation should be permitted without the expectation of a commensurate benefit.

But the BEIR report did not end the row over low-level radiation. It simply made it more acrimonious. Eight years later, in 1980, the BEIR committee published another report whose drafting had produced much heated dissension among the committee's own members. Its chairman, Professor Edward Radford, an epidemiologist of Pittsburgh University, issued a separate statement saying he believed the latest BEIR report had underestimated the cancer dangers from low-level radiation, while another member claimed publicly the report had overestimated them.

The International Commission on Radiological Protection (ICRP) had effectively abandoned the 'threshold' concept in formulating its recommendations by the late 1950s. But in the debate that has raged since then, the ICRP's risk estimates, although often cited as the most authoritative, have come under considerable fire and have been often criticised for underestimating the risks. Dr Alice Stewart, by then in her late seventies, appeared before the Australian royal commission in London in 1985 where she said the ICRP risk estimates had understated the incidence of cancers produced by low doses of radiation by as much as 40 times; certainly, in her view, the latest ICRP figures had understated it by 10 times.

One criticism of the ICRP has centred on its claims to be a dispassionate, international watchdog on radiation exposure standards, supposedly detached from any governmental or commercial affiliation. In fact, the ICRP has proved to be quite a conservative body on the question of public exposure to radiation. During the 1950s, for instance, it never spoke out as an organisation against testing nuclear weapons in the atmosphere. One analysis has suggested that the clues to this are to be found in the composition of the ICRP's membership.

In early 1985 a British scientist, Patrick Green, completed a long study of radiation protection standards which formed the basis of a submission to the Australian royal commission from Greenpeace in Britain. Green analysed in some detail the composition of the ICRP between 1959 and 1984, when the row over low-level radiation really took off. He found, first, what he called a scientific imbalance among the ICRP's members. Of the 37 scientists who had been members since 1959, some 14 were physicists, a discipline which tends to be very pro-nuclear energy, 10 were doctors and eight were radiologists. The biological and environmental sciences, by contrast, had been very poorly represented.

Second, Patrick Green discovered a low turnover rate among ICRP members. The membership, he suggested, had circulated among a small elite of people who had remained in control since 1959, creating a closed system. The average time members spent with the ICRP was eight years. Two physicists, a Frenchman and an Englishman, had actually been members of the ICRP, or one of its committees, for 26 years. Both had also been members of government atomic energy authorities, in Britain and France.

Third, Green also found a domination among the ICRP's members of scientists who were affiliated to government or commercial organisations concerned with commercial exploitation of nuclear energy and to government nuclear regulation bodies. Green concluded that this was a clear conflict of interest:

• NO CONCEIVABLE INJURY

Far from being primarily concerned with researching the fundamental principles related to radiological protection, the ICRP has shown itself to be an organisation concerned with the commercial exploitation of nuclear energy.

Edward Radford, the American professor who was a former chairman of the BEIR committee in the US, took a similar view. He told the Australian royal commission that by the early 1970s, the ICRP and several other radiation protection bodies had provoked

concern on the part of some people that they were not independent – they were viewed as government agencies, and equivalent, and made up largely of representatives who worked for government agencies.

Much of the evidence on which ICRP and other studies are made has come from the histories of those actually exposed to large doses of radiation, such as the Japanese atomic bomb survivors and patients and medical workers involved in radiation medicine. The studies of high doses have then been extrapolated back to low doses using the 'non threshold' philosophy, namely that incidence of cancer is likely to be proportional to the dose received.

By the mid-eighties, a significant re-evaluation was under way of the effects of radiation on the Hiroshima and Nagasaki survivors. The results were anticipated to produce still higher estimates of cancer risks. Edward Radford was involved in the revised study at Hiroshima between 1982 and 1984. He told the Australian royal commission he believed the results would show a cancer incidence rate which was 10 times higher than the figures on which the latest ICRP protection standards are based. Sir Edward Pochin, himself a former ICRP chairman, and not a man to overemphasise radiation dangers, also forecast a change, but a more conservative one. When Pochin appeared before the Australian royal commission in Sydney in July, 1985, he expected that the risk estimates for some cancers may be increased by a factor of two when the latest Japanese studies were over.

Pochin explained how some of the revisions of the Japanese data stemmed from uncertainties about such things as the actual explosive yield of the weapons dropped on Hiroshima and

Nagasaki (the 'nominal' yield of 20 kilotons has often been used for both bombs, although some later estimates put the Hiroshima weapon at about 13 kilotons); the amount of radiation that escaped from the metal containment of the weapons; and the amount of radiation that was actually transmitted to people rather than being absorbed into the atmosphere between the detonation points and the ground. 'There is good estimation of the absorption in body tissues before the radiation reaches certain organs', Pochin explained. 'What has not been done yet is the heavy and laborious job of examining the resultant estimate of doses to individuals according to the position they were in – houses – and it is that reallocation of individuals into dose groups which is taking time.'[3]

More than 20 000 British servicemen were involved in the British nuclear tests in Australia and the Pacific and more than 15 000 Australians took part in the tests in Australia between 1952 and 1963. The veterans, and their families, from both countries who have lodged claims against their governments for compensation over cancers and other illnesses, and even death, which they attribute to radiation exposure during the tests, have faced three main difficulties.

First, governments of whatever political colour have a natural propensity for denying culpability over some controversial decision of the past, even though the events may have been the work of an entirely different generation of politicians. Apart from governments' instincts for defending themselves against assaults on the governmental decision making process, there is also a large element of financial self protection involved: bureaucracies are always afraid of setting precedents for a flood of litigation, whether the complaint involves a government bus slamming into the back of a motor car or radioactivity from an atomic cloud drifting over a population centre.

Second, the controversy that has prevailed over low-level radiation dangers, outlined above, has enabled the British and Australian governments to maintain that safeguards were implemented and that they were in accord with standards and recommendations of the time – even though many of those standards have since been abandoned internationally as inadequate in the light of present opinions.

Third, the records of radiation doses received by servicemen at the British tests have been shown in may cases since then to be at best incomplete and, at worst, inaccurate. It appears from the evidence that no more than a few servicemen at the tests in Australia were exposed to high or excessive radiation doses; but the governments in both countries have always refused to release the exposure records to the servicemen themselves.

Exposures to the servicemen were measured by film badges, which everyone on the range was required to wear, and, in a smaller number of cases, by dosimeters. Fallout measurements to the Australian population were also made, but not until the tests had been going for a few years. For the first two tests, Totem and Hurricane, there were no official measurements recorded of fallout across the Australian continent. It was not until the Australian safety committee was set up in 1955 that the scientists decided to install a number of monitoring stations around Australia, the number of which rose to 86 for the final two bomb trials, Buffalo and Antler. At these ground stations, fallout was measured by means of air filters and sticky-paper samples designed to catch fine, contaminated particles tumbling to the ground. But there were problems with both the personal film badges and the sticky paper system.

Many servicemen in Britain and Australia told stories to the Australian royal commission of how the film badge system broke down: badges were worn incorrectly or not worn at all, thrown away or kept as souvenirs. Doug Rickard, the Australian service-man who discovered the secret cobalt 60 on the Maralinga range several months after the 1957 Antler tests, described what appeared to be a typical story: servicemen who were keen to work overtime would often deliberately remove their film badges when they entered a forward area so as not to exceed their dose limits; and, in some cases, the doses recorded were simply estimated or made up if the film badges appeared not to be working properly or had become 'saturated'.

In most cases, the men wore the film badges at chest level. But it was not until after Buffalo, the second last round of bomb trials in 1956, that the British scientists discovered that these chest readings were probably underestimating radiation doses received by other parts of the body. At Buffalo, they conducted a little experiment by building a life-size dummy out of mahogany wood, dressing it in protective clothing and attaching dosimeters in the positions of various organs, including the lungs, spleen, testicles and intestine. Then they put the dummy in a spot contaminated with fission products after one of the bomb blasts. They concluded that the intestine and testicles received about a 40 per cent higher dose than those recorded by the devices worn on the upper half of the body.

The sticky paper system at the ground stations around Australia was unreliable for several reasons. If it rained, the radioactive material suspended on the samples would just wash away. But on more than one occasion, the sticky paper samples were placed out in the field and never collected again. Frank Smith, a member of the Australian radiation detection team who installed the sticky papers at cattle stations north of Maralinga for the first Buffalo bomb, One Tree, in 1956, described to the royal commission how his unit was ordered to skip collecting them afterwards and to go to Coober Pedy instead. 'Nothing would have surprised me', said Smith. 'And I am quite candid.'

At the Australian royal commission's hearings in Britain and Australia, some 92 witnesses gave evidence of having been involved as servicemen in the largest British bomb trial, Buffalo, in 1956, where four bombs were exploded. Only 26 of these men did not complain of ill health in the years since, although the royal commission drew no conclusions about whether their health problems were directly related to the tests. Until now, the onus of proof has always been on the servicemen to show that any cancer they suffered was directly linked to their radiation exposures – an uphill task, since it is impossible to distinguish between cancers induced by radiation and any other cancers. John Coulter, an Adelaide doctor who has specialised in medical research in genetics, described to the Australian royal commission how he saw the risks of connecting low-level radiation with cancer:

The situation is that in most Western countries approximately 25 per cent of the population will get cancer at some stage in their life, and I think in Australia the figures indicate that about 19 per cent of the population currently will die of cancer. The causes of that cancer are a multiplicity of factors: background radiation, exposure to naturally occurring chemicals, exposure to man made chemicals – a whole host of factors, any one of which may give rise to the genetic damage which then subsequently could give rise to a cancer. We must ask the question: does an additional exposure to a mutagenic agent such as radiation cause an additional expectation of developing cancer or any of these other consequences? I think the answer quite clearly is yes.

By the time the Australian royal commission had presented its report in December 1985, there had been no completed epidemiological study in Britain or Australia comparing test veterans with others in a bid to determine how much the risks Coulter described may have affected their health. In the United States, one such study had been completed in 1980, although even that generated much controversy. Scientists at the centre for disease control, Atlanta, examined the histories of 3224 men who had taken part in field experiments at the test explosion of a 44 kiloton nuclear weapon in Nevada in August 1957, codenamed Smoky. Nine of the men had since contracted leukaemia, which the researchers reported was three times the expected rate for the ordinary male population. Film badge records were available for eight of the nine men, and all had received low average doses of a little more than 1 r.

The Smoky researchers cautioned that more follow-up studies were needed of people involved in other nuclear tests before any conclusions could be drawn. A follow-up study was commissioned by the Defence Nuclear Agency, an American government body. It involved about 50 000 people who had taken part in one or more of five US tests in Nevada and the Pacific. The results were reported in May 1985, and confirmed the excessive leukaemia rate among Smoky participants. But the researchers found no significant excess of leukaemia or other cancers among those who took part in other tests, although they warned that several aspects of the study again limited the scope of any conclusions.

In the same year as the initial Smoky study in the US, 1980, Neal Blewett, a prominent member of Australia's Labor party opposition, was making a call for exactly a study of this sort to be made among Australia's Maralinga veterans. Blewett told parliament in

Canberra in April that year:

There seems now to be enough evidence to enable us to make a presumption that the Australians in and around Maralinga were exposed to radiation considerably in excess of that experienced by the average Australian.

Blewett dismissed assurances from previous governments that monitoring procedures at the tests in Australia had been stringent. He asked for a study to be set up of cancer incidence among Maralinga veterans, and measured against a similar group of Australians who had not been exposed to radiation.

Three years later, Blewett became minister for health in Bob Hawke's government when Labor came to power. But the sort of 'control' study which Blewett had suggested has never been undertaken. Instead, a survey of health among Australian veterans, commissioned under Malcolm Fraser's conservative government, was presented in 1983. This study was called the Donovan report, after its author, Dr John Donovan, but it has been widely criticised over its methodology. As Donovan explained to the Australian royal commission, he identified from records more than 15 300 Australians who were involved in the British nuclear tests, and was able to find addresses for 8000. He sent out questionnaires, but finally received replies from only 2440.

Donovan's study was in two parts: a questionnaire to veterans seeking their health histories and possible indicators of their exposure to radiation at the tests, such as the tasks they performed and the sites they visited; and an analysis of causes of death based on death certificates of those who had since died. The Donovan report found that there were no grounds for concluding that Australian personnel suffered significant adverse health effects from the tests.

But Donovan himself expressed reservations about his study when he was asked at the Australian royal commission if it was possible to reach such a conclusion after 30 years, in the light of the limitations on medical records. He replied: 'It is an impossible task to do so at the standard that I would like to have applied. The data were just not of sufficient quality for me to do so.'

John Coulter, the Adelaide medical researcher quoted earlier, expressed surprise at one aspect of the Donovan report when he gave evidence to the royal commission:

it passes over the observation that in the main survey group there were only four respondents with a history of lung cancer, nine with leukaemia. It simply allows that statement to go by default. In any population, if one finds a substantial increase in leukaemia relative to lung cancer when lung cancer is so much more common, one should be, I believe, very suspicious. The figures may be too small to prove anything statistically, but that is a most unusual observation.

The Australian royal commission concluded that the Donovan report, while a valid and useful survey, could not be regarded as an adequate epidemiological study because of the paucity of relevant information on which it was based. It called for a national register to be set up of nuclear veterans, Aborigines and others who may have been exposed to radiation. But, strangely, it said nothing in its recommendations about a need for the sort of full-scale, rigorous epidemiological survey of such people which may have gone some way towards shedding light on the long-running radiation health controversy.

In Britain, after pressure from test veterans, supported by a handful of MPs, notably David Alton and Gavin Strang, the Thatcher government ordered a health survey of 20 000 British ex-servicemen and civilians who took part in the fifties nuclear tests in Australia and the Pacific. The survey had not been finished by the time the Australian royal commission presented its report at the end of 1985. The British survey, too, was limited in scope, although more extensive than anything undertaken in Australia.

It sought to compare cancer and death rates among the test veterans with a similar 'control' group of people who did not take part in any tests. The study was being conducted on behalf of the UK Ministry of Defence by the National Radiological Protection Board, NRPB, the main body concerned with monitoring and advising on radiation protection standards in the UK. The NRPB, set up in 1970, has come under similar criticism as the ICRP over its independence, namely that its members have been too consistently linked to the nuclear industry to give the body the true image of a nuclear watchdog. Some critics of the British study believe it should have been commissioned from an independent, academic institution instead. Many British veterans have also criticised the limited scope of the NRPB's study, particularly its focus only on cancer and not on other radiation linked illnesses such as cataracts. The British government, however, placed great authority in the study and argued that the Australian royal commission should have waited for its completion so as to take account of the findings – a move that would have extended the life of the royal commission by at least a year, and possibly more.

One non-government survey of British veterans from the hydrogen bomb tests in the Pacific had already commenced before the launching of the NRPB study was announced in October 1983. The previous year, Alice Stewart, the pioneer of research on radiation effects on unborn children, began looking at reports of death and illness among the H-bomb test veterans after a BBC television program, 'Nationwide', had invited firsthand accounts of the Pacific tests from viewers. Stewart and two colleagues from Birmingham University reported their findings in April 1983 in a letter to the *Lancet*, the authoritative British medical journal. Although they had examined only 330 cases by then, they found an abnormally high number of leukaemias and lymph gland cancers. There were also ten reported cases of cataracts. Stewart said the findings indicated either that the veterans were exposed to much higher radiation doses than hitherto supposed or that there were much higher cancer risks from small radiation doses than hitherto supposed – or both.

Governments in Britain and the United States have always refused to accept compensation claims from veterans of nuclear weapons tests in the fifties and sixties, citing legislation in both countries which prevents servicemen from suing over alleged injuries received during government service. Similar legislation exists in Australia, although as the number of compensation claims reaching Canberra began to mount in the eighties the Australian authorities have not sought to invoke it. This does not mean, however, that Australia has been bountiful or generous towards its nuclear veterans. By early 1986, some 204 compensation claims had been lodged in Australia over illnesses or death allegedly suffered from the British nuclear tests. Only six had been found in favour of veterans' claims that their ill health was caused by radiation.

Another 87 were decided in favour of the Australian government – in other words, the government was not liable. The rest of the cases were still plodding on.

These cases all came under the federal compensation system for government employees, rather than the ordinary courts of law. Australia's compensation system sets strict limits on cash awards: the highest of the six compensation awards was $30 000. One widow, Peggy Jones, whose husband, William, died of cancer in 1966 at the age of 39, received just $8600. Jones had served at Emu Field during the Totem trials, and, according to his family, had spent several days in a 'hot' area where he was sent to recover a tank following an atomic bomb blast.

Some Australian veterans and their families have begun going beyond the compensation system and taking their cases directly to the courts, where, theoretically, there is no limit on the amount of compensation that could be awarded. By 1986, five civil court actions in Australia had been commenced or foreshadowed. They came from Colin Bird, of Brisbane, who had worked on decontaminating Lincoln aircraft used in atomic cloud tracking, and who is now suffering from throat cancer; the family of Robert McLean, also involved in aircraft decontamination, who died of cancer in 1983; Ric Johnstone, of Sydney, who was a driver with the Australian air force at Maralinga involved with decontaminating vehicles, and who claims that his subsequent health breakdown, including agoraphobia, was a result of radiation exposure; Peggy Jones; and Yami Lester, the Aborigine who alleges his blindness was due to fallout from the Black Mist after the Totem One bomb.

The Australian royal commission in its final report made no comments on these cases, or their validity. With regard to the Black Mist affair generally, the royal commission found that such a phenomenon passing over Wallatinna and Welbourn Hill could have happened and that there was no reason to disbelieve Aboriginal accounts of it.

Given the historical uncertainties and the current state of scientific knowledge, the evidence presented does not enable the royal commission to decide one way or the other whether the Black Mist caused or contributed to the blindness of Yami Lester.

The most dramatic legal decision in favour of plaintiffs from nuclear tests of the fifties came in the American federal district court judgment of May 1984, mentioned at the beginning of this chapter. Here, for the first time, was a court deciding that cancers among a group of people exposed to nuclear fallout had been caused by radiation. Judge Bruce Jenkins ruled in favour of 10 out of 24 people whose actions were heard as 'bellweather' cases on behalf of 375 cancer victims in Nevada, Utah and Arizona.

All the litigants had lived near the Nevada Test Site where the US tested more than 90 nuclear weapons above ground up to 1962, sometimes at the rate of four a month. The ten successful cases included the families of eight people who had since died of leukaemia, one woman who died of breast cancer after the close of the trial and a 38-year-old woman still living but suffering from thyroid cancer. The judge ordered the US government to pay $2.66 million to compensate the families and the surviving victim.

In the 14 unsuccessful cases – involving cancers of the pancreas, stomach, kidneys, ovaries, prostate, bladder, lungs, lymph system and skin – the judge accepted the government's argument that radiation from the tests had not been a cause. Nevertheless, the judgment appeared to have opened the way for a flood of litigation or out of court settlements in other cases.

The American judgment, more than 400 pages long and some 19 months in preparation, was interesting because many cases of negligence which the judge identified in the conduct of the American tests were similar to allegations about the British tests heard before the Australian royal commission. Judge Jenkins introduced his findings on negligence with this philosophical comment:

Atmospheric nuclear testing has expelled more radioactive material into the world under far less human control than any other human activity to date. Finding a small corner of the earth which as yet remains wholly untouched by radioactive fallout would be a match for even the most seasoned of explorers.

Ounce for ounce, the risks associated with that dispersal are far greater than the relative risks of any other human enterprise. Extraordinary risk demands extraordinary care.

The standard of care, of course, is tempered in this case by the limits of human control. Once loosed in the air, the nuclear fireball engulfs and annihilates the devices of direct restraint and control available to humans; its cloud of lethal debris may be predicted, traced and monitored, but it is never confined. Failure to prevent the inevitable may not be negligence. Failure to take the best, most stringent protective measures to warn of, lessen and mitigate its risks may very well be negligence.

The American judge went on to argue that by 1951, when the Nevada tests began, the American authorities had a good deal of knowledge about radioactivity, fallout and the real and potential effects on human health: a body of experience had already built up from the Alamogordo test in 1945, the Hiroshima and Nagasaki bombs and five atomic tests already held at Bikini and Eniwetok in the Pacific in 1946 and 1948. The point could also be made that British scientists were also privy to information from most of these explosions.

Jenkins found that up to the end of 1958, when the moratorium on tests began, at least 29 Nevada tests deposited significant, measured fallout in Utah, 16 in northern Arizona and 18 in northern Nevada, while between three and 10 shots delivered fallout to Las Vegas and to cities and towns in California. The American judge found it 'astounding' that between 1951 and 1962, no-one made any concerted effort to monitor and record internal contamination or dosage to residents who lived near the test sites. Random samples among residents using film badges did not start until the 1957 series codenamed Plumbbob, when 28 nuclear bombs (including Smoky) were exploded at Nevada in one year. Even then, few exposure records were kept for civilians, in contrast to servicemen working on the bomb sites. Jenkins commented:

The negligence reflected in the monitoring program is highlighted by the fact that even now we have more direct data concerning the amount of strontium 90 deposited in the bones of the people of Nepal, Norway or

Australia than we have concerning residents of St George, Cedar City or Fredonia.

Finally, the American judge found a series of cover-ups at the Nevada tests with an uncanny similarity to those alleged at the British tests in Australia. Among them:

The public education program in off-site communities was consistently heavy with confident reassurances. Important information concerning both risks and effective precautions was scarce at best, and largely ineffective as a rule; [the residents near Nevada] were never fully and accurately informed of what it was they were exposed to, what it might entail in terms of long term consequences, or how to keep the additional risk as low as was possible at that time. Consequently, many people were exposed to more radiation, and greater risk, than ever needed to be.

The American judge also issued a warning about film badges, the main method of monitoring exposures to servicemen at Nevada, as at Maralinga, Emu Field and the Monte Bellos:

Film badge data are not perfect. Badges may be damaged or lost. Film badges provide little information about beta exposure, less about beta/gamma ratios and almost nothing about internal exposure due to inhalation or ingestion of alpha-and-beta-emitting radionuclides. Hair, hands and shoes may collect more contamination than the shirt pocket where a badge may be clipped.

In one of his most damning findings of government behaviour towards the public at the American tests in the fifties, Jenkins declared:

The public pronouncements as given do not really warn and do not sufficiently educate. They reassure. They don't talk of potential long term dangers. They talk of how effectively the program is being managed . . . They demonstrate that responsible persons at the operational level of continental nuclear testing neglected an important, basic idea: there is just nothing wrong with telling the American people the truth.

In the fifties there were big problems from the perspectives of the American, British and Australian governments about telling their respective publics about the sorts of dangers which the American judge identified. If the governments had been as frank with the public as it now seems clear they should have been, the whole nuclear testing program could well have ground to a halt. Secrecy and public reassurance thus became primary tools of governments and their scientific advisors in Australia as much as in the US.

There were, of course, differences between the Nevada case and the British tests in Australia. The Nevada court judgment covered civilians, not servicemen actually involved in the tests. Civilians lived in much larger concentrations near the Nevada tests than they did near Maralinga. And yet, there were Aborigines living under close exposure to the Maralinga tests who were treated with the same contempt as the much larger white populations around Nevada: they were never warned about the tests, monitored for radiation or advised of the consequences.

The Australian royal commission, of course, had no power to award compensation, nor did it spend as much time as the American district court examining specific claims of links between radiation and cancer. But it did identify similar cases of negligence in the conduct of the tests in Australia (see Appendix One). When it reported in December 1985, it did not rule out radiation from the tests as a cause of cancer among the British and Australian veterans and the Aborigines. 'The royal commission has accepted that in the present state of knowledge it must be assumed that any exposure to ionising radiation, however small the dose, gives rise to an increased risk of a cancer or heritable defects', it concluded.

The royal commission took an open view on these dangers, towards both servicemen and the Australian population at large. With the servicemen it noted that recorded film badge doses were an imperfect guide and likely to be underestimates of the doses actually received, endorsing the American judge's conclusion on this monitoring method. For some at the tests in Australia, radiation doses were not even recorded: the Australian air and ground crews involved with air sampling flights at the first two trials, Hurricane and Totem One, were not issued with personal film badges or dosimeters for the aircraft.

As for the Australian public, the royal commission decided not to be bound by two earlier scientific studies which had sought to estimate the actual numbers of cancers which may have been caused by fallout among the population. The first, by the Australian Ionising Radiation Advisory Council, AIRAC, came in 1983 in a controversial report known as 'AIRAC 9'. The AIRAC scientists took fallout data from the monitoring stations set up around Australia in 1956 and estimated a collective dose for the Australian population. They then used risk factors suggested by the ICRP in 1977 and came up with the conservative estimate that the maximum number of cases of cancer in the Australian population which could be attributed to the nuclear tests was no more than one and may have been zero.

In 1985, two scientists from the Australian Radiation Laboratory re-evaluated the fallout data, using different methods from AIRAC's, and produced a somewhat larger collective dose estimate for the Australian people. The ARL scientists concluded there could have been as many as seven cancers and seven serious hereditary effects among Australians at large from the British nuclear tests – although they warned that their estimates could be too high by a factor of ten or too low by a factor of two.

The Australian royal commission did not accept either of these conclusions, but it failed to provide an alternative. It believed the data were insufficient to estimate a collective radiation dose to the Australian population. And because the risk factors were in a state of flux with the revised studies of the Japanese atomic bomb survivors, it said, 'no useful assessment of likely numbers of health effects in the Australian population, due to the tests, is possible'.

The royal commission recommended that the compensation system for federal employees, mentioned earlier, be opened up to people besides military servicemen and government employees, such as university scientists, civilian workers at the test sites and Aborigines who may have been exposed to the Black Mist. The legislation under which the compensation scheme is conducted allows for the onus of proof to be shifted from the claimant to the government for diseases which can be shown to be generally associated with certain types of employment, including employment involving exposure to radioactive substances. The royal commission urged that the same shifting of the onus of proof apply to non-government employees who may seek compensation: 'By their very nature, the diseases and injuries upon which claims will be based will be life threatening or will have resulted in fatalities. Justice demands that such claims be processed as expeditiously as possible'.

So by the mid-eighties, in Australia at least, the whole question of radiation and health had been turned over to be fought through the legal tribunals and courts. The outcome in Britain was even more vague. Yet the governments in both countries were not about to shift their ground and admit liability for radiation damage from the fifties. The openendedness of the Australian royal commission's conclusions foreshadowed a flood of litigation; but it was also typical of the way in which legal and scientific opinion has been consistently unable to come to grips with one of the most harrowing and bitterly contested public health issues of our time.

Chapter Eight
DIAMOND JIM GOES
TO LONDON

'Only one question remained to be answered – would anything, after all, be done? Or would the royal commission, like so many other royal commissions before and since, turn out to have achieved nothing but the concoction of a very fat blue-book on a very high shelf?' – Lytton Strachey, *Eminent Victorians*.

When the Australian government decided in July 1984 to set up a royal commission into the British nuclear tests, the man it chose as president of the inquiry was James Robert McClelland, then the chief judge of the New South Wales land and environment court, and a former federal Labor government minister. In most respects, McClelland was not like other judges. He courted publicity. Few lawyers, British or Australian, had come across a judge quite like McClelland. Often he appeared to feel totally unconstrained by the conventions of his role, and to relish the headlines surrounding his inquiry as much as the substance of it. He turned 70 in the middle of his inquiry, although he looked younger, and he maintained a taste for being photographed, quoted and seen on television at a time of life long after most public figures and former public figures had tired of it. McClelland's overriding publicity consciousness was to be crucial to the royal commission's success in unleashing thousands of documents in Britain and Australia which had been locked up in secret government archives for more than 30 years. In November 1985, shortly before his royal commission's report was released, McClelland described his stand against the British government to an Australian magazine this way: 'Frankly, my attitude was "fuck you bastards, we'll get what we can out of you, even if we have to shame you into it by going public and showing what you're about". And it worked.' [1]

He is known as Diamond Jim because of his stylish way of dressing: he was once selected as one of Australia's ten best-dressed men. The judge was certainly free with his comments on government leaders, and other public figures. He called the Australian prime minister, Bob Hawke, the man whose government gave him his commission, a 'pygmy' compared with Hawke's predecessor as Labor prime minister, Gough Whitlam, in whose government McClelland himself had once served as a minister.

But his most controversial remarks came in an interview he gave to the London magazine, *Time Out*, a few days before he left for Australia in March 1985, at the end of his commission's hearings in London. Looking back on his impressions of life as experienced from the British capital over the previous ten weeks, the judge was quoted describing Margaret Thatcher, the prime minister, as 'that silly woman' and said:

In Australia, Thatcher's regarded as a figure of fun. When she stands in front of the camera and puts on what seems to us a terribly phoney accent we rub our eyes and wonder how can the British people cop this one as leader!

McClelland also made a swipe at what he called Britain's 'lickspittle bureaucracy' and had some thoughts on British government secrecy as highlighted in a recent scandal over telephone tapping by the security service, MI5: 'I'd say that you are getting pretty close to needing a new Magna Carta in this country'. *Time Out* published the interview with a drawing of McClelland wearing his judge's wig, and a hat on top with corks dangling from it.

Soon after he returned to Australia at the end of March, and with several months of hearings still ahead, McClelland gave a national television interview in which he said the royal commission's inquiry in London had showed the British had something to answer for, and that he hoped the inquiry would help to prevent 'the same awful mistakes in the future'. He also criticised Thatcher's dress sense. These were unusual remarks coming from a royal commissioner in the middle of a complex inquiry. In each of the many royal commissions Australians had experienced in recent years, on organised crime, drug trafficking, agent orange and corruption in trade unions, the judges in charge had maintained a stony silence until their reports were delivered, and then, for the most part, had faded quietly back into obscurity.

Some of McClelland's colleagues at the royal commission, and in Canberra, believed he had gone too far with his uninhibited interviews, and that he risked opening up the royal commission to the charge of bias and lack of objectivity. Indeed, the British government did not let the opportunity pass to make just this point five months later when it presented its final submission to the royal commision the following September. Under a special heading, 'Objectivity of the Commission', the British government noted:

There have been widely reported comments made by the President outside the proceedings of the Commission which suggested an attitude hostile to the UK, to its conduct of the tests and to the UK attitude to the matters being investigated by the Commission.

The British nuclear tests royal commission had given an unexpectedly dramatic finale to McClelland's career. He had retired from parliament in Canberra in 1978, having quickly lost interest in life as a politician when Whitlam's Labor party went back into opposition after the drama of its sensational dismissal from office by the governor general, Sir John Kerr, three years earlier.

McClelland returned to the world he knew best, the Sydney law, settled into the comfortable and less volatile round of a judge on the industrial court, and then chief judge of the land and environment court, and, in the normal course of events, could have expected to end his working life on the bench, a forgotten figure from the seventies.

McClelland's high-profile performance during the royal commission's hearings in Britain and Australia brought out the strange contradictions in his character: a mixture of liberal and conservative, traditionalist and iconoclast, Anglophile and Pom basher. Part of McClelland's feistiness towards Britain sprang from his Irish working-class origins in Melbourne. Like others of his generation, he harboured a mixture of admiration and resentment towards Britain, made more pertinent in his case by his perceptions of himself as a literary figure (his first ambition, he always said, was to be a journalist, not a lawyer). While he bristled at Britain's social system, he wallowed in its theatrical and artistic life, and he enjoyed flaunting his verbal dexterity and wit during the royal commission's hearings, often at the expense of witnesses. During a hearing in London, he told the counsel assisting the royal commission: 'You must remember that you are present in a country where there exists a lingering doubt whether the plays of Shakespeare were written by Sir Christopher Marlowe'. Later, during a long answer from Sir Ernest Titterton in Sydney, McClelland cut in contemptuously: 'I think the needle is stuck'.

A key factor in the success of McClelland's outbursts was that they were taken up by the British press, which supported the inquiry and reported it extensively, at least in the early days of its London appearance. When the royal commission opened its London hearings in January 1985, the *Times* called for full British government co-operation: 'This is not principally an issue of science or medicine, but of whether Britain can convince a friendly ally to whom we owe a debt that when we say we will help we mean what we say'. At the close of the London hearings, almost three months later, the *Guardian* referred to 'the persistently inquisitive and refreshingly informal Australians' who had managed to prise loose 38 tons of documents from the death grip of the Official Secrets Act: 'The whole sorry story amounts to another swingeing indictment of British official secretiveness, and it is to our shame that it was left to the Australians to expose it'.

On another level, though, McClelland clearly amused the British. After a party in March 1985, to farewell the Australian lawyers at the Wig and Pen club, a chic Fleet Street watering hole for lawyers and journalists, the *Listener's* gossip columnist reported:

McClelland is rough and tough and wants you to know it: he gives a performance like John Wayne in *True Grit*. He despises the people 'who run Britain', but he is sentimental about cockneys: 'I love their accents'. . . . As I left, he called out: 'The *Listener* is a real class paper – Don't let that Murdoch get hold of it'. Or words to that effect.

McClelland's two fellow royal commissioners could hardly match him in flamboyance, but their backgrounds were diverse enough and well suited to the royal commission's inquiry. Dr Bill Jonas, a lecturer in geography at the University of Newcastle, New South Wales, had emerged from a poverty stricken, Aboriginal background, and devoted much of his spare time to Aboriginal welfare work in and around Newcastle. The third royal commissioner, Jill Fitch, was a senior health physicist with the health commission of South Australia, specialising in radiation medicine. (The royal commissioners are discussed further in Appendix One.)

About thee months before she took up her role on the royal commission, Fitch had joined the Australian Ionising Radiation Advisory Council (AIRAC). This body of eminent scientists had already produced several reports on the conduct of the British nuclear tests, reports which were to become a key focus of attention and attack at the royal commission. Fitch had not been with AIRAC when the reports were prepared; but her membership of AIRAC was enough to provoke a challenge to her role on the royal commission, in October 1984, from Greg James, QC, the counsel appearing for the Australian nuclear veterans, and supported by Geoff Eames, the senior counsel for the Aborigines. They charged that Fitch's membership of both the royal commission and AIRAC was a clear conflict of interest. Fitch promptly quit AIRAC and stayed on the royal commission.

AIRAC's role, in fact, had been pivotal to the setting up of the royal commission in the first place. AIRAC had been formed in 1973 after the Whitlam Labor government dissolved the two bodies which had remained in existence since the days of the British nuclear tests – the Australian safety committee and the National Radiation Advisory Committee. Titterton had remained chairman of the Australian safety committee since 1957, but he was not asked to join the new body, AIRAC. Its functions were similar to those of the old National Radiation Advisory Committee, namely to advise and make recommendations to the government about the various sources of ionising radiation to which Australians were exposed and their likely dangers.

The people appointed to AIRAC were leading figures from

Australia's scientific and medical establishment. But the body eventually suffered from criticisms similar to those levelled against the International Commission on Radiological Protection, the ICRP, and Britain's National Radiological Protection Board, namely that many of its members were too closely linked to the nuclear industry for AIRAC to be a truly independent watchdog.

By the late seventies, the British nuclear tests had begun to emerge as a controversial issue in Australia, with the row over the return of the half kilogram of plutonium to Britain, reports by Yami Lester and other Aborigines about the Black Mist and growing numbers of stories from Australian nuclear veterans about cancer deaths among their members allegedly caused by radiation exposure at the tests 25 years earlier. The press in Australia took up the stories and some newspapers, particularly the *Adverstiser* in Adelaide, began conducting their own investigations. Similar allegations among veterans in Britain followed. Fleet Street began to take the claims of some British veterans seriously and ran big stories about them.

As the controversy developed, the Australian government relied increasingly on AIRAC for advice and began to use the organisation in a similar manner to that which the Menzies government had used the Australian safety committee 30 years earlier, to instil an atmosphere of public reassurance. In November 1980, Prime Minister Fraser's minister for national development, Senator John Carrick, wrote to a ministerial colleague asking for AIRAC's help to investigate allegations about the Black Mist and the exposure of the Australian population to high fallout levels from the nuclear tests. Carrick noted that, in calling for AIRAC's help, he wanted 'an independent assessment' of the charges.

AIRAC eventually responded in January 1983, with a report, known as 'AIRAC 9', on the safety measures taken at the nuclear tests and the possible after effects. The report, in effect, gave the British nuclear tests a clean bill of health. In some cases, the 'AIRAC 9' report employed language which obscured the facts or accepted at face value official information which has since been proved wrong. It said, for example, that none of the British bombs exploded in Australia had a yield much more than 20 kilotons, when the second Mosaic bomb was three times that strength. The

AIRAC report also dismissed the possibility of the Black Mist, and of the nuclear tests having caused any short-term illnesses or early deaths among Aborigines in South Australia. It barely mentioned the minor trials, and said nothing about plutonium contamination on the range as a result of the trials.

Malcolm Fraser's conservative government was defeated at the polls in March 1983, shortly before the 'AIRAC 9' report was tabled in parliament in Canberra. By now, any government would have found the build-up of claims and counterclaims about events at the British nuclear tests impossible to ignore. But the new Labor government, headed by Bob Hawke, was in a particularly delicate position. For the rest of 1983 and during early 1984, Hawke's government proceeded to do a U-turn on a number of Labor's nuclear policies. Many Labor supporters were angered by the government's approval of new uranium mining contracts and by its reluctance to take a stronger stand than the previous conservative administration on Australian control over American defence bases in Australia. Some of Hawke's critics thus interpreted his eventual appointment of the British nuclear tests royal commission as a sop to the anti-nuclear lobby.

Just over a year after the Hawke government took office, in May 1984, the *National Times* published an article on plutonium contamination at Maralinga based on a leaked copy of the full Pearce report (see Chapter Six). Two weeks later, Hawke's minister for resources and energy, Senator Peter Walsh, responded to the controversy this disclosure generated by setting up a special committee to review all the data on atmospheric fallout from the British nuclear tests. It was given the daunting task to report in just two weeks. This committee was headed by Charles Kerr, professor of preventive and social medicine at the University of Sydney, and himself a former member of AIRAC, and included three other scientists from Melbourne University, the Australian Radiation Laboratory and the Commonwealth Institute of Health.

Given the limitations of its inquiry, Kerr's committee focused its attention on the 'AIRAC 9' report, the most comprehensive public account of the British tests so far. It demolished the report, concluding that it 'could not be regarded as an authoritative scientific account nor as an informative public record of important aspects of the British nuclear tests'. From its reading of official documents, The Kerr committee disagreed with AIRAC on many fundamental issues, including interpretation of information on fallout levels, progress of radioactive clouds, dosage estimates, risks of radiation exposure and aspects of management during the tests. 'Most of all', Kerr's committee said:

it disagreed with the philosophy used to construct 'AIRAC 9' – the use of simplified assumptions which do not accurately reflect the complexities of what took place and the constant endeavour to present the best possible case which results, to quote the *Canberra Times*, in a comfortable picture of the British nuclear tests.

It recommended a public inquiry into the conduct and consequences of the tests, and cited, in particular, the Black Mist story as something worthy of full investigation.

The Kerr report infuriated AIRAC. Its chairman, Professor Maxwell Clark, a geneticist of Flinders University in South Australia, wrote to Hawke's government: 'We take great exception to the unsubstantiated criticisms by Professor Kerr and his committee'. Clark and his AIRAC colleagues stood by the 'AIRAC 9' report, and, in doing so, Clark invoked the authority of science over decisions reached from anecdotal and other non-scientific evidence: 'We are satsified that there is no reason to amend the scientifically based conclusions in 'AIRAC 9'.'

This was at the heart of the affair. By the time Clark's letter of protest arrived, the Hawke government had decided to set up a royal commission to inquire into the conduct of the British nuclear tests, with wide terms of reference. [3] Meanwhile, public attention had focused dramatically on the issue once again when an Australian test veteran, Jack Burke, gave a harrowing television interview from his deathbed, a day before he died of stomach cancer, alleging, among other things, that the bodies of four Aborigines were found in a bomb crater at Maralinga (this story was later repeated in evidence to the royal commission by another witness, but the royal commission eventually found there was not enough evidence to accept it).

The royal commission's appointment was announced in July

1984, two weeks after the premier of South Australia, John Bannon, had written to Hawke asking for a full public inquiry and expressing his deep concern 'at the potential for unauthorised persons to be able to recover lethal materials left as residue at the Maralinga sites'. In April, Bannon had also written to Margaret Thatcher of his concern about various aspects of the British nuclear tests. Bannon's demand for a public inquiry reinforced a similar call which Don Dunstan, a previous premier of South Australia, had made to the federal government some years earlier.

Although royal commissions are not courts of law and do not have power to charge or convict witnesses, they are run by lawyers who stick to the conventions and quaint mannerisms of courtroom behaviour. The lawyers still defer to the judge in charge as 'your honour' and to their fellow barristers as 'my friend' or, in the case of Queen's counsels, 'my learned friend'. All that are missing are the wigs and gowns. The lawyers run the show very much as if the proceedings are taking place in some vast, impersonal court, seeking to impress their colleagues and the judge by working relentlessly on tricky witnesses and getting them to confess the truth. In this case, the entity on trial from beginning to end was the profession of science.

This was fairly inevitable. Lawyers and scientists have diametrically opposite ways of looking at the world, of judging right and wrong, truth and fiction. The United States district court judgment in 1984 on the Nevada tests noted this fundamental difference when it quoted from the contemporary observations of an American judge:

Science normally evolves a new, general physical principle from hypotheses proven by numerous specific experiments. The normal judicial process is precisely the reverse, for, when properly conducted, it applies an existing, generally accepted moral or social value, an ethical principle, a rule of law, to a specific problem . . . Judges and lawyers must approach with great care the idea that court decisions can be justified solely on the findings of science, lest the quest for justice be lost along the way. For the particular 'scientific truth' relied upon may prove transient indeed. [4]

The tensions and suspicions which had characterised Anglo-

Australian relations towards the end of the British nuclear testing in the early sixties were carried through to the royal commission's inquiry more than 20 years later. There had been, according to one story, a garage at Maralinga outside which an Australian serviceman had painted a sign: 'Hop in for service – Everyone welcome – No poms'. By the end of the royal commission's hearings in September, 1985, it was almost as if 'Diamond Jim' McClelland himself could have nailed up the same sign outside his commission's hearing rooms on the ninth floor of a skyscraper overlooking the harbour in East Sydney.

The royal commission had gotten off to a somewhat hurried start in Sydney on 22 August 1984. Margaret Thatcher's government pledged its full co-operation to Bob Hawke, but from the very beginning there was a great deal of uncertainty about what this meant. The royal commission had begun questioning witnesses without having access to the mountains of documents which lay in British archives or, indeed, without securing the release of all the documents from the Australian files in Canberra. The British government ignored the royal commission's hearings for the first four months by deciding not to send a barrister to represent it.

Even the Australian government debated whether it should be represented, the argument in Canberra being that they had been British nuclear tests and, although the Australian government had set up the inquiry, this was no implicit admission that Australia had done anything wrong. In the end, the Hawke government elected to be represented from the first day through a Sydney barrister, James McIntyre, who took a low key approach during the entire proceedings.

The counsel assisting the royal commission was Peter McClellan, a 37-year-old Sydney barrister who had appeared in several cases before Justice James McClelland over the past four years in the New South Wales land and environment court. (The similarity of their names often caused confusion.) The judge had been impressed enough with McClellan's courtroom performance to nominate him for the role of counsel assisting – in effect, leading the questioning of witnesses on behalf of the royal commission, and making sure the commission's inquiry stayed on the right track.

Peter McClellan's style was almost the antithesis of the judge's. He was ordinary rather than flashy: he smoked a pipe and played golf in his spare time. He had a keen attention for detail and his courtroom manner was dogged and persistent without fluster or drama. While the judge was making headlines with his speeches and interviews, Peter McClellan was tirelessly sifting through thousands of documents to unravel the thread of events in the fifties which gave the inquiry its substance. His job called for him to become an instant expert in many aspects of nuclear physics, medicine and political history, and he handled it brilliantly. The judge and McClellan began the proceedings with an obvious warm personal regard for each other. But as the pressures and strain mounted, and as Peter McClellan's role as a marshaller of documents and an organiser of witnesses became more dominant, the relationship came under stress.

When the royal commission visited Maralinga in April 1985, to inspect the extent of plutonium contamination and to take evidence from Aborigines, the two men disagreed openly. Three days had been set aside for the Maralinga visit, which Peter McClellan argued were needed to assess the key question of the future of the range; the judge, however, was impatient to cut the visit short. To bystanders who witnessed the disagreement, it appeared to be a dispute over who was really in charge. In November 1985, shortly before the royal commission handed down its report, the New South Wales government appointed Peter McClellan a Queen's counsel.

The counsel appearing for several Australian veterans' groups was Greg James, a Sydney barrister who had specialised in criminal law and had become a QC three years earlier – like Peter McClellan, before he was 40. The nuclear veterans in Australia, as in Britain and the United States, were not unified and had split off into several different factions. Greg James represented two of the groups: the Maralinga and Monte Bello Atomic Ex-servicemen's Association and the Australian Nuclear Veterans' Association, South Australia Inc.

The nuclear test veterans of Britain, covering several thousand ex-servicemen from the tests in Australia and Christmas Island, were represented at the London hearings of the royal commission by Mark Mildred, a tall, courteous London solicitor with a background in community legal work on behalf of minority groups. Mildred appeared before the royal commission when it reached London, and again during the closing days in Sydney a few months later, courtesy of the Australian legal aid office. Mildred acknowledged this financial support before the royal commission in Sydney. The British veterans, he said,

will remember the gratuitous assistance they have received from the [Australian] attorney-general's department and contrast it with the gratuitous pleasure with which the then responsible British official in London was able to deny their request for financial assistance to be represented in these proceedings.

Mildred's brief was a difficult one: the Australian royal commission was a foreign body which was taking evidence in Britain simply under an agreement with the host country, the first time this had happened. It had no powers to call witnesses in Britain – that privilege remained with the Treasury Solicitors of Whitehall and the barrister whom the British government eventually briefed to represent it. Nor was the British government obliged to take any account of the royal commission's findings. So the most Mark Mildred's clients could hope for was public relations value from his appearance, in the hope of using the royal commission's disclosures and findings to exert further political pressure for their cases after it was all over.

Mildred at least was able to use his appearance to exercise his wit on behalf of the British veterans against the secrecy in Westminister and Whitehall. At one point, he referred to an incident in which the British authorities had denied him access in London to radiation dose records of British veterans, then sent the same records to the royal commission in Sydney. Mildred remarked: 'Since you will appreciate there are no longer any left arms still attached to the British body politic, I can only conclude this was another case of the right hand not knowing what the right hand was doing'.

Acknowledging the royal commission's success in dislodging thousands of secret documents from British archives, Mildred said:

We reflect with pleasure, but with no surprise, that the disgorging of all this information, until so recently adorned with various badges of secrecy, has not brought so much as a single brick, let alone the entire walls, of Whitehall tumbling down. I hope we shall in due course hear counsel for the United Kingdom acknowledging the foolishness of his client's ways thus far, confirming that the breeze of open government and the public's need, and right, to know is now blowing down the corridors of power and thanking the royal commission for bringing his clients to this painless state of grace.

The Aborigines of South Australia, Western Australia and the Northern Territory could not have hoped for more able representation than from the two Adelaide barristers who appeared on their behalf, Geoff Eames and Andrew Collett. Both men had a long understanding and experience of Aboriginal legal problems. Eames had worked for several years in the seventies for Aboriginal legal aid services in Alice Springs and Darwin, and as a counsel in some of the first Aboriginal land rights battles in the Northern Territory. Collett had founded an office in Port Augusta, South Australia, of the Aboriginal legal rights movement and had travelled in this job through most of the Pitjantjatjara lands around Maralinga.

Eames conducted most of the cross-examination for the Aborigines at the royal commission. He was tall and swarthy and had a courtroom manner that was tough, penetrating and lucid. He shone best when confronting as witnesses the men of the fifties, now well into their seventies, and had an ability to carefully tear down the veils which shrouded their almost complete ignorance, then and now, of Aboriginal life and the relics of their colonial attitudes.

It was Andrew Collett who spotted among the torrent of documentary material produced in London one of the most revealing documents to come out of the royal commission's inquiry. This was the document with the innocuous title, 'High Explosives Research A32', which, together with later evidence, disclosed how the first Totem bomb at Emu Field – the Black Mist bomb – had been fired in exactly the conditions which scientists had warned were the least advisable for radiological safety.

In their final, outstanding submission on behalf of the Aborigines in September 1985, Eames and Collett presented a challenging attack on the manner in which scientific wisdom had been allowed to escape public scrutiny at the time of the nuclear tests, and on the authority of scientific bodies appointed to advise governments 30 years later such as the Australian Ionising Radiation Advisory Council, producers of the controversial 'AIRAC 9'. 'The "AIRAC 9" report has been so thoroughly discredited as a document of scientific integrity that we believe detailed attention to its terms is unnecessary', they wrote. '[AIRAC's] conduct in investigating the British nuclear test program has been so inadequate and unbalanced that its advice should not again be sought by government. In short, it should be disbanded forthwith.'

And they concluded their 500-page submission to the royal commission with these words:

The public has a right to know at what point scientific knowledge ceases to be conjecture and at what point subjectivity replaces science. The public were never placed in this position of wisdom during the British nuclear test program. The scientists cannot be heard to complain if the wisdom gained through this royal commission causes the public to be harsh in its criticism of the scientists, who did so little during the program to inform them of the risks to public safety that were being taken.

When the royal commission opened its hearings in London on 3 January 1985, after more than three months spent taking evidence in Australia, a new face appeared at the bar table of lawyers in the hearing rooms in Little St James Street, in the heart of London's clubland. This was Robin Auld QC, a 47-year-old barrister whom Thatcher's government had briefed to represent it for the rest of the inquiry. Auld had had an eminent career, much of it spent in the service of government inquiries. In the sixties, he had been a member of a commission of inquiry into alleged corruption of gambling casinos in the Bahamas involving the Mafia. In the seventies, he had chaired an inquiry into schools in Britain at a time of raging debate between traditional and progressive education. In the early eighties, he had been counsel to an inquiry into race riots in Brixton, London. Just before the Australian royal commission, he had conducted a government inquiry into Sunday shop trading in Britain.

Auld was assisted by a junior barrister and briefed by three lawyers from the Treasury Solicitors. Clearly, the British government had decided, somewhat belatedly, to take the royal commission seriously. Auld had a polite, co-operative manner which impressed the Australians in the early days of the London hearings, but which masked a professional thoroughness and shrewdness. The judge commented informally that he found Auld 'gracious and very British'. But underneath the initial bonhomie that prevailed, as the two sides gingerly felt each other out, was a minefield of tension between the British lawyers and the royal commission that was to erupt into total war as the months unfolded.

Even before the royal commission arrived in London a public quarrel had broken out between the British and the judge. During the early days of the hearings in Australia, in October 1984, the new British high commissioner to Australia, Sir John Leahy, announced his unhappiness at the way allegations before the royal commission about the conduct of the British nuclear tests were being made public straight away: 'Obviously one can't feel happy when the name of one's country is called into question', Leahy said. Judge McClelland reacted with characteristic tetchiness to this, and lambasted the high commissioner. Shortly afterwards, the two men patched up their disagreement when they met, for the first time, over a discreet lunch at the Union Club in Sydney at the invitation of Sir John Leahy.

The drama over the release of documents did not really begin until the royal commission reached London. Peter McClellan and his staff arrived just before Christmas and encountered a distinctly cool reaction at the Ministry of Defence when they sought to put into practice Thatcher's earlier offer to the Australians of full co-operation. He was welcome to go to inspect the index of files in the vaults at Aldermaston, he was told; but he would find so much paper there that he would go away and probably never want to come back.

By the time the hearings were due to begin, this standoffishness had produced almost nothing from the British files. So the judge decided to take a calculated gamble and, as he later put it, shout the

Australians' case from the rooftops in a somewhat contrived outburst. On the opening day, the air temperature outside was below zero. Inside, the diplomatic heat rose with television crews jostling for position, the press table spilling over with reporters and the public gallery packed as the judge slowly read from his carefully prepared opening address:

It is only in recent weeks that the British government has decided to be represented before the commission. There are grounds for believing that this decision was taken reluctantly and only after the commission had publicly suggested that the British government was dragging its feet.

The nuclear tests were carried out by the British and the evidence which has already been adduced suggests to us that they told the Australian authorities almost nothing about what they were doing in Australia during the tests.

Since the British know so much more than we do about what they did in our country at that time, co-operation now, if it is to mean anything, involves not simply telling us that we are free to delve into the mountain of documents which are in British hands, but positive assistance in bringing to light anything of relevance which those documents may disclose.

Secrecy, in the national interest, has always been a convenient alibi for failure of disclosure. But today it is hard to believe that Britain is in possession of any atomic secrets unknown to the great nuclear powers. We're not here to poke our noses into British technical secrets, but there is a certain minimum of information to which, as the host country to nuclear tests, we feel entitled to have access.

As an exercise in tactics, it was Judge McClelland's finest hour because the outburst, reported as it was that night on the BBC and ITN television news and on the front pages of many Fleet Street newspapers next morning, produced results. Over the next few days and weeks, civil servants in the Ministry of Defence, the Foreign and Commonwealth Office and at Aldermaston worked overtime to declassify and copy thousands of documents among the 38 tons of documentary material on the nuclear tests. They began arriving at the royal commission in a series of avalanches.

The decision to hold back the documents had been made by the bureaucrats in Whitehall, not the politicians at Westminister. As the royal commission gathered a momentum of public interest, it was Sir Michael Havers, Thatcher's attorney general, who advised the prime minister that Britain had nothing to gain politically from hiding from the Australians secret information about the nuclear tests any longer, provided the information had nothing to do with weapons design. Thatcher agreed, and the order went out to Whitehall to change course. Havers had also recommended to Thatcher earlier on that the British government should stop ignoring the royal commission and send a barrister to represent it when the commission reached London.

Havers, fortuitously, had developed a personal interest in Australian affairs at this time. His son is Nigel Havers, the prominent British actor, and, while the row was brewing in Britain about the production of documents, Nigel Havers had been working on location in South Australia as the co-star of a feature film about two famous nineteenth-century explorers in Australia, Burke and Wills. A few weeks after the royal commission opened in London, in early January, Peter McClellan received an invitation to what was billed as a late Christmas drinks party at the Treasury Solicitors' offices near Buckingham Gate. On his arrival at the party, McClellan was taken straight to meet Sir Michael Havers, who was hovering in a corner. The British attorney general and the Australian barrister chatted amicably for half an hour about Australia and the royal commission's work. Then Sir Michael Havers politely made his excuses and left, without speaking to any other guests. Clearly, it had been an exercise in diplomatic fence-mending.

Soon afterwards, the Australians put out feelers across the Whitehall divide that an informal meeting with Adam Butler, the British minister for defence procurement, might be equally efficacious. Butler, whose father was the famous Conservative MP, R.A. 'Rab' Butler, had come in for an attack from both Peter McClellan and the judge on the opening day of the royal commission's London hearings over remarks Butler had made in the House of Commons just before Christmas, in which he appeared to raise some question about the royal commission's objectivity.

Adam Butler responded to the Australians' overtures by agreeing to an informal meeting with Peter McClellan and the judge. The meeting took place over a drink in the billiards room of the St James's club, the comfortable Mayfair establishment where the judge lived during his London sojourn. It was friendly enough, both sides listening and talking intently about politics in Britain and Australia, with the judge making a bid to upstage Butler over his knowledge of British political history. But when Butler stood up and shook hands to depart, neither he nor the Australians had given anything away on the vital issue at hand. Sadly, it was to be the final amicable meeting of any substance between the royal commission and the British.

More than 40 witnesses appeared before the royal commission in London. The star figure was Lord Penney, who gave evidence on two occasions (see Chapter Two). The others included some of Penney's ageing colleagues from Aldermaston in the fifties, who had come out of retirement in the counties for the occasion, and who, in many cases, clearly resented their lives' work being questioned by lawyers half their ages. No civil service veterans who had been in charge in Whitehall at the time were called, a curious omission. Because the Australians had no power to summon witnesses in Britain, most of the witness list had been drawn up by the British government's lawyers, who had then showed it to each of the Australian parties for approval and had invited them to nominate any further witnesses. Early on, the Australian government's lawyers sought the addition of a small number of military, scientific and service veterans; but when the British declined to disclose the locations of these people, on grounds of confidentiality, the Australian government's lawyers hired a private detective to track them down so they could interview them before the hearings.

At the end of March 1985, with thousands of British documents, disclosing a completely new picture of the nuclear tests, in its hands, the royal commission returned to Australia to take vital evidence from Australian scientific witnesses and to inspect the test ranges at Maralinga and the Monte Bello Islands. Then in Sydney on 26 June, less than a month before the formal hearings were due to end, the uneasy amity that had prevailed so far was finally shattered when Robin Auld rose to make a blistering attack on the manner in which the royal commission had been conducting its business. The British government's counsel, in effect, accused the royal commission of the same crime which the judge had levelled at the British six months earlier: of failing to have declassified and presented in evidence large bundles of documents from the Australian government's own files.

The brunt of Auld's complaint was that the royal commission's staff had failed to prepare a proper collection of documents gathered from 3000 files in federal government, South Australian and West Australian archives, or to declassify hundreds of other secret Australian documents. Auld also accused the royal commission's staff of frustrating a British Ministry of Defence official who had flown out from London to declassify British documents held in Australian files, and of choosing for presentation in evidence mostly the Australian files which were potentially adverse to the British. 'The mismanagement of the commission's documents is at risk of undermining this inquiry and the resulting report', Auld declared.

Auld's long attack was received with stunned silence. When the British QC sat down, the judge turned to him and said: 'It is news to me that there are so many documents which you seek, Australian documents, which have not yet been declassified. Don't you think it might have been a good idea to bring this publicly to the notice of the commissioners earlier than today?'

'I always took the view that it would be wrong for me, an outsider, to attempt at any stage to tell the royal commission how to do its job', Auld replied. 'I find it strange, if I may say so, that your honour is unaware of the rate of declassification of Australian files. I have no doubt that Mr McClellan, as part of his duties, has made it his busines to keep you and your fellow commissioners informed.'

'Well, that is news to me that you are aggrieved by the belated attempts to declassify Australian documents', snapped the judge. Auld: 'Well, forget for the moment whether I am aggrieved and take the position of the commission . . . I find it astonishing that the commission has been unaware of the late stage of preparation of bundles to be put in evidence and declassification of hundreds of Australian files.'

While there was an element of tactics in Auld's attack, preparing the ground for possible British government criticism that the royal commission's inquiry was biased and incomplete, there was also some substance to his complaint about documents. While the royal commission had been in London demanding British documents, the Australians back home had been remarkably slow in gathering together and organising their own files. The eventual full collation of Australian documents, comprising material extracted from some 3000 files, was not tendered in evidence until the closing days of the royal commission's hearings in July 1985. Some of the Australian legal counsel obliquely acknowledged Auld's complaint. 'In a sense, I am accepting some of the matters which are put forward by Mr Auld', said Geoff Eames, for the Aborigines. 'Your honour, there is a problem with the documents', said Greg James for the Australian veterans.

Over the next few weeks, the level of Robin Auld's attacks on the royal commission's handling of the documentary evidence mounted, and they became the source of rapidly deteriorating relations between him and Peter McCellan. In early July, Auld revived his accusations:

I have been involved in commissions and tribunals of inquiries in various capacities in the United States, the United Kingdom, Europe, Africa and the Far East and in all of them there has been a common fund of documents amassed from the beginning by the controlling body and circulated to all parties . . . The real evil of what has happened is this: that from the beginning of this inquiry, witnesses have been examined by Mr McClellan without the assistance of documents which would have enabled him to have examined in a more informed and balanced way. That is the evil and that cannot be undone.

'Who do you blame for that evil, Mr Auld?' asked the judge.

I have to say that I blame the commission for taking the course that it did . . . My readings of the Australian files have been very interesting in the information that they revealed was available to the commission at the outset and which it left for London leaving unread. In my respectful submission, the proper course when a tribunal of inquiry or a royal commission sets about its task is to get control of the documents first and then examine the witnesses.

Peter McClellan defended the manner of presentation of the Australian documents, and vigorously denied that the royal commission had been biased against Britain. 'It is a gross assertion', McClellan said. 'Mr Auld, in my submission, has demeaned his clients by the remarks he has made.' He added: 'I should say on my own behalf, notwithstanding the criticism which Mr Auld has directed to me, I do not carry any colonial chip, even though he may have adopted the tone of the whingeing Pom'.

'I wondered how long I would get through this inquiry without somebody calling me that', Auld replied. Peter McClellan called on Auld to withdraw his charges. But by now, relations between the two men had become almost irretrievable.

In late September, the seven legal counsel and their advisers gathered together for the last time in the Sydney hearing rooms to reply to each other's final submissions before the judge and his two fellow commissioners. In the packed public gallery sat nearly a dozen Pitjantjatjara Aborigines from Maralinga, whom Geoff Eames and Andrew Collett had invited to Sydney in a symbolic gesture for the occasion.

The final submissions are a written summary of each party's arguments, a last opportunity to persuade the royal commissioners before they retire to write their report. The replies are thus a grand finale, in which each counsel stands up and points out why his submission should be given more weight in the report than everyone else's. As counsel assisting this royal commission, Peter McClellan had also put in a final submission even though he did not technically represent any group affected by the nuclear tests. As it turned out, the occasion was highlighted by a trenchant attack from Robin Auld, lasting almost two days, on McClellan and his submission.

The tenacity of Auld's final attack surprised many people in view of the nature of McClellan's final submission. McClellan had been deeply critical of the conduct of many of the British bomb tests, and of the minor trials. He argued that four of the bombs – Totem One; and three in the Buffalo series: One Tree, Breakaway and Kite – should not have been fired in the weather conditions prevailing at the time. But on another key question, the link between radiation exposures from the tests and health, he was very cautious in his advice to the royal commissioners. Indeed, in this respect there was little to choose between McClellan's argument and that of the British government, as contained in Robin Auld's submission.

This is what the British government said in its final argument:

The wide ranging and detailed investigations of the royal commission do not show that the health of anyone in Australia has been harmed by the nuclear tests or minor trials. In particular, the commission has found no evidence upon which it could conclude that any Aborigine has suffered harm from any of the tests or minor trials, including Operation Totem One, at which the 'Black Mist' occurred. The weight of the evidence is that the low levels of ionising radiation to which people may have been exposed as a result of the nuclear tests or trials have not exposed them to any greater risk of harm than that to which the general population is subject.

Peter McClellan's final argument said:

The regulations with respect to permissible levels of radiation exposure at each test were carefully prepared and reflected contemporary scientific knowledge. In general the organisation of radiation protection was well administered although it is likely that some accidents and isolated breaches of the regulations did occur . . .

By reason of the detonation of the major trials and the deposition of fallout across Australia it is possible that cancers which would not otherwise have occurred have been caused in the Australian population. The number caused could be as high as 14 or as low as one. The best estimate is that the number caused is seven. By reason of their exposure to radiation as participants in the trial program there may be an increased incidence of fatal cancer among 'nuclear veterans' of perhaps one cancer.

Robin Auld recalled how the judge had recently indicated to him that the British government's role was something rather more than to simply assist the royal commission with documents and witnesses: Britain was, in the judge's view, a defendant, there to defend its position. So the British government had responded with a final submission of its case running to more than 700 pages with a detailed analysis of each of the bomb trials.

The Australian government, by contrast, whose predecessors had allowed the tests to take place, but which the judge did not cast in the role of a defendant, produced a very slim final submission of less than 150 pages, simply drawing the royal commission's attention to several key points of evidence.

Robin Auld's attack built to a climax. 'Where is this royal commission going?' he asked. 'Is it looking at words you can slice in order to impale witnesses with them?' He demanded that any British witnesses whose credibility the royal commission intended to criticise in its report should have been notified beforehand so they could prepare a reply. And, in this respect, Auld came close to characterising the Australian royal commission's inquiry as something of a roughneck exercise: 'In all civilised proceedings of this sort with which I have had anything to do, that basic courtesy has been extended to all persons likely to be criticised'. The anger rising visibly in his face, the judge sat silently and impassively, staring at the wall beyond where Auld stood, as these words were uttered.

So the royal commission ended as it had begun, with an apparently unbridgeable gulf between the British and the Australians. Many of the more lurid claims about events at the British nuclear tests, which had helped to spark the inquiry – for example, that dead Aborigines were found in a bomb crater; that mental patients had been secretly installed in a bunker as human guinea pigs and were heard screaming as an atomic bomb exploded; and that servicemen had been ordered to bury atomic bombs in the desert – were not substantiated in the evidence. To that extent, the royal commission ended with a sense of spectacular anti-climax.

As the judge and his fellow commissioners went away to prepare their report, and as Robin Auld and Peter McClellan parted without speaking to each other again, one fact appeared to have escaped most people in the heavy drama of the final days. The royal commission had been not just an inquiry into the health and safety aspects of nuclear weapons testing, but an exercise in Australia of the post-Menzies Anglomania era examining the legacies of its recent history. The British civil service establishment, steeped in a world of secrecy, never really understood this two-dimensional nature to the inquiry and, to the end, bitterly resented this outside challenge to its own private rules. To that extent, at least, little had changed since the fifties. One British official privately described the royal commission as 'a blunt instrument' used for digging up the past. This attitude was certain to continue as the royal commission's report, finally delivered in December 1985, seemed destined to become a source of diplomatic wrangling between Britain and Australia for the rest of the eighties.

The royal commission had taken evidence from 311 witnesses over 118 days. It had sat in London, Sydney, Melbourne, Brisbane, Adelaide, Perth, Marla Bore, Wallatinna and Maralinga. The transcripts of its hearings ran to more than 10 000 pages. It had received in evidence more than 10 000 documents which had remained top secret in British and Australian government archives for the previous 30 years.

The British nuclear tests in Australia from 1952 to 1963 were the story of a once great power seeking to adjust itself to its changed position in a new and different world. When the key decisions of the 1940s were made to build a British nuclear bomb, many of those who took them perceived Britain as a nation which should develop her own independent nuclear deterrent as a perfectly natural outcome of her long leadership in science and technology and her great power status of the past. At the end of the Second World War, Britain, indeed, could still claim to be the most significant power after the world's two emerging economic and military giants, America and Russia; the great economic success stories that were to overtake Britain and render her a middle-level power over the next 30 years, Japan and Germany, still lay in ruins.

As Britain sought to cope with its rapidly reducing power status during the fifties, its nuclear weapons tests became an instrument of policy in order to ensure its position at the top level of the Western alliance. In this sense, the tests were enormously successful. By exploding its first atomic weapon in the Monte Bello Islands in 1952, and its first hydrogen weapon in the Pacific five years later, Britain succeeded in persuading the United States to ditch the restrictions on information sharing which had begun with the McMahon Act in 1946 and to restore the atomic collaboration between the two countries to its former level. Britain's position as the world's third nuclear power enabled her to exert influence over American nuclear policy and strategy and to play a leading role in the formulation of American policy towards Europe. Moreover, Britain had managed to enter the nuclear league relatively cheaply: the cost of developing the British atomic bomb, from 1946, when work began, to early 1953, just after the first successful weapon test, was, according to the official figures, just under 160 million pounds sterling (at the currency value of the time), or 1.5 per cent of the total defence expenditure in the same period. [5]

In later years, as the cost of Britain's nuclear deterrent escalated, her strategic policy and position became more blurred. [6] From the early 1960s, Britain began testing both tactical and strategic nuclear weapons jointly with the Americans in Nevada. She gradually came to depend on American technology for the delivery systems for her extended nuclear arsenal, through to the Polaris submarine force and its Trident replacement planned by the Thatcher government in the eighties. At the same time Britain, along with several other West European nations, accepted American cruise missiles aimed at the Soviet Union to be stationed on her soil. In all these measures, Britain had lost a large degree of the strategic sovereignty and independence which she had set out to achieve with her first atomic explosion just 30 years earlier.

Australia, by contrast, gained little, if anything, from the British nuclear tests. Although Australian political leaders at the time often presented the tests to the public as joint exercises, the reality was different. Britain was in charge of them, and only a handful of Australian scientists were vouchsafed information which was largely limited to safety criteria for the firing of the bombs. In the case of the minor trials, the Australians were not even involved to this limited extent. At various points in the early days of the British nuclear tests, an Australian domestic atomic energy program had been mooted as a possible spinoff from any Australian knowledge gained through its peripheral involvement with the British nuclear program; by the 1980s, however, Australia remained a non-nuclear country.

Yet it had never really been a consideration of the Menzies government, in approving the nuclear tests, that Australia may gain a significant amount of nuclear know-how from them. Menzies simply did not care about the tests, apart from exploiting them as a show of Commonwealth solidarity with Britain's contribution to the Cold War against communism. He was content to leave Australia's representation to the safety committee of scientists which, in turn, largely identified itself with the British scientific effort rather than with an independent Australian role.

It has often been too easy to explain the British nuclear tests as a case of Britain exploiting one of her former colonies, a view that often came through at the Australian royal commission. If there was any exploitation, then Australia was a willing exploitee. The royal commission in its report, for example, spoke of a British plot to 'plant' Titterton on Menzies in 1951, before the British nuclear tests began in Australia, so that the British would have, again to quote the royal commision, 'their man' on the Australian side. The need for plots and plants usually arises only when there is opposition from the other side. In Australia in the early fifties, there was no opposition to the British project whatsoever. When Britain turned to Australia to conduct its nuclear tests, after failing to secure Nevada on its own terms, it fully expected questions to be asked and demands to be imposed from Canberra, as they had been from Washington. It was pleasantly surprised when there were none. The Menzies government asked for nothing in return for holding the tests in Australia and was prepared to agree to them informally for as long as Britain wanted. With Menzies at the helm, plots and plants became unnecessary.

In one of the few aspects of the testing program that was actually committed to a written agreement between the two countries, the 1956 memorandum setting up the Maralinga test range, the terms were extremely open-ended and asked only that Britain provide 'sufficient information' to satisfy the Australian authorities that the tests could be carried out safely. When the trials were over Canberra signed an agreement in 1968, on the recommendation of the Australian safety committee of scientists, releasing Britain from further liabilities and responsibilities at Maralinga. The agreement was reinforced in these terms in 1979 after the row over the repatriation of the half kilogram of plutonium to Britain. Justice James McClelland's remark in January 1985, at the opening of the

London hearings of the royal commission, about Australia, as host country to the nuclear tests, being entitled to access to information about them, may have been true enough; but it was a cry that came 35 years too late.

The Anglophile personality and pro-British policies of Menzies were crucial to the holding of the British nuclear tests in Australia. Under the wartime leadership of John Curtin's Labor government, Australia had begun to shake loose its old deference towards Britain and had made an historic foreign policy turn towards the United States. Under Menzies' dominant leadership in the fifties the British nuclear tests represented a final episode in Australia's traditional foreign policy subservience to the mother country.

They also represented a consistent theme in Australian foreign policy since the Second World War. Apart from Menzies' emotional loyalties to Britain, his government saw Australia's agreement to the nuclear tests as an insurance policy which would help to link Australia to the defence umbrella of, to use Menzies' own phrase, her 'great and powerful friends'. The 1950s were years when many scientists and politicians believed the 'atomic genie' would unleash all sorts of benefits to the world. It was only in the later years of the British nuclear tests, when the public's response to the supposed magic of atomic energy began to grow more informed, critical and alarmed, that the British tests in Australia faced any threat of closure.

The same insurance policy argument accompanied Australia's decisions to send combat troops to support the Americans in Vietnam in the sixties and to agree to the stationing of vital American defence communications bases in Australia in the seventies and eighties. In all three cases, the decisions were taken secretly by the government of the day and announced without public debate. The American defence communications bases at Pine Gap, Nurrungar and North West Cape in Australia represented the frightening speed and technological sophistication with which the arms race had progressed in the short time since the British tests of the fifties. They differed from the British nuclear defence project, however, in two significant respects: they would prove far more difficult to terminate and they drew Australia more ineluctably and permanently into the nuclear war strategies of the superpowers. On a broader scale, the British nuclear tests were a story of government secrecy – then and now. They were about the issue of what governments knew or should have known and what they told or should have told the public.

It was a significant historical coincidence that the Australian royal commission's inquiry had occupied the whole of 1985. This was the centenary year of the birth of Niels Bohr, the great Danish physicist whose theory of nuclear fission using uranium was published just before the outbreak of the Second World War. Bohr, as we saw in Chapter One, had been the first scientist who was involved in the birth of the atomic bomb during the Manhattan Project to realise the frightening dangers that lay ahead if nuclear weapons were to proliferate without control after the war.

He made it his mission to persuade the wartime leaders, President Franklin Roosevelt and Winston Churchill, to initiate an early control arrangement over the use of atomic energy before it was too late. Part of Niels Bohr's memorandum to the two leaders, in July 1944, is worth recalling in the mid 1980s. He wrote it before he was received by Roosevelt at the White House on 26 August 1944:

The fact of immediate preponderance is, however, that a weapon of an unparalleled power is being created which will completely change all future conditions of warfare.

Quite apart from the question of how soon the weapon will be ready for use and what role it may play in the present war, this situation raises a number of problems which call for most urgent attention. Unless, indeed, some agreement about the control of the use of the new active materials can be obtained in due time, any temporary advantage, however great, may be outweighed by a perpetual menace to human security.

Ever since the possibilities of releasing atomic energy on a vast scale came in sight, much thought has naturally been given to the question of control, but the further the exploration of the scientific problems concerned is proceeding, the clearer it becomes that no kind of customary measures will suffice for this purpose, and that the terrifying prospect of a future competition between nations about a weapon of such formidable character can only be avoided through a universal agreement in true confidence.

As we saw earlier, Churchill had also granted Bohr an audience, before the Danish scientist met Roosevelt, but the meeting was a disaster. Churchill had abruptly ended it after half an hour when he stood up, turned to his scientific adviser, Lord Cherwell, and asked: 'What is he really talking about? Politics or physics?' [7]

Ever since then, politics and science have continued to march hand in hand as the nuclear arms race, which Niels Bohr feared so much, has accelerated. The alliance of politics and science was never so successful as in the 1950s, when it laid the ground for that arms race which will continue to haunt our lives unless the 'agreement in true confidence' which Bohr begged for just 40 years ago is ever achieved.

Appendix One

THE AUSTRALIAN ROYAL COMMISSIONERS AND THEIR REPORT

The royal commission members

James McClelland, the president of the Australian royal commission, was born in Melbourne in 1915, the son of a railways painter. He won scholarships to St Kevin's, a leading Roman Catholic boys' school in Melbourne, and to the University of Melbourne, where he studied for an arts degree. At 19, money worries forced him to interrupt his course to take a job as a clerk for his father's old employer, the Victorian railways. In the meantime, he had ditched his Roman Catholicism, and later took the credit for gradually disabusing the rest of his family, including his God-fearing mother, of the need for religion as well. 'It bored me', he said.[1]

At St Kevin's College, McClelland had shared a desk with B.A. Santamaria, who, in the 1950s, was to emerge as a leading Catholic and conservative intellectual in Australia. During these, the years of the British nuclear tests, McClelland himself settled down to building a successful and lucrative Sydney legal practice, specialising in industrial law. He had had a brief intellectual flirtation with Trotskyism following the depression of the thirties, served in the Australian armed forces during the Second World War, then studied law at the University of Sydney on a returned serviceman's scholarship. He elected to settle in Sydney after the war because he found it more to his flamboyant tastes than his home city, where, no doubt, he and the famous Melbourne establishment would have been destined to have a mutual antipathy towards each other.

McClelland's work as an industrial lawyer, involving a number of successful battles against Communist takeovers in trade unions, brought him into close contact with the Labor party, although he was always careful to avoid becoming readily identified with either the Left or the Right of Labor politics. If anything, he was a liberal on most social issues: he was against censorship or any other constraints on free speech, but he also strongly opposed laws which invaded the privacy of citizens.

McClelland won a seat in the Senate, the upper house in Canberra, in 1971, and arrived in parliament, at 56, just in time for the election of Gough Whitlam's Labor government the following year, which brought to an end the long rule by the conservative Liberals stretching back to the beginning of the Menzies era in 1949. But he had to wait until 1975, the last year of Whitlam's administration, before gaining a place in the ministry, first as minister for manufacturing industry and then as minister for labor and immigration.

The sensational dismissal of Whitlam's government on 11 November 1975, by Sir John Kerr, the governor general, the Queen's representative, had a profound impact on McClelland. Kerr had been a friend and colleague from their days together in the Sydney legal world of the fifties. McClelland felt Whitlam and the Labor government had been betrayed by a man whom, he believed, had used the office of governor general to ingratiate himself with the establishment. The trauma turned McClelland into a strong advocate of republicanism in Australia. In 1978, he described Kerr as 'a lickspittle from the wrong side of the tracks who always wanted to get to the big end of town, moved to the Right and charmed the Sydney Establishment to get there'. [2] His attacks on Kerr have never diminished, and in 1985 he said of the former governor general: 'He had a scintillating intellect, but he was lazy, self indulgent and he had no guts. His judgment had been impaired by the pretensions of office and by the company he kept'. [3]

When Whitlam's party lost power in Canberra, McClelland lost interest in staying there as an opposition MP. He resigned from parliament, returned to Sydney and became a judge on the New South Wales industrial court and then, in 1980, chief judge of the

• NO CONCEIVABLE INJURY

land and environment court of New South Wales, a post he held until Bob Hawke's government appointed him head of the royal commission into British nuclear tests in July 1984.

William Jonas, the second member of the royal commission, was an academic in geography, who had emerged from a tough and poverty stricken upbringing in a tiny town called Alworth, near the New South Wales city of Newcastle. His grandfather was an Aborigine who had gone to England at the turn of the century and joined a circus. Jonas's grandfather met his future wife there, and the pair teamed up to join the famous American wild west troupe of Buffalo Bill Cody, then touring England: Jonas's grandfather would startle the crowds by standing on the backs of cantering horses and cracking lighted cigarettes out of his wife's mouth with a stockwhip.

Back in Australia, William Jonas's own parents separated when he was a schoolboy, leaving Jonas and his older sister to fend for themselves. Eventually, Jonas was left in the house alone, free from the distractions of family tensions to get on with his real love, schoolwork, supported by his grandmother who lived nearby. Jonas won a scholarship to university, where he completed an arts degree, and later took a PhD for which he began work while teaching geography at the University of Papua New Guinea.

Jonas's Aboriginal blood stemmed only from his grandfather, himself a part-Aborigine. His sense of his own 'Aboriginality' came years afterwards when he had settled into his teaching job back at the University of Newcastle: a relation got into trouble with the law and was defended by the Aboriginal Legal Service of New South Wales. This impressed Jonas, who began devoting much of his spare time to Aboriginal welfare projects in his own city. Jonas was the member of the royal commission who took on the Aborigines' story in the nuclear tests as his own special interest.

The third royal commisioner, Jill Fitch, was qualified in another big area of the royal commission's inquiry, radiation and its effects. She had had an outstanding career as a health physicist in England and Australia. Fitch's father had become head of the state railways of New South Wales after starting out as a porter, and she always cited his influence on her for achieving results through hard work. At St George's Girls' High School, in the Sydney beachside suburb of Kogarah, Fitch became head girl and dux, or top pupil, then went on to Sydney University for a science degree. She began working at the Royal Prince Alfred Hospital in Sydney, and later, in London, studied for a master's degree in radiation biology and radiation physics while working at St Mary's Hospital, Paddington. When she returned to Australia in 1963 it was for less than a year, because St Mary's asked her to go back to London where she eventually became the hospital's principal physicist, working in nuclear medicine.

Later, back in Australia, Fitch joined the health commission of South Australia in a job to oversee the administration of regulations covering radiation exposure for health workers. The job took her to Maralinga several times, including during the preparation work for the secret repatriation of the half kilogram of plutonium to Britain in early 1979. Fitch actually flew out of Maralinga on the same aircraft as the plutonium.

The findings
[The Australian royal commission presented 201 conclusions, some of which are quoted here:]

At the Hurricane trial Australian scientists did not have sufficient information to advise the Australian government whether the weapon could be fired in conditions which would represent no hazard to the Australian mainland.

The Australian government was placed in a position where it was forced to accept UK assurances on the safety aspects of the test without any critical examination by its own scientists.

There was virtually complete government control of the Australian media reporting of the Hurricane test and the lead up to it, thus ensuring that the Australian news media reported only what the UK government wished.

The decision to use the mainland for atomic tests was made without specific consideration by Australian scientists or others of whether weapons could be safely fired. Consideration was limited to the fact that Emu was a remote location.

Information available to the Australian scientists on the movement and location of people in the vicinity of Emu was inadequate.

The establishment of the atomic weapons tests safety committee [AWTSC - referred to in the text as the Australian safety committee] was an important, albeit tardy, step in providing the Australian government with the opportunity to obtain independent scientific advice on the safety aspects of the tests.

Although the AWTSC was established by the time of Mosaic and had an effective power of veto, it was not provided with sufficient information to discharge its function properly for the Mosaic tests.

The AWTSC was provided with adequate information and was able properly to advise the government about the safety of the proposed Buffalo tests.

The Australian government had sufficient information to make an informed decision as to the criteria for safe firing for the Buffalo tests.

Significantly greater attempts were made to inform the public about the Buffalo testing program with a view to allaying public concerns about safety. The public was not, however, informed of the true nature of the hazards involved.

The AWTSC was provided with adequate information and was able properly to advise the government about the safety of the proposed Antler tests.

The Australian government had sufficient information to make an informed decision as to the criteria for safe firing for the Antler tests.

The AWTSC failed to carry out many of its tasks in a proper manner. At times it was deceitful and allowed unsafe firing to occur. It deviated from its proper charter by assuming responsibilities which properly belonged to the Australian government.

Titterton played a political as well as a safety role in the testing program, especially in the minor trials. He was prepared to conceal information from the Australian government and his fellow [safety] committee members if he believed to do so would suit the interests of the United Kingdom government and the testing program.

The fact that the AWTSC did not negotiate with the UK openly and independently in relation to the minor trials was a result of the special relationship which enabled Titterton to deal with the atomic weapons research establishment [AWRE - referred to in the text as Aldermaston] in a personal and informal manner. He was from first to last 'their man' and the concerns which were ultimately voiced in relation to the Vixen B proposals and which forced the introduction of more formal procedures for approving minor trials were a direct result of the perceived inadequacies in the manner in which he had carried out his tasks.

Radiation protections standards

The policy on exposure to radiation laid down for participants in all the major trials, the code of practice for application of the policy, and the maximum radiation doses specified, were reasonable and compatible with the international recommendations applicable at the time.

There were departures, some serious and some minor, from compliance with the prescribed radiation protection policy and standards during the test program.

The measures taken before and at the time of the tests for protecting persons against exposure to the harmful effects of radiation, based as they were on the concept that any dose below a certain level was 'safe', must be regarded as inadequate in the light of radiation protection standards at the present time.

By reason of the detonation of the major trials and the deposition of fallout across Australia, it is probable that cancers which would not otherwise have occurred have been caused in the Australian population.

Their exposure to radiation as participants in the trial program has increased the risk of cancer among 'nuclear veterans'.

The royal commission has been unable to quantify the probable increase in the risk of cancer among the participants in the trial program or among the Australian population in general.

The Hurricane test

The Monte Bello Islands were not an appropriate place for atomic tests owing to the prevailing weather patterns and the limited opportunities for safe firing.

There was fallout on the mainland following Hurricane,

although most of the activity fell in the sea to the north and west, as was intended. The fallout probably did not begin falling on the mainland until 30 hours after the burst. Hence it is unlikely that the fallout exceeded the no risk level proposed in the report prepared prior to the test.

There was a failure at the Hurricane trial to consider the distinctive lifestyles of Aboriginal people. As no record was made of any contamination of the mainland it is impossible to determine whether Aborigines were exposed to any significant short or long-term hazards.

Air crew of the [RAAF] Lincoln aircraft at Hurricane should have been supplied with radiation monitoring devices and given instructions as to their behaviour when in the cloud or a contaminated aircraft. The failure to provide this equipment and instructions was negligent. Ground crew should have been similarly equipped and instructed.

The failure to make provision for personal monitoring of air and ground crews was an omission which fortuitously did not result in exposure of those personnel to high levels of radioactivity. The RAAF should have been informed of the risks and provided with equipment to monitor the crews.

The royal commission finds convincing the recurring evidence given by servicemen who were at the Hurricane test in positions close to the site of the explosion that after a person had entered an active area decontamination procedures were tediously and thoroughly carried out.

The Totem tests
The Totem One test was fired under wind conditions that the study in Report A32 had shown would produce unacceptable levels of fallout. Measured fallout from Totem One on inhabited regions did exceed the limits proposed in Report A32.

The firing criteria used for the Totem One test ignored some of the recommendations of Report A32 and did not take into account the existence of people at Wallatinna and Welbourn Hill downwind of the test site.

The weather conditions at the time of firing Totem Two satisfied the criteria for firing.

There was a failure at the Totem trials to consider adequately the distinctive lifestyle of Aborigines and, as a consequence, their special vulnerability to radioactive fallout.

Meteorological, mathematical and statistical modelling indicates that a black mist passing over Wallatinna and Welbourn Hill could have happened.

There is no reason to disbelieve Aboriginal accounts that the Black Mist occurred and that it made some people sick. Both radiation exposure and fear can lead to vomiting. At Wallatinna, the vomiting by Aborigines may have resulted from radiation, it may have been a psychogenic reaction to a frightening experience, or it may have resulted from both of these.

The royal commission believes that Aboriginal people experienced radioactive fallout from Totem One in the form of a black mist or cloud at and near Wallatinna. This may have made some people temporarily ill. The royal commission does not have sufficient evidence to say whether or not it caused other illnesses or injuries.

Given the historical uncertainties and the current state of scientific knowledge, the evidence presented does not enable the royal commission to decide one way or the other whether the Black Mist caused or contributed to the blindness of Yami Lester.

Radiological safety procedures at Emu, including decontamination, were well planned and executed. The royal commission cannot exclude the possibility that some unplanned incidents occurred, including the loosening or removal of respirators by participants in the forward areas.

It was negligent to allow aircrew to fly through the Totem One cloud without proper instructions and without protective clothing.

Aircrew of Lincoln aircraft at Totem One should have been supplied with radiation monitoring devices and given instructions as to the behaviour of these devices when in the cloud or a contaminated aircraft. The failure to provide this equipment and instructions was negligent. Ground crew should have been similarly equipped and instructed.

The Mosaic tests

The Monte Bello Islands were not a suitable site for the Mosaic tests G1 and G2 because the chances of obtaining suitable occasions to fire were too low.

The Mosaic tests were conducted in a hurry under marginal meteorological conditions.

The theoretical predictions were incorrect for both Mosaic tests and parts of the clouds passed over the mainland of Australia.

The AWTSC [Australian safety committee] report to the prime minister following the Mosaic tests was misleading and did not properly inform the government of the difficulties experienced with meeting the firing criteria, the unexpected winds that brought some of the stem and cloud over the mainland and the higher than expected levels of fallout on the mainland.

For the chairman of the AWTSC to advise the minister for supply that conditions for firing G2 were ideal from the point of view of safety of the mainland was grossly misleading and irresponsible.

The presence of Aborigines on the mainland near the Monte Bello Islands and their extra vulnerability to the effect of fallout was not recognised by either AWRE [Aldermaston] or the safety committee. It was a major oversight that the question of acceptable dose levels for Aborigines was recognised as a problem at Maralinga but was ignored in setting the fallout criteria for the Mosaic tests.

The royal commission concludes that the precautions taken for the health and safety of the servicemen at Mosaic were generally adequate.

The Buffalo tests

Buffalo round 1 (One Tree) was fired at a time when the fallout was predicted to violate the firing conditions that had been proposed by the AWTSC and agreed to by the government. Measurements after Buffalo round 1 confirmed that fallout exceeded Level A at locations beyond Coober Pedy and exceeded the Level B for nomadic people where Aborigines could be expected to be living.

Round 2 (Marcoo) was fired in conditions which violated the

firing criterion that there should be no forecast of rain except in areas remote – interpreted as 500 miles (800 kilometres) from ground zero. Rain was forecast within 250 miles (400 kilometres) and actually fell within 100 miles (160 kilometres) of ground zero.

Round 3 (Kite) was fired under conditions which led to contamination of Maralinga village. Although, in the event, the contamination was minor, the round should not have been fired under the conditions prevailing at the time.

Round 4 (Breakaway) was fired under conditions for which the fallout was predicted to exceed Level A beyond a distance of 100 miles (160 kilometres) and into the inhabited region. In addition, the condition that there should be no overlap of fallout exceeding the Level A at distances more than 100 miles (160 kilometres) from the site was violated.

Overall, the attempts to ensure Aboriginal safety during the Buffalo series demonstrate ignorance, incompetence and cynicism on the part of those responsible for the safety. The inescapable conclusion is that if Aborigines were not injured or killed as a result of the explosions, this was a matter of luck rather than adequate organisation, management and resources allocated to ensuring safety.

The Pom Pom incident demonstrated that flaws existed in the security system at Maralinga. Those responsible for security seemed at least as concerned about the exposure of such flaws as the welfare of the Milpuddie family.

For the Milpuddies the experience caused great concern and it distresses Edie Milpuddie today. The royal commission cannot exclude the possibility that the Milpuddies' entry into the contaminated area resulted in injury to them.

Radiological and physical safety arrangements for participants during the Buffalo tests were well planned and sound. Security was strictly policed during the major tests but was relaxed afterwards. Unplanned incidents and exposures may have occurred during this time. Breaches of safety regulations may also have occurred when participants loosened or discarded respirators.

Operation of the 'need to know' principle and the minimal amount of information given to participants has been a factor contributing to participants' concerns and fears regarding what might have resulted from their experiences at Maralinga. Nevertheless, such participation at the tests, including residence in the village during the Kite explosion, has increased the risk of cancer to those participants who were exposed to radiation but the royal commission has been unable to quantify the probable increase.

The royal commission rejects the allegation that mentally defective people were used in nuclear experiments at the Buffalo tests.

The Antler tests

The extent of the fallout was predicted reasonably well for the two tower bursts (rounds 1 and 2), but the intermediate distance fallout from the air burst (round 3) was seriously underestimated.

Inadequate attention was paid to Aboriginal safety during the Antler tests. People continued to inhabit the prohibited zone as close to the test sites as 130 kilometres.

Air and ground patrols for Antler were neither well planned nor well executed.

The Antler series of tests was clearly better planned, organised and documented than any of the previous test series. Nevertheless, it was not entirely without unplanned incident.

The procedures adopted for the decontamination of aircraft at Mosaic, Buffalo and Antler were based on experience gained at Hurricane and Totem and were, for the most part, well developed and managed.

The weapon exploded at Tadje had associated with it cobalt 60 to be used as a tracer. The technique used proved to be unsuccessful and the resultant dispersal of the active pellets was only discovered accidentally many months after the explosion.

The Australian health physics representative (AHPR) and those personnel who helped collect the pellets for subsequent disposal were exposed to radiation as a result.

The British scientists should, as had been agreed, have informed the AHPR of the existence of the pellets, before they left the range at the end of the Antler series. By their failure to do so, an unnecessary radiation hazard was created.

The royal commission believes that Titterton was the only

member of the [Australian safety committee] who knew of the use of cobalt 60 at the time of the Tadje test. In not informing other members of the [safety committee] and the AHPR, he also contributed to an unnecessary radiation hazard.

The Minor Trials
In view of the known long half life of plutonium (24000 years), the Vixen series of minor trials should never have been conducted at Maralinga.

Clean-up of the ranges
The Australian government failed to set adequate policy guidelines or give adequate direction to the [Australian safety committee] regarding future plans for the Maralinga range.

Operation Brumby was based on wrong assumptions. It was planned in haste to meet political deadlines and, in some cases, the tasks undertaken made the ultimate clean up of the range more difficult.

The Maralinga range is not acceptable in its present condition and it must be cleaned up.

The aim of the clean-up should be to allow Aborigines access to the test sites without restriction.

The hazard from radiation at the [bomb trial] ground zeros is not excessive. The concrete plinths with their warning messages are an adequate indication to people not to camp permanently at these sites. The level of radiation will decay to one of no significance during the lifetime of the younger people now returning to the area.

The most significant hazard to Aborigines using the test sites is from the plutonium contamination. The hazard from the inhalation of dust raised by winds appears to be acceptable. However, three other pathways – inhalation by children digging and playing, ingestion through bush foods and injection of plutonium – do produce unacceptable levels of risk. From the range of estimates of the level of this risk in the evidence tendered to the royal commission, it is clear that more information is needed on the possible Aboriginal lifestyles in the area, the dust conditions in

Aboriginal camps, the types and amounts of specific food items and the amounts of plutonium in these food items. Information on the particle size distribution of plutonium contamination is also very important and needs to be determined.

The plutonium-contaminated areas must be cleaned up. However, more work is needed to develop realistic hazard assessments so that criteria can be derived for the clean up otherwise it is impossible to specify what areas must be cleaned, to what depth and to what level of residual contamination.

The pits containing plutonium waste at Taranaki and TM101 must be treated by either immobilising the plutonium in the debris or by removing the material from the pits.

Various options for clean-up were considered but the royal commission has not been able to make detailed recommendations because insufficient data were tendered on the levels of risk, options for clean-up and the associated costs. Nevertheless, the royal commission would suggest that any clean-up should include additional fencing in the short term, an emu parade to collect plutonium-contaminated fragments, the removal and burial of the plutonium-contaminated soil at Taranaki and action to immobilise or exhume the waste pits at Taranaki.

The traditional owners of the Maralinga lands were denied effective access to these lands for over 30 years as a result of the British nuclear test program. This denial has contributed to their emotional, social and material distress and deprivation.

The royal commission concludes that responsibility for compensation to those people who have been denied use of their lands because of the nuclear test program should be assumed by the Commonwealth government.

The cost of clean-up of the Maralinga range should be borne by the UK government because the previous clean-up in 1968 was clearly inadequate and based on insufficient information.

AIRAC 9 *and other reports*
The report, AIRAC 9, prepared by the Australian Ionising Radiation Advisory Council, is not an adequate scientific account of the testing program. In particular AIRAC failed to make

adequate inquiries before offering its conclusions. This failure may have been due to an agreement with the relevant minister to limit its inquiries. If so, it should have indicated this in its report. Rather than give the impression of a thorough investigation it should have clearly indicated that it had not investigated and sought out evidence of ineffective controls.

AIRAC with one exception spoke only to persons with an interest in advancing the view that the safety measures taken were adequate and effective. This had led to an apparent bias in the material before it. As a consequence the report cannot be described as an objective and impartial assessment of the situation.

Because of the paucity of relevant information on which it is based, the Donovan report cannot be regarded as an adequate epidemiological study of the health of atomic test personnel.

Because of the deficiencies in the available data, there is little prospect of carrying out any worthwhile epidemiological study of those involved in the tests nor of others who might have been directly affected by them.

Recommendations

1 The benefits of the Compensation (Commonwealth Government Employees) Act 1971, including the shifting of the onus of proof from the claimant to the Commonwealth should be extended so as to include not only members of the armed forces who are at present covered by the act, but also civilians who were at the test sites at the relevant times, and Aborigines and other civilians who may have been exposed to the Black Mist.

2 To assist the commissioner for employees' compensation in the performance of the additional duties recommended in recommendation 1, a national register of nuclear veterans, Aborigines and other persons who may have been exposed to the Black Mist or exposed to radiation at the tests should be compiled.

3 Action should be commenced immediately to effect a clean-up of Maralinga and Emu to the satisfaction of the Australian government so that they are fit for unrestricted habitation by the traditional Aboriginal owners as soon as practicable.

4 A Maralinga commission, comprising representatives of the traditional owners, the UK, Australian and South Australian governments should be established to determine the clean-up criteria, oversee the clean-up and co-ordinate all future range management.

5 Action should be taken immediately to ensure that all areas of the Monte Bello Islands where the radiation levels are above the limits recommended for continous exposure of members of the public are suitably signposted until safe for permanent occupation. Small pieces of debris should be collected to avoid them being removed as souvenirs. The large structures remaining on Trimouille Island that are relics of the test programs could remain for historic interest.

6 All costs of any future clean-ups at Maralinga, Emu and the Monte Bello Islands should be borne by the United Kingdom government.

7 The Australian government should make compensation to those persons and descendants of those persons who have a traditional interest in sites at the former Maralinga prohibited area for loss of enjoyment of their lands since the beginning, and as a result of the atomic tests program. This should take the form of technology and services which Aboriginal people regard as necessary for them to re-establish their relationships with their land as rapidly as possible and with minimal hardship.

Appendix Two

AGREEMENTS BETWEEN THE UNITED KINGDOM AND AUSTRALIA ON FUTURE RESPONSIBILITIES AT MARALINGA

As noted in Chapter Six, Australia agreed on two occasions, in 1968 and again in 1979, to absolve Britain of further responsibilities for the range at Maralinga. On each occasion, the governments of both countries had information through the Pearce report of January 1968, that the range was contaminated with plutonium, although they are unlikely to have known the full extent of the contamination which was revealed by the Australian Radiation Laboratory's survey in 1984-85.

On 7 March 1956, Britain and Australia agreed to a memorandum of arrangements for the operation of the atomic weapons proving ground at Maralinga for the next ten years. The memorandum provided, among other things, that:

The United Kingdom Government accepts liability for such corrective measures as may be practicable in the event of radioactive contamination resulting from tests on the site.

On 23 September 1968, British and Australian representatives in Canberra signed an agreement to terminate this memorandum of arrangements. It said, among other things:

(a) The United Kingdom Government have completed decontamination and debris clearance at the Atomic Weapons Proving Ground Maralinga to the satisfaction of the Australian Government.

and

(c) With effect from 21 December 1967, the United Kingdom Government are released from all liabilities and responsibialities under the Memorandum of Arrangements. . .

(It then mentioned, as an exception, the compensation clause in the memorandum of arrangements over death or injury to people from the tests. This clause, however, defined Britain's obligations narrowly, saying Britain would indemnify the Australian government for 'valid claims', *except* those from Australian government employees or servicemen. This did leave open the technical possibility of Britain being responsible for meeting compensation for claims from Aborigines who could prove their health was harmed by the tests.)

On 23 November 1978, after Australia had asked Britain to take back half a kilogram of plutonium from a burial pit at Maralinga, the British high commissioner in Canberra handed the following note to the Australian minister for national development:

NUCLEAR WASTE AT MARALINGA
British Ministers have agreed to the Australian request for repatriation to the United Kingdom of the half a kilogram of potentially recoverable plutonium buried at Maralinga, subject to Australian written acceptance of the four points listed below:

1. In the light of the joint team's findings, no basis now remains for any further request for repatriation of nuclear waste and there is, therefore, no question of the United Kingdom having any further responsibility to repatriate waste. The United Kingdom will need a clear statement that the Australian government accept this. The United Kingdom would however be willing, as in the past, to provide technical advice if requested on any further on-site operations which may be undertaken by the Australian Government at Maralinga to reduce surface contamination.

2. It will be for the United Kingdom to decide the timing and modalities of the transport of the six drums containing the half kilogram of

plutonium from Australia to the United Kingdom. These depend on the availability of a suitable means of transport which can ensure safe transit and avoid possible international complications of overflying or port entry.

3. To protect the means and timing of repatriation, the United Kingdom will need a firm undertaking from the Australian Government that the operations will be conducted with maximum secrecy. Any leak of information before completion of repatriation could jeopardise the deal because of the port entry difficulties this would cause.

4. The Australian Government should meet all costs of the operation within Australia and should be responsible for the provision of anti-terrorist protection while the material remains on Australian soil. The United Kingdom would be prepared to take responsibility for safe and secure transport of the material from Australia to the United Kingdom, including the cost. This being so, the United Kingdom would wish to be involved in supervising the packaging of the material at Maralinga to ensure that it meets appropriate containment standards both for its transport within Australia and subsequently.

Only when all these points are agreed would the United Kingdom Government think it right that any public statement should be issued. It is proposed that this should take the form of a joint press statement to be released simultaneously in the two countries. A draft is attached on which Australian views would be welcomed. Once a text is agreed between officials, it will need to be submitted to the United Kingdom Ministers for approval.

The United Kingdom Government requires written confirmation of agreement between the two Governments on the four points listed above and this should precede the issue of any press release.

MARALINGA: PROPOSED JOINT PRESS RELEASE (SUBJECT TO AGREEMENT BY UNITED KINGDOM MINISTERS)

The Australian Government has reviewed with the help of British experts the status of the nuclear waste buried in the South Australian desert following the British nuclear tests at Maralinga in the 1950s. Although it was concluded that the burials are safe and secure the existence in a single burial of a small quantity of plutonium in a potentially recoverable form was high-lighted. The Australian Government considered that the best long-term solution would be to return this potentially recoverable material to the United Kingdom. The British Government has agreed exceptionally that, in this specific instance, the plutonium in question should be returned to the United Kingdom, and this will now be arranged.

On 29 November 1978, the Australian minister for national development replied to the above British note:

Australian Ministers have considered the Bout de Papier passed by the British High Commisioner to the Minister for National Development on 23 November, and appreciate the agreement of the United Kingdom to the Australian request for repatriation to the United Kingdom of the half a kilogram of recoverable plutonium buried at Maralinga.

Australian Ministers have agreed that the British proposals contained in points 2, 3 and 4 of their paper are acceptable to the Australian Government, subject to detailed discussions on apportionment of costs.

In relation to point 2, the Australian Government shares the concern of the United Kingdom Government that the matter be resolved speedily.

With regard to point 1 of the British paper, the Australian Government accepts, on the basis of the agreed joint Australian/British assessment of the position at Maralinga, set out in the Pearce report that there is no question of the United Kingdom having further responsibility to repatriate waste from Maralinga.

The Australian Government agrees with the British proposal for a joint simultaneous press statement, and should the above be acceptable to the United Kingdom Government, would wish to agree the terms of such a statement quickly.

The above correspondence between the British and Australian governments was made the basis of a formal agreement on 4 January 1979. On 11 January 1979, the Australian minister for national development, Kevin Newman, issued a press statement from Canberra, whose wording was identical with the press statement above, which Britain had proposed earlier. The statement was issued simultaneously in London.

In December 1985, the Australian royal commission made the following remarks in its report about the above agreements of 1968 and 1979 between Britain and Australia:

Both the 1968 and 1979 agreements were intended to operate as a general release of the UK with respect to the obligation imposed under the original Memorandum. As such, their affect may be limited and will only operate with respect to the matters in the contemplation of the parties at the time when the release is given. . .

In the opinion of the Royal Commission, it is clear that, at the time of the execution of both releases, matters now relevant were not in the contemplation of the parties. It would appear that no one was aware, and certainly not the Australian authorities, of the nature and extent of the contaminated fragments. This was almost certainly due to the technical difficulty of detecting them. Furthermore, no one seems to have appreciated the significance of the movement toward the granting of land rights to Aboriginal peoples. It is certain that no thought was given to the problem of establishing the safety of the land over many thousands of years. All that appears to have exercised the minds of the decision makers at the time of execution after release was an immediate need to alleviate the obvious problem. No one gave thought to control of that problem beyond a period of about twenty years.

As a consequence, neither of the purported releases would operate to excuse the UK from a responsibility to eliminate the present problems. In the opinion of the Royal Commission, the UK remains liable for the total cost of rendering the contaminated areas safe without fences or patrols.

The Royal Commission also believes that there is an overwhelming moral obligation on the UK. It has become clear to everyone that Operation Brumby was neither prudent or effective. It was poorly conceived, carried out without proper consideration being given or a decision made with respect to its objective. It exacerbated the hazard rather than alleviated it.

It would, in the opinion of the Royal Commission, be grossly irresponsible of the UK Government if it did not now accept that it has a continuing obligation to clean up the contaminated areas so that they are acceptable for unrestrictive access. No one can foresee how the area will be used over the coming thousands of years. It is incumbent on the UK to accept the responsibility which it undertook in return for being allowed to use Australian land for its weapons development program.

CHAPTER NOTES

Chapter One: From Hiroshima to Hurricane

1. *Diary of the Exploration in South Australia of W.H. Tietkens Esq, F.R.G.S., 1879*, Department of Supply, Weapons Research Establishment, Salisbury, South Australia, 1961.
2. Quoted in Gowing, Margaret, *Britain and Atomic Energy, 1939-45*, Macmillan, London, 1964, Appendix One, pp. 392-93.
3. Gowing, ibid. p. 42.
4. Gowing, Margaret, 'Britain, America and the Bomb', in Dilks, David (ed.) *Retreat from Power, Volume 2*, Macmillan, 1981.
5. Gowing, *Britain and Atomic Energy, 1939-45*, p. 354.
6. Gowing, ibid. p.353.
7. Gowing, with Lorna Arnold, *Independence and Deterrence: Britain and Atomic Energy 1945-52, Volume 1*, Macmillan, London, 1974. pp. 407-8.
8. ibid. p. 20.
9. At the official level, apart from Sir Henry Tizard, only Professor Patrick Blackett, a member of the government's advisory committee on atomic energy, appears to have put his opposition to the bomb on record. Blackett's dissent is discussed in Chapter Three.
10. ibid. p. 337.

Chapter Two: Penney

1. *Transcript of the Royal Commission into British Nuclear Tests in Australia*, p. 4432. (Future references from the royal commission transcript will be made in the following form: T. 4432.)
2. Margaret Gowing, the official historian of the British atomic project, has written that 22 years later Penney still had no idea about the secret

January decision; he still 'believed that the decision was not actually made until May, and only then was he told to do something about it'. Gowing, *Independence and Deterrence: Britain and Atomic Energy, 1945-1952*, Volume 2, p. 442.

3. Gowing is left with the conviction 'that if it had not been for the extraordinary competence of three men at the working level – John Cockcroft, Christopher Hinton and William Penney – the project might have been an expensive fiasco. Instead it was to prove in this period of the Labour government, within the objectives set for it, one of the most successfully executed programs in British scientific and technological history.' Ibid. Volume 1, p.57.

4. Quoted by Chapman Pincher, *Daily Express*, 16 May 1957.

5. T. 4454.

6. Gowing, Volume 2, p.474.

7. Gowing, Volume 1, p.52.

8. The *Times*, 23 May 1952.

9. Gowing, Volume 2, p.478.

10. Cameron, James, *Point of Departure*. Panther, London, 1967, p.69.

11. T. 4312.

12. Gowing, Volume 2, p.492

13. Statement to royal commission, 1985.

Chapter Three: Menzies and Titterton

1. Transcript of a meeting between Sir Ernest Titterton and members of the Australian Ionising Radiation Advisory Council, March 1981.

2. Menzies, *The Measure of the Years*, Cassell, Australia, 1970, p. 212.

3. Statement by Menzies on foreign affairs to the House of Representatives, Canberra, 7 March 1951.

4. The cabinet agreed with Menzies that the title should be the same throughout the Commonwealth: 'Elizabeth the Second, by the Grace of God of the United Kingdom of Great Britain and Northern Ireland, Canada, Australia, New Zealand, South Africa, Pakistan, Ceylon and of all other Her Realms and Territories Queen, Head of the Commonwealth, Defender of the Faith'. In October 1973, the Whitlam government changed the royal style and title, in relation to Australia and its territories, to: 'Elizabeth the Second, by the Grace of God Queen of Australia and Her

other Realms and Territories, Head of the Commonwealth'.

5. *Century*, Sydney, 25 January 1957.

6. Beale, *This Inch of Time*, Melbourne University Press, 1977, p. 109.

7. ibid.

8. Blackett's memorandum is reproduced in Gowing, Volume 1, p.194.

9. Gowing, Volume 1, p.116.

10. Gowing, Volume 1, p.113. Gowing gives the figure of 19 British scientists working at Los Alamos during the war in *Britain and Atomic Energy, 1939-45*, p. 262. There were more British scientists stationed at other vital wartime atomic research locations in the US, such as Oak Ridge and Berkeley.

11. Statement to Royal Commission, 1985.

12. T.4401.

13. For biographical information on Martin and Butement, the author is grateful to Tim Sherratt, of the history and philosophy of science department at the University of Melbourne. Sherratt, 'A Political Inconvenience: Australian Scientists at the British Atomic Weapon Tests, 1952-3', HPS department, University of Melbourne, 1984.

14. A documentary film in 1985 called *Half Life*, by Dennis O'Rourke, argues from recently declassified American documents and official film that those conducting the Bravo test made no attempt to evacuate Marshall Islanders who were living in the path of the fallout, and that the victims have been used by the US authorities as guinea pigs ever since to study the long-term effects of radiation on human beings who have to live in a contaminated environment.

15. T. 7619.

16. T. 7648.

17. T. 7637.

18. T. 4375.

19. T. 7620.

20. T. 7627.

21. T. 7634.

22. T. 7841.

23. Quoted by Stewart Cockburn and David Ellyard, *Oliphant*, Axiom Books, 1981, p. 187.

24. Statement by Sir Mark Oliphant to the author, August 1985.

25. Letter from Oliphant to Dr Hedley Marston, September 1956, quoted by Cockburn and Ellyard, op. cit., p.194.

26. T. 7643.

27. Correspondence quoted by Sherratt, op. cit., appendix two.

28. Titterton. T. 7671a.

29. John Moroney, scientific secretary of the safety committee from 1957, told the royal commission in 1985: 'The minor trials did not fall within the [safety committee's] terms of reference. . . In its work on the minor trials, the [safety committee] was responding to requests by the Australian government for advice, rather than fulfilling a function under its terms of reference.'

30. T. 7072.

Chapter Four: Edie and Darlene – the story of the Aborigines

1. T.3548.

2. T.6637.

3. T.4385.

4. T.2396.

5. T.6646.

6. T.2399, 2441, 2460.

7. Transcript of a conversation between Penney and Butement at a location 65 kilometres north of Ooldea, 20 October 1953.

8. Transcript of a meeting between Titterton and members of the Australian Ionising Radiation Advisory Council, 20 March 1981.

Chapter Five: 1956 'She Shook Them'

1. Stockholm International Peace Research Institute, *Nuclear Radiation in Warfare*, Taylor and Francis, London, 1981. p.8.

2. Symonds, J. L. *A History of British Atomic Tests in Australia*, Department of Resources and Energy, Canberra, 1985. p.142.

3. Statement to royal commission, October 1984.

4. Statement to royal commission, February 1985.

5. T.5889.

6. Gowing, Volume 1, p.437.

7. Recording of a conversation between Penney and Butement at a location 65 kilometres north of Ooldea, 20 October 1953.

8. Symonds, p. 237.

9. op. cit., p. 234.

10. op. cit., p.310.

11. Hole's accounts from T. 5164, 5165, 5166, 5168, 5178, 5191 and 5264.

12. Statement to royal commission, December 1984.

13. In evidence to the Australian royal commission in London in January 1985, Bernard Perkins, a radio operator on the HMS *Narvik*, said in a statement widely reported in the press: 'I went on duty at 4 pm. This time I was sending press releases from the journalists who were on board. Suddenly a signal came in direct from Sydney. It was written down on a pad in manuscript by the operator who took it. It was from the Australian prime minister to the prime minister of Great Britain. It simply said, "What the bloody hell is going on, the cloud is drifting over the mainland?" It was a very short message and everybody stood there looking at it.'

Among the thousands of pages of documents declassified at the royal commission in 1984-85, no copy of this alleged message was found. Fadden was acting prime minister of Australia at the time in Menzies' absence.

14. Beale, *This Inch of Time*, Melbourne University Press, 1977, p.83.

15. Symonds, p.337.

16. T.7061.

17. T.2425.

18. Statement to royal commission.

19. Statement to royal commission.

20. Carter, Melvin W. and Moghissi, A. Alan, 'Three Decades of Nuclear Testing', in *Health Physics*, Pergamon Press, 1977, Vol. 33.

21. Quoted in Pierre, Andrew J. *Nuclear Politics*, Oxford University Press, London, 1972.

22. The *Times*, 31 October 1956.

23. Statement to royal commission.

Chapter Six: 'Minor Trials'

1. Symonds, *A History of British Atomic Tests in Australia*, Department of Resources and Energy, Canberra, 1985, p.555. This may not be necessarily a complete figure of the plutonium used and still at Maralinga. Symonds points out that this plutonium data is from information 'available and reviewed' up to 24 September 1984.

2. Rotblat, Joseph (for the Stockholm International Peace Research Institute) *Nuclear Radiation in Warfare*, Taylor and Francis, London, 1981, p. 55.

3. Symonds, ibid. p. 506.

4. The above account of Anglo-Australian negotiations over approvals for the minor trials is based largely, but not entirely, on material in Symonds, ibid. p. 500-532.

5. The use of the term Maralinga Experimental Programme in this British report, in the absence of any qualifying remarks, is taken to refer to all the minor trials from 1955 to 1963, not just the more controversial Vixen series.

6. Symonds, ibid. p. 525.

7. 'Radiological Safety and Future Land Use at the Maralinga Atomic Weapons Test Range, AIRAC 4', January, 1979.

8. 'Killen Warns on Plutonium Pile', by Brian Toohey, *Australian Financial Review*, 5 October 1978.

9. Australia had recently ratified the Nuclear Non Proliferation Treaty, thereby giving an undertaking to adopt a system of safeguards, to be agreed with the International Atomic Energy Agency, designed to stop the diversion of fissionable material from peaceful purposes to nuclear weapons.

10. 'The Terrible Legacy of Maralinga', by Brian Toohey, the *National Times*, 4 May 1984.

11. T. 1925 and T. 8033.

12. T. 8180.

13. T. 7808a.

Chapter Seven: No Conceivable Injury?

1. 'Ionising Radiation: Sources and Biological Effects.' Report by UNSCEAR, the United Nations scientific committee on the effects of atomic radiation, 1982.

2. Rotblat (for the Stockholm International Peace Research Institute), *Nuclear Radiation in Warfare*, Taylor and Francis, London, 1981. pp. 97-99.

3. The description of the nature and effects of radioactivity and the growth of radiation protection standards is drawn largely from the

following sources: Rotblat, ibid; Pochin, Edward, *Nuclear Radiation: Risks and Benefits*, Clarendon Press, Oxford, 1985; Gowing, Margaret, *Independence and Deterrence, Volume Two*; Patterson, Walter, *Nuclear Power*, Penguin, 1976; Moss, Norman, *Men Who Play God*, Penguin, 1968; Green, Patrick, 'The Controversy Over Low Dose Exposure to Ionising Radiations', submission by Greenpeace UK to the Australian royal commission, 1985; Submissions and evidence to the Australian royal commission by Lord Penney, Sir Edward Pochin, Edward Radford, Alice Stewart, David Barnes, John Dunster and others; Judgment of the United States district court by Judge Bruce S. Jenkins, May 1984. A comprehensive account of the Marston controversy is in 'Our Atomic Cover Up', by Deborah Smith and Deborah Snow, the *National Times*, 4 May 1980.

Chapter Eight: Diamond Jim Goes to London

1. *Matilda*, November 1985, p.37.
2. The *National Times*, 16 February 1976.
3. The royal commission's terms of reference asked it to examine the measures that were taken for protection against the harmful effects of exposure to ionising radiation and the dispersal of radioactive substances and toxic materials from the tests and minor trials, as judged by the standards applicable at the time and with reference to the standards of today. They asked it to look in particular at the effects of the tests on Australian service personnel and civilian employees at the test sites, Aborigines and other civilians in the test regions. They also asked it to make recommendations about the future management and use of the test ranges.
4. Address by chief judge Howard T. Markey, quoted in the United States district court for the district of Utah, central division, judgment on Irene Allen et al. v. United States of America, 10 May 1984, p.7.
5. Margaret Gowing, Volume 2, pp.37 and 85.
6. One writer, Andrew J. Pierre, has estimated total expenditure on Britain's nuclear defence force between 1945 and 1970 as 3200 million pounds sterling, including nuclear facilities, warheads, bombers, missiles and cancelled projects. Pierre, *Nuclear Politics: The British Experience with an Independent Strategic Force 1939-1970*, Oxford University Press, London, 1972.
7. Jungk, Robert, *Brighter Than a Thousand Suns*, Pelican, 1965, p.160.

Appendix One

1. Interview with the author, 1985.
2. Quoted by George Negus, the *Australian*, March 1978.
3. Interview with the author, 1985.

BIBLIOGRAPHY

Beadell, Len. *Blast the Bush*. Rigby, 1967.

Beale, Howard. *This Inch of Time: Memoirs of Politics and Diplomacy*. Melbourne University Press, 1977.

Bertell, Rosalie. *No Immediate Danger*. The Women's Press, London, 1985.

Bertin, Leonard. *Atom Harvest*. Secker and Warburg, 1955.

Bradley, David. *No Place to Hide, 1964-84*. University Press of New England, 1983.

Cameron, James. *Point of Departure*. Panther, London, 1969.

Cockburn, Stewart, and Ellyard, David. *Oliphant*. Axiom Books, Adelaide, 1981.

Fuller, John G. *The Day We Bombed Utah*. New American Library, New York, 1984.

Gowing, Margaret. *Britain and Atomic Energy 1939-1945*. Macmillan, London, 1964.

Gowing, Margaret with Arnold, Lorna. *Independence and Deterrence: Britain and Atomic Energy 1945-52*. Two volumes. Macmillan, London, 1974.

Malone, Peter. *The British Nuclear Deterrent*. St. Martin's Press, New York, 1984.

Mandle, W.F. *Going It Alone: Australia's National Identity in the Twentieth Century*. Penguin, Melbourne, 1980.

Martin, Brian. *Nuclear Knights*. Rupert Public Interest Movement Inc., Canberra, 1980.

Menaul, Stewart. *Countdown: Britain's Strategic Nuclear Forces*. Hale, London, 1980.

Moss, Norman. *Men Who Play God: The Story of the Hydrogen Bomb*. Penguin, London, 1970.

Patterson, Walter C. *Nuclear Power*. Penguin, London 1976.

Pierre, Andrew J. *Nuclear Politics: The British Experience with an Independent Strategic Force*. Oxford University Press, London, 1972.

Pochin, Edward. *Nuclear Radiation: Risks and Benefits*. Clarendon Press, Oxford, 1985.

Pringle, Peter, and Spigelman, James. *The Nuclear Barons*. Sphere Books, London, 1983.

Rotblat, Joseph (for the Stockholm International Peace Research Institute). *Nuclear Radiation in Warfare*. Taylor and Francis, London, 1981.

Saffer, Thomas H. and Kelly, Orville E. *Countdown Zero*. Putnam, New York, 1982.

Simpson, John. *The Independent Nuclear State: The United States, Britain and the Nuclear Atom*. Macmillan, London, 1983.

Southall, Ivan. *Woomera*. Angus and Robertson, Sydney, 1962.

Symonds, J.L. *A History of British Atomic Tests in Australia*. Department of Resources and Energy, Canberra, 1985.

Tame, Adrian, and Robotham, F.P.J. *Maralinga*. Fontana, Melbourne, 1982.

INDEX